# Immunology

# Immunology

**Lars Å. Hanson**

Professor of Clinical Immunology, University of Gothenburg
and Physician-in-Chief, Sahlgren Hospital, Gothenburg, Sweden

**and**

**Hans Wigzell**

Professor of Immunology, Karolinska Institute, Stockholm, Sweden

**Butterworths**
London · Boston · Durban · Singapore · Sydney · Toronto · Wellington

Swedish sixth edition published 1983
© Almqvist & Wiksell Förlag AB, Stockholm 1983

English first edition, revised and updated 1985
© Butterworth & Co. (Publishers) Ltd 1985

---

**British Library Cataloguing in Publication Data**

Immunology.
  1. Immunology
  I. Hanson, Lars Ake    II. Wigzell, Hans
  616.07'9      QR181

  ISBN 0-407-00372-X

---

**Library of Congress Cataloging in Publication Data**

Main entry under title:

Immunology.

  Translation of: Immunologi. 6th ed.
  Includes bibliographies and index.
  1. Immunology.  I. Hanson, Lars A.  II. Wigzell,
Hans, 1938–    . [DNLM: 1. Allergy and Immunology.
QW 504 I326i]
QR181.I41813  1985      616.07'9      85-4185
ISBN 0-407-00372-X

---

Filmset by Mid-County Press, London SW15
Printed and bound by Robert Hartnoll Ltd, Bodmin, Cornwall

# Preface

There are at least three good reasons to study immunology. The first is that man cannot survive without immunological defence against foreign material, especially micro-organisms. The second is that these same immunological defence mechanisms can cause various forms of tissue damage which result in different diseases. The third is that some immunological reactions can be used as sensitive and highly specific methods for analytical and diagnostically useful determinations of low molecular substances alike drugs, and high molecular components such as serum proteins, enzymes and micro-organisms.

Against this background interest in immunology has increased dramatically during recent years. Research is continuously adding useful and exciting new discoveries.

This is a translation into English of the sixth Edition of the Swedish Textbook of Basic and Clinical Immunology. In its first part it provides a treatise of basic immunology primarily aimed at students of medicine, and natural sciences. The second half is more clinically orientated and illustrates to students of medicine and clinicians the importance of immune mechanisms for health and disease.

Lars Å Hanson and Hans Wigzell

# List of contributors

Alm, Gunnar, MD   Division of Clinical Immunology, Academic Hospital, Uppsala University, Sweden

Bennich, Hans, MD   Associate Professor, Department of Immunology, Biochemical Center, University of Uppsala, Sweden

Grubb, Rune, MD   Professor, Department of Bacteriology, University of Lund, Sweden

Hammarström, Sten, PhD   Department of Immunology, University of Stockholm, Sweden

Hanson, Lars Å, MD   Professor, Department of Immunology, University of Gothenburg, Sweden

Holm, Göran, MD   Professor, Department of Clinical Immunology, Huddinge Hospital, Karolinska Institute, Stockholm

Laurell, Anna–Brita, MD   Professor, Department of Clinical Immunology, University of Lund, Sweden

Löw, Bengt, MD   Associate Professor, The Blood Bank, Central Hospital, Lund, Sweden

Möller, Erna, MD   Professor, Department of Clinical Immunology, Huddinge Hospital, Karolinska Institute, Stockholm

Norberg, Renée, MD   Associate Professor, Department of Immunology, National Bacteriologic Laboratory, Solna, Sweden

Norrby, Erling, MD   Professor, Department of Virology, Karolinska Institute, Stockholm

Perlmann, Peter, PhD   Professor, Department of Immunology, University of Stockholm, Sweden

Sjögren, Hans Olof, MD   Professor, Institute of Tumor Immunology, University of Lund, Sweden

Wigzell, Hans, MD   Professor, Department of Immunology, Karolinska Institute, Stockholm, Sweden

# Contents

# Chapter 1

# Anatomy of the immune system

Gunnar Alm and Hans Wigzell

The word immune means 'exempt from burden'. Its connection with modern day immunology stems from the old observation that when an epidemic disease returned to a society some people were exempt, i.e. immune to that disease. These, of course, were the people who had contracted but had survived the disease when it appeared for the first time. We now know that our immune system not only functions as a protective mechanism against infection but that this is probably the main function of the system. The term immunology is thus still an appropriate one. However, we should realize that our immune system can react in a manner disadvantageous to our own body by way of allergic and autoimmune ('self' immune) diseases. It is also likely that immune reactions to a certain degree may protect us against the appearance of malignant tumours.

There is a need for a highly sophisticated immune system in higher animals in order to achieve safe and efficient elimination of foreign material and organisms. In order to understand how this system functions one needs to know the components of the system and how these are coordinated within our own body into a functioning unit.

## The construction of the immune system: some common principles and concepts

The cellular capacity to sense a difference between self and non-self serves as a fundamental basis for immune reactions. In unicellular organisms this capacity may become expressed as an ability to form complicated colonies, while in multicellular individuals it can be displayed, for example, in the creation of organs during ontogeny. Unicellular organisms have defence mechanisms through which they may manage, in a more or less non-specific manner, to inactivate foreign organisms. Such a defence mechanism has been further developed into sophisticated immune systems in the vertebrates, where a number of specialized cell types can be shown to collaborate. During an immune response there is normally participation of cells as well as of humoral molecules. Some of these cells can be highly selective, i.e. can have a unique capacity to react with a specific structure but not with other foreign substances. Others are of a more non-specific nature but can be recruited in a selective manner to places where specific immune reactions occur. Through this collaboration it is possible for the immune system of vertebrates to produce a large number of cells and molecules of specific as well as non-specific nature allowing a highly varied attack against a foreign substance or organism. In the following chapters we will describe in brief the various isolated components of the immune system followed by a description of the build-up and physiology of the lymphoid system.

## Cell types of the immune system

### Lymphocytes

Foreign substances which, in vertebrates, induce immune reactions are called immunogens or antigens (inducers of immune reactions). The lymphocytes are the only cells in the body which have an inbuilt unique capacity to recognize selectively immunogenic substances. The basis of this ability is the fact that they carry antigen-specific receptors on their outer cell surface. These receptors or cell-bound antibodies are normally produced by the same cell on which they are located. When lymphocytes react against an immunogen they may release specific antibodies and also other substances (lymphokines), whereupon other cells or humoral factors are recruited into the immune response. The key cells of the immune response are these antigen-specific lymphocytes. They constitute a heterogeneous cell population as far as function, production and distribution in various tissues and organisms are concerned. Lympho-cytes can be subdivided into two major groups which according to the organ of maturation, are called B or T lymphocytes. The two groups of lymphocytes have distinctly different functions. One lymphocyte of one type cannot change to become a lymphocyte of the other group. In a human adult there are roughly equal numbers of T and B lymphocytes. They constitute one of the most numerous cell types of the body.

B lymphocytes are so called because they mature in birds in a specific organ named the bursa of Fabricus. If this organ is removed during the embryonic period it will result in a bird with comparatively normal T but no B lymphocytes. The counterpart in the mammals to this bursa has not been clearly delineated but the liver would seem to function during the embryonic period like the bursa of Fabricus in birds (*see also below*). The sole known function of the B lymphocyte is to produce humoral antibodies. These antibodies or immunoglobulins (*see* chapter 2) are produced at a high rate for export to the bodily fluids by B cells after activation, normally through contact with antigen. Under such conditions small resting B lymphocytes are changed into larger cells, lymphoblasts, which later turn into specialized cells called plasma cells. The latter represent the most highly differentiated cells within our body with regard to production of humoral antibodies.

T lymphocytes received their name due to their dependence on the thymus to achieve full differentiation (*Figure 1.1*). Removal of the thymus early in life may thus lead to an individual with comparatively normal B lymphocytes but lacking functional T lymphocytes. The earlier such a removal of thymus is carried out the more complete is this deficiency of immunocompetent T cells. Antigen-reactive T lymphocytes have, like the immunocompetent B lymphocytes, specific receptors for antigen on the outer cell surface through which they can recognize foreign structures. Like the B lymphocytes, T cells can be activated to proliferation and differentiation through contact with a suitable immunogen. However, in contrast to B cells, T lymphocytes can never produce humoral antibodies in response to such activation. The functions that T lymphocytes can exert are called specific cell-mediated immunity (*see* chapter 7). This requires a presence of cells but not of humoral antibodies in order to function. Included within this term are T cells with different abilities such as cytolytic function or the capacity to induce delayed-type hypersensitivity reactions. T lymphocytes have also, however, an important role in the activation of B lymphocytes to produce large amounts of

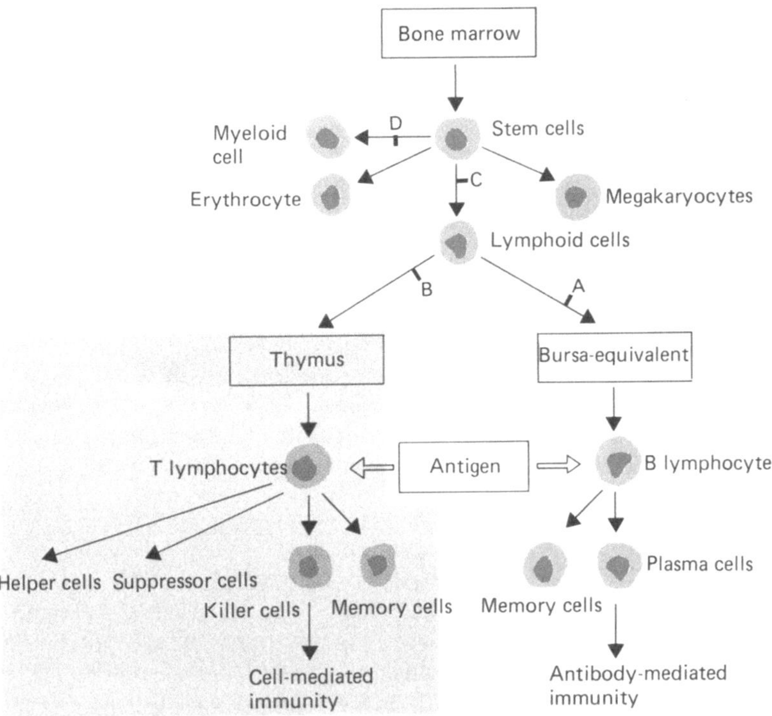



*Figure 1.1* Scheme of the development of the cells of the immune system. Stem cells from the bone marrow can differentiate into antibody-forming cells through the development of B lymphocytes. Thymus directs the development of T lymphocytes responsible for specific cell-mediated immunity and also has the ability to regulate the function of B lymphocytes. The specific immune response is induced by foreign material, immunogen. The specific effector components of the immune system, i.e. the antigen-reactive T cells and the humoral antibodies are characterized by selective affinity towards the inducing immunogen

antibodies after contact with the proper immunogens. There is thus often a requirement for a cellular collaboration (T–B collaboration) in order for fullblown antibody production to be induced with the T cells functioning as specific 'catalysts' for the B lymphocytes (T cells are functioning as helper T cells). Both T and B lymphocytes can be carriers of the immune memory, demonstrable by the fact that a second contact with the same immunogen is frequently recognized by the immune system in a more efficient manner than on the first encounter.

Undefined lymphocytes which are not easily classified as either B or T type are also present. These cells may represent immature stages that eventually become B or T lymphocytes. It is, however, quite possible that there exist as yet undefined subgroups of lymphocytes outside the large B and T groups. Of particular functional interest within this group are the cells with the capacity to exert selective cytolysis (cell killing capacity), termed natural killer (NK) cells (*see* chapter 7).

The different lymphocyte groups are not easily separable using conventional light microscopy. Reagents specific for various cell surface structures are normally used to differentiate between the various lymphocyte subgroups. B cells are most easily detected through the use of fluorescent antibodies directed against the immuno-

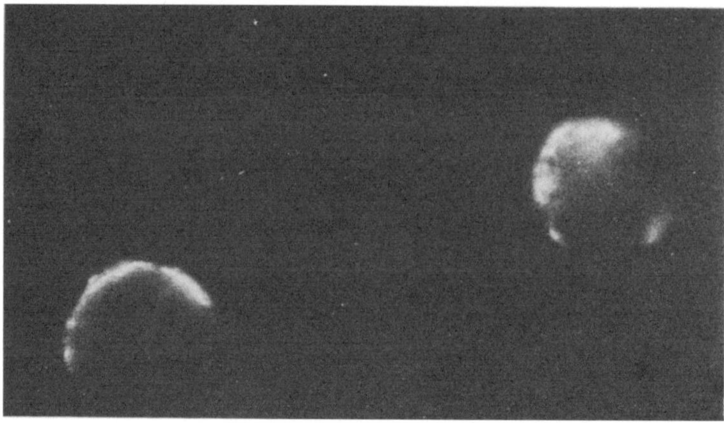

*Figure 1.2* Demonstration of immunoglobulin on the surface of a **B** lymphocyte through the use of fluorescein-labelled anti-immunoglobulin antibodies produced in another species

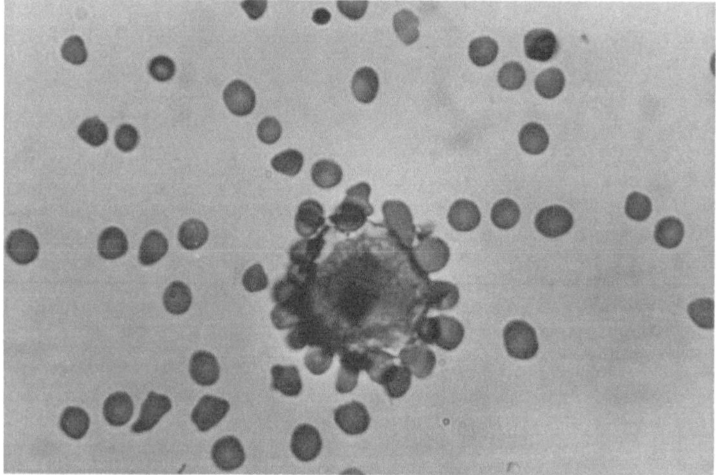

*Figure 1.3* Human T lymphocytes all express ability to bind sheep erythrocytes to the other cell surface

globulins present on the surface of the B lymphocyte (*Figure 1.2*). T lymphocytes of human origin have the capacity to bind sheep erythrocytes to the surface where rosettes are formed which can easily be counted. (*Figure 1.3*). Specific antibodies of monoclonal origin directed against unique differentiation antigens on lymphocyte subsets are now frequently used to further identify the cells being studied.

## Macrophages (monocytes)

Like lymphocytes, macrophages and monocytes are produced within the bone marrow but then repopulate various organs in the body. In the present context monocytes can be considered to represent certain differentiation steps among the macrophage groups. Certain macrophages are stationary while others are moving around in the tissues. These cells are characterized by the capacity to take up, to phagocytose, molecules or organisms perceived by the cells as foreign (macrophage = big eater). One efficient way to identify a substance as 'foreign' to the macrophages is to allow antibodies to react with it. Besides having a phagocytic capacity the macrophages are also important participants in the induction of immunity, in particular with regard to the T lymphocytes. It is only when an antigen is presented on the surface of a macrophage that this substance can be used to activate specific T lymphocytes into an active immune response (*see* chapter 7). Monocytes and macrophages can also be activated by antibodies to serve as killer cells against relevant target organisms. It is likely that macrophages, like lymphocytes, can be subdivided into subsets with distinct differentiation pathways but this is not clear as yet. As a group these cells can normally be separated from lymphocytes by conventional light microscopy to which may be added histochemical staining or tests of phagocytosis.

**Granulocytes**

Granulocytes exist in three forms, neutrophil, basophil and eosinophil. They normally exist in the bone marrow, the spleen and peripheral blood, but can occur in large amounts in any tissue where inflammatory processes are occurring. Like macrophages these cells lack their own antigen-specific receptors but may receive them passively through humoral antibodies. Granulocytes are pharmacologically extraordinarily potent cells. Their participation in the immune process is often of vital importance in providing enough force for the immune response to combat an infection. Like macrophages, neutrophil granulocytes have an excellent capacity to phagocytose antibody-coated organisms where the strong intracellular enzymes of the granulocytes can digest most organisms. Eosinophil granulocytes can function as killer cells against antibody-coated parasites. Basophil granulocytes and mast cells are capable of releasing histamine and other pharmacologically active substances and may thereby cause a local inflammatory condition (*see* chapter 2). The granulocytes have a characteristic morphology and stainability and can be separated from other cell types by conventional light microscopy.

# The lymphoid system

The immune system takes advantage of a complicated collaboration between different cell types and humoral factors in order to achieve the largest possible impact of an immune response. The anatomical relationship between the distinct cell types in the tissues is here of great importance. The lymphocytes in vertebrates constitute a dominating cell group in many immune reactions and their specific reactions can then bring the other more non-specific cell types and humoral systems into action. It is of importance for the understanding of the function of the immune system to know how the different cell types, in particular lymphocytes, are produced, differentiated and distributed in various tissues. The organ system within which lymphocytes can for the most part be found is called the lymphoid system. It consists, in principle, of a reticular or epithelial basic tissue frame creating a net in the meshes of which lymphocytes, but also macrophages and monocytes, are localized. Such lymphoid tissue can constitute whole organs or components of an organ. Lymph nodes, spleen (the white splenic pulp), appendix, Peyer's patches, tonsils and lymphocyte-rich tissue in bone marrow, in the lamina propria of the gut mucosa and in the liver are examples of such lymphoid tissue. Epithelial tissue such as that in the intestine and in the skin may also contain many lymphocytes. The lympho-epithelial tissue of certain organs such as the thymus and, in the birds, the bursa of Fabricus are unique and have, as will be discussed later, specific functions. The macro- and microanatomy of the particular structures of the lymphoid systems cannot be discussed here in detail due to lack of space. Readers interested in such information should consult any modern textbook on histology and cell biology.

The lymphoid system is a highly complex structure in the higher vertebrates, e.g. birds and mammals. This is naturally related to the manifold functions it has to fulfil. It contains the majority of the micro-environmental niches which the lymphocytes require for their proper differentiation and function.

## Central and peripheral lymphoid organs

Experimental studies on rodents and chickens and analyses of immune defects in humans have shown that T and B lymphocytes, from the point of differentiation, belong to distinct parts of the lymphoid system. This has produced our present concept of the compartmentalization of the lymphoid system as delineated in *Figure 1.1*. What does not clearly project from such a static figure is the dynamics within the lymphoid system. From early ontogeny and during the whole life-span of the individual there is a production and movement of lymphocytes in various stages of differentiation between distinct lymphoid organs and tissues. This cellular migration may take place via the lymph or the blood. In a highly schematic summary the lymphoid system functions as follows. Lymphoid stem cells which, in adult individuals are produced in the bone marrow, migrate with the blood to either of the two 'central' lymphoid organs, namely the thymus and the bursa of Fabricus of the birds (the question of the bursa-equivalent organs in mammals will be discussed later). Within this organ differentiation of the immigrant stages of lymphocytes will take place. This differentiation, which occurs during rapid cellular proliferation in the thymus, will produce T lymphocytes and in the bursa of Fabricus (and respectively the bursa equivalent) B lymphocytes. From these central lymphoid organs lymphocytes then migrate into the peripheral lymphoid tissues. They can also recirculate between peripheral lymphoid organs via the blood or the lymph.

### *Lymphoid stem cells*

The lymphoid stem cells differentiate originally from the same pluripotent haemo-poietic stem cells that give rise to the rest of the cells within the blood (granulocytes, erythrocytes, etc., *see Figure 1.1*). During embryonic life they are in the yolk sack and the liver whereas late during ontogeny they are found in the red bone marrow. The stem cells for the T lymphocytes are predestined to go to the thymus to further develop into typical T cells.

### *The thymus as a central lymphoid organ*

Before discussing the mechanism behind the function of the thymus during the development of the lymphoid organs it is relevant to repeat the essential features of the morphology of the thymus (*Figure 1.4*). The basic morphological entity within the thymus is the thymus lobulus. It is separated by walls of connective tissue and contains

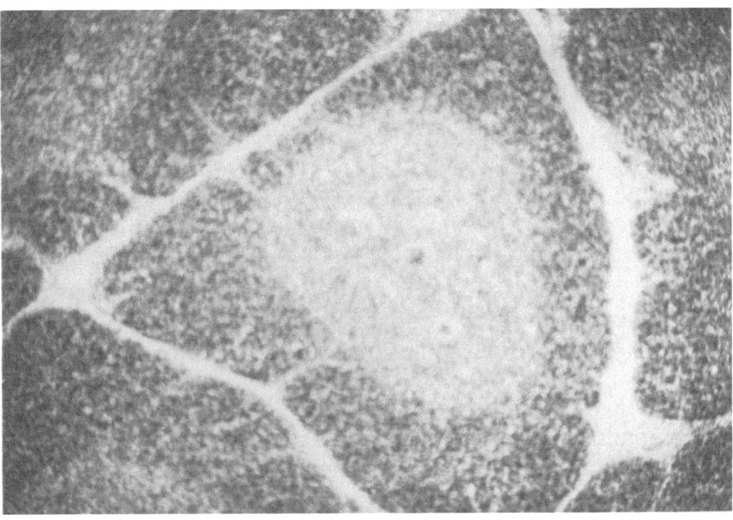

*Figure 1.4* Histology of the thymus showing the compartmentalization of one lobulus with the outer cortex with high cell density and the interior medulla with low cell density. The thymus is composed of a great number of such lobuli

a lymphocyte-poor medulla (containing around 10% of the cells) surrounded by a lymphocyte-rich cortex (around 90% of the cells). The thymus is composed of epithelial cells, lymphocytes, macrophage-like cells and blood vessels.

The epithelial part of the thymus develops during the embryonic period from the epithelium of the third and fourth gill pouch. The final organ is created through expansion and separation of the epithelial anlage from the gill pouches followed by an invasion of blood-borne lymphoid cells into the anlage. The major proliferation of T cells and differentiation towards small lymphocytes occurs in the thymic cortex. The thymus is the organ of the body which, next to the epithelium of the intestine, expresses the most rapid cellular proliferation. It has been calculated, for example, that the entire lymphocyte population in the thymus of a child is replaced within four to six days.

The regulation of the cellular proliferation within the thymus is, to a certain degree, a built-in function of this organ. It can, however, be regulated in part by hormones, and will be stimulated by growth hormone and thyroxine but will be inhibited by corticosteroids. Cellular division within the thymus is not influenced by stimulation with immunogen in the same manner as are the lymph nodes and the spleen. In contrast to such peripheral lymphoid tissue the thymus also lacks normal lymphoid follicles and germinal centres (*see below*).

The thymus will go through marked changes in size in relation to age. Similar but less pronounced changes are also displayed by the peripheral lymphoid organs. During ontogeny the thymus is the first organ to contain lymphocytes. It grows rapidly in young individuals after birth and will reach maximum size at puberty. After puberty has been established the thymus will rapidly shrink followed by a slow involution during the rest of life. Information exists to indicate that this involution is at least in part determined by temporary changes in the non-lymphoid elements of the thymus, i.e. epithelial cells.

In situations of stress rapid diminution of the thymus weight may occur within 24 hours. This so-called accidental involution is probably caused by the high sensitivity of the cortical thymus cells to the action of corticosteroids. Recovery of the thymus weight can subsequently occur within one to two weeks.

*Function of the thymus*

Certain functions of the thymus are still unclear but we already know several important details. As stated before, the bone marrow contains prothymocytes which can move to the thymus. Such cells are not immunologically competent. These cells will start to divide rapidly after arriving at the cortex of the thymus. This proliferation is independent of exogenous antigen and is thought to reflect differentiation steps of prothymocytes towards mature immunocompetent T lymphocytes. Parallel to cellular divisions there appear changes in the cell surface structures of the thymocytes. Several new structures related to differentiation can be demonstrated. Experimental evidence exists to indicate that the thymocytes, during this period of life, are selected for, or may receive, imprints for immunological specificity (*see* chapter 7) in such a manner that they become especially efficient at recognizing changes within the tissues of the same individual. It is likely that this latter specific differentiation process may occur via a direct contact between thymocytes and other cell types within the thymus. In addition, several thymic hormones and their amino acid sequences are now known to exist and some are available in synthetic form. These hormones have, to a varying degree, the capacity to enhance the differentiation of thymocytes, but there is no single thymic hormone which alone is able to induce a prothymocyte to become a fully mature and immunocompetent T lymphocyte.

Calculation of the number of cells which are generated within the thymus through cellular proliferation in relation to the number of cells which leave the thymus indicates that a large fraction of the cells within the cortex of the thymus probably die *in situ*. After the differentiation process has been concluded in the cortex some immunocompetent T cells migrate to the medulla of the thymus while other cells leave the organ. A certain fraction of the T cells which leave the thymus are probably still not fully immunocompetent. It is likely that they can undergo further differentiation in the peripheral lymphoid organs. Such cells may also play a particularly important role in the induction of certain cell-mediated immune reactions.

*Bursa of Fabricus as a central lymphoid organ*

The bursa of Fabricus has so far only been found as a morphologically well defined organ in birds. It has certain similarities to the thymus with regard to differentiation and morphology. During embryonic life it is developed from the intestinal epithelium of the cloaca. The epithelial bursa anlage is invaded by blood-borne lymphoid stem cells which develop during proliferation to so-called bursa lymphocytes. These cells are generally somewhat larger than the corresponding cells within the thymus and have certain other morphological dissimilarities. Like the thymus the bursa has a lymphocyte-rich cortex while the medulla contains fewer cells (*Figure 1.5*).

*Function of the bursa of Fabricus*

It has been possible to demonstrate that immunoglobulin-producing lymphocytes develop within the bursa of Fabricus from blood-borne stem cells. Immunoglobulin (Ig) exists in various classes (*see* chapter 2). During the embryonic development IgM-producing cells appear first followed by IgG- and IgA-producing lymphocytes.

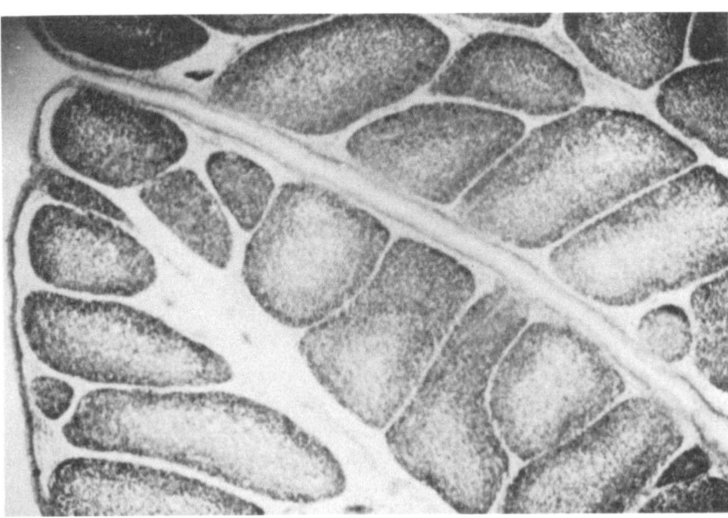

*Figure 1.5* Histology of the bursa of Fabricus in a chicken. The lobuli of cortex and medulla are in close contact with the intestinal epithelium in the folds created by the epithelium, in the pouch-like bag in the dorsal part of the cloaca

Evidence also exists for a direct change of cells from IgM to IgG synthesis. The mature bursa lymphocytes leave the organ and emigrate to the peripheral lymphoid organs, in particular to the so-called bursa or B-dependent (*see below*) areas in these organs. Here they constitute the B lymphocytes which, after immunogen stimulation, will proliferate and differentiate into the typical antibody-forming lymphocytes or plasma cells.

No evidence exists as yet for specific bursal hormones.

From the above it can be understood that if a chicken is bursectomized before or just after hatching when relatively few lymphocytes have been able to leave the bursa, this will result in a selective lack of immunoglobulin and antibody production.

### Bursa equivalent in mammals

Several reasons exist to suggest that mammals have one or more structures which functionally correspond to the bursa of Fabricus of birds. However, such organs are as yet not clearly defined. Some evidence exists to indicate that Peyer's patches and the appendix in rabbits may have a bursa-like function. In animals which have tonsils, such tissue may also serve as a partial bursa equivalent. It is also possible that in mammals, as in lower vertebrates, the whole epithelium of the gut with its lymphocytes and some of the lymphocytes in the lamina propria of the gut can serve as a diffuse kind of bursa of Fabricus. B lymphocytes develop in the liver and spleen during embryogenesis in mice. These organs could thus serve as a bursa equivalent during the embryonic period.

### Differentiation of B lymphocytes in mammals

Studies of B cell differentiation in mammals have been made more difficult through the lack of a particular organ serving as a defined bursa of Fabricus. Experiments using tissue culture to study B cell differentiation have already clearly indicated that they develop in a stepwise manner with regard to immunocompetence. Thus it is clear that B lymphocytes in their capacity to produce different forms of immunoglobulins develop this competence in a defined sequence with IgM as the first immunoglobulin (*see* Chapter 6). Likewise the ability of B lymphocytes to be inactivated rather than activated upon antigen contact (development of immunologic tolerance instead of immunity, *see* chapter 8) would seem to be limited to a critical period early during differentiation. Other features linked to different stages of B cell differentiation are the capacity to make antibodies against certain immunogens without the help of T lymphocytes, the ability to bind certain complement components to the cellular surface (chapter 4), etc. The production of B lymphocytes occurs via a number of discrete differentiation steps. Genetic defects or other factors can lead to a select lack of B lymphocytes (*see* chapter 13).

*Peripheral lymphoid organs*

The central lymphoid organs serve as production and differentiation sites for lymphocytes. They are then spread out into the peripheral lymphoid tissues. In the latter organs there is most likely a continuation of cellular division leading to an increased differentiation linked to or occurring in the absence of specific antigenic stimulation. The various lymphoid tissues are often compartmentalized into areas rich in T and B lymphocytes respectively. In order to optimize the 'division of labour' during an immune response, the organ or tissue may in addition have some specific feature which allows the accumulation of a special subgroup of lymphocytes in that particular tissue.

In a schematic manner one can subdivide peripheral lymphoid tissue into the following groups:

(1)  gut-associated lymphoid tissue: Peyer's patches, appendix and tonsils. These organs often have close contact with the contents in the oral cavity and intestinal tract via specialized gut epithelium;
(2)  lymph nodes which receive antigen through afferent lymphatic vessels, especially from the large surface area, but which can also exert a localized effect by connection with internal organs;
(3)  diffuse or only partly organized lymphoid tissue is richly represented in the liver, the bone marrow or the mucosa of the gut. It is partly organized as to primary and secondary follicles (*see below*). In addition there are large numbers of lymphocytes in various epithelial tissues such as the skin.

When an immunogen reaches peripheral lymphoid tissue this normally leads to an immune response. The character of this reaction is determined in part by the immunogen itself and in part by the particular lymphoid tissue. It is well known how the immunogen is handled and recognized in lymph nodes. It is likely that similar reactions take place in the other kinds of peripheral lymphoid organs and tissues.

The lymph nodes are surrounded by a lymphatic sinus into which the afferent lymphatics open (*Figure 1.6*). Within this there is a cortex rich in cells which contains round groups of tightly packed small lymphocytes, primary lymph follicles. The lymph follicles contain primarily B lymphocytes and macrophages of a special kind with long, dendritic-like extensions which are in close contact with the lymphocytes.  The deepest part of the cortex is called the paracortical area. T lymphocytes dominate in this area. Inside the cortex is the medulla of the lymph node. It consists of multiple lymphatic sinuses which contain macrophages with long, dendrite-like extensions. In the medulla there are groups of lymphocytes sometimes orientated into strings

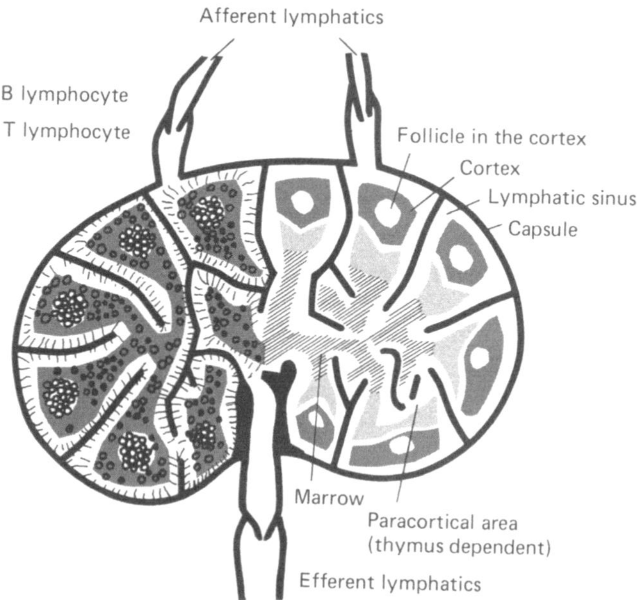


*Figure 1.6* Diagram of the structure of a lymph node. Note that **B** lymphocytes (○) dominate in the follicles whereas T lymphocytes (●) dominate in the deep parts of the cortex, i.e. the thymus-dependent paracortical area

connected to the cortex. The efferent lymphatics leave the lymph node via the hilus, i.e. the central part of the medulla.

The lymph nodes are highly dynamic organs and constitute a site for a considerable production of small lymphocytes. In addition there is a continuous flow of cells through the lymph nodes. Small lymphocytes enter the lymph node through endothelial cells in the postcapillary venulae and leave the lymph node through the efferent lymphatics and reach the blood circulation via the major lymphatic vessels (*Figure 1.7*).

Stimulation by an immunogen giving rise to an antibody response in the lymph node will cause characteristic morphological changes in that node. The antigen is first taken up by macrophages in the medulla and primary lymph follicles. A few days later secondary lymph follicles are developed in close contact with the follicular antigen carrying macrophages. The centre of a secondary lymph follicle is often called the germinal centre and contains a large number of antibody-forming cells (*Figure 1.8*). Some antibody-forming cells will then leave the germinal centres and migrate down into the cellular strings of the medulla of the node.

A lymph node which is engaged in a cell-mediated immune response (chapter 7) will display a different morphological picture upon immune activation. In such a lymph node there is no creation of germinal centres but instead a massive increase in the number of small lymphocytes in the T cell dominated paracortical areas will occur.

Many immunogens require, for proper activation of B lymphocytes, that T lymphocytes and macrophages also participate in the immune reaction. Such immunogens are called thymus-dependent immunogens. Other immunogens, on the

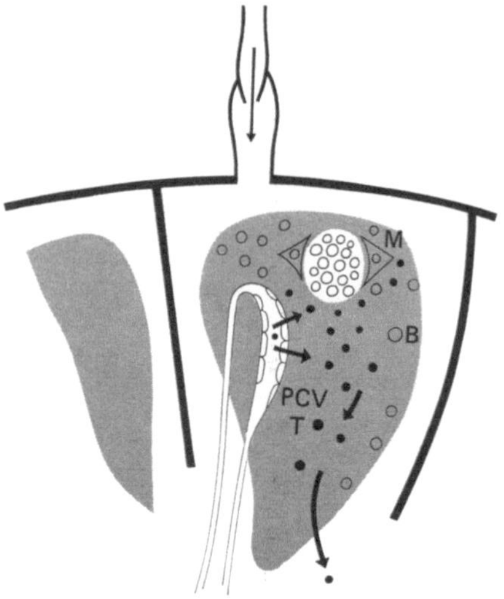

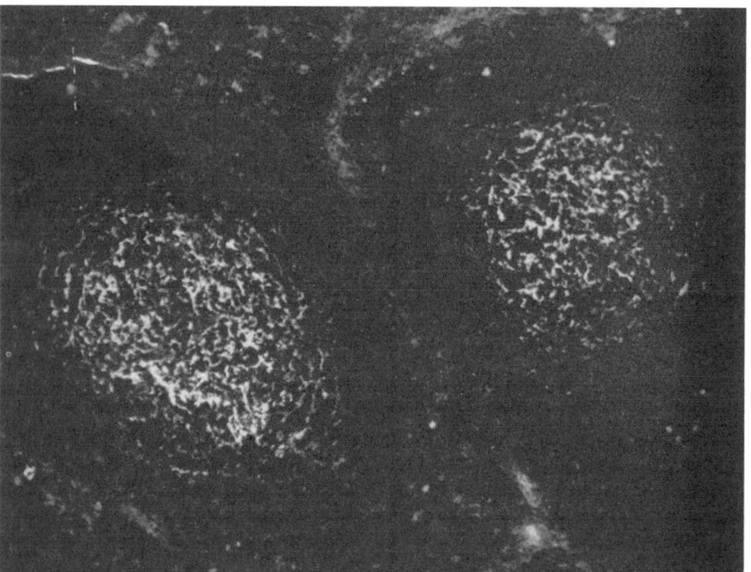

*Figure 1.7* T lymphocytes (T) migrate into the cortex of the lymph node through endothelial cells in the postcapillary venules (PCV). They leave the lymph node via lymphatics which start from the medulla of the lymph node. Antigen is brought to the lymph node through afferent lymphatics and will be localized on macrophages (M) in the follicles. B lymphocytes (B) are probably influenced by such macrophage-bound antigen

*Figure 1.8* Two germinal centres containing antibody-forming cells in a lymph node. The antibody forming cells can be seen as brighter areas. No such cells are seen outside the germinal centres. (After Mellors and Korngold, 1963)

other hand, can activate the B lymphocytes directly without requiring the presence of specific T lymphocytes. They are therefore called thymus-independent immunogens.

The lymphocytes circulate in the body through the various peripheral lymphoid organs by travelling in lymphatic vessels or in the peripheral blood. The advantage of such a circulation is obvious. It allows a large number of lymphocytes to pass through various locations in the body where immunogenic foreign substances are most likely to be captured.

This will significantly enhance the possibility of a single immunocompetent lymphocyte encountering that immunogen against which the cell is able to react in a specific manner.

**Ontogeny of the lymphoid system**

We have so far dealt with the development of single lymphocytes within the lymphatic system. It is also important to know something about the development of the lymphoid system during ontogeny (the development of the individual). Several important parameters exist here.

(1)   The development of the central lymphoid organs demands firstly that epithelial anlagen of the thymus and bursal types are created. Such epithelial anlagen are developed very early during embryonic life. Only then is it possible for immature cells to enter the organs and start to differentiate into conventional lymphocytes for further export into the peripheral lymphoid organs.

(2)   The non-lymphocytic part of the peripheral lymphoid organs is also of great importance for correct presentation of antigen immunocompetent lymphocytes. As stated before it is likely that a certain differentiation of the lymphocytes may also occur through contact with such cellular elements in the peripheral tissues. Phagocytosis by macrophages develops early during ontogeny while their ability to act as effective presenters of antigens to lymphocytes is only expressed in later life. For example, it is clear that macrophages from newborn mice are defective as antigen-presenting cells while cells from the same mice a few weeks later are as efficient as macrophages from adult animals. Whether macrophages from newborn human beings function in a mature way is not clear but the immune system of the human at birth is generally speaking much more developed than that of the newborn mice.

(3)   Invasion and proliferation of lymphocytes into peripheral lymphoid organs of course play an important role in the build-up of the lymphoid system. It is of interest to know that germfree (gnotobiotic) animals display atrophic peripheral lymphoid tissue while the central lymphoid organs are of normal size and structure. However, these animals respond in a comparatively normal manner when confronted with new immunogens which demonstrates that the small number of lymphocytes which exist in the peripheral tissue is enough for a normal immune response. The large number of peripheral lymphocytes which exists in normal but not in gnotobiotic animals probably represents memory cells induced by contact with immunogens in the environment.

During ontogeny in most species specific cellular immunity precedes the humoral antibody-mediated immunity. This is normally compensated by the fact that the neonate will receive or has already received antibodies from its mother. In the human being this will take place through the transfer of immunoglobulin of a certain class (IgG) through the placental barrier. In other species, such as the cow and the pig, this will occur in the first milk of the mother (colostrum), while in birds immunoglobulin is received from the mother through the yolk of the egg. After birth and with increasing age the individual will become gradually better equipped to react immunologically to combat infections. This depends in part on better functioning of the various components of the immune system and in part through a gradual accumulation of immune memory via natural infections or vaccination. It is believed that in the human being an optimal immune defence exists at around ten years of age after which it will slowly decline (*Figure 1.9*).

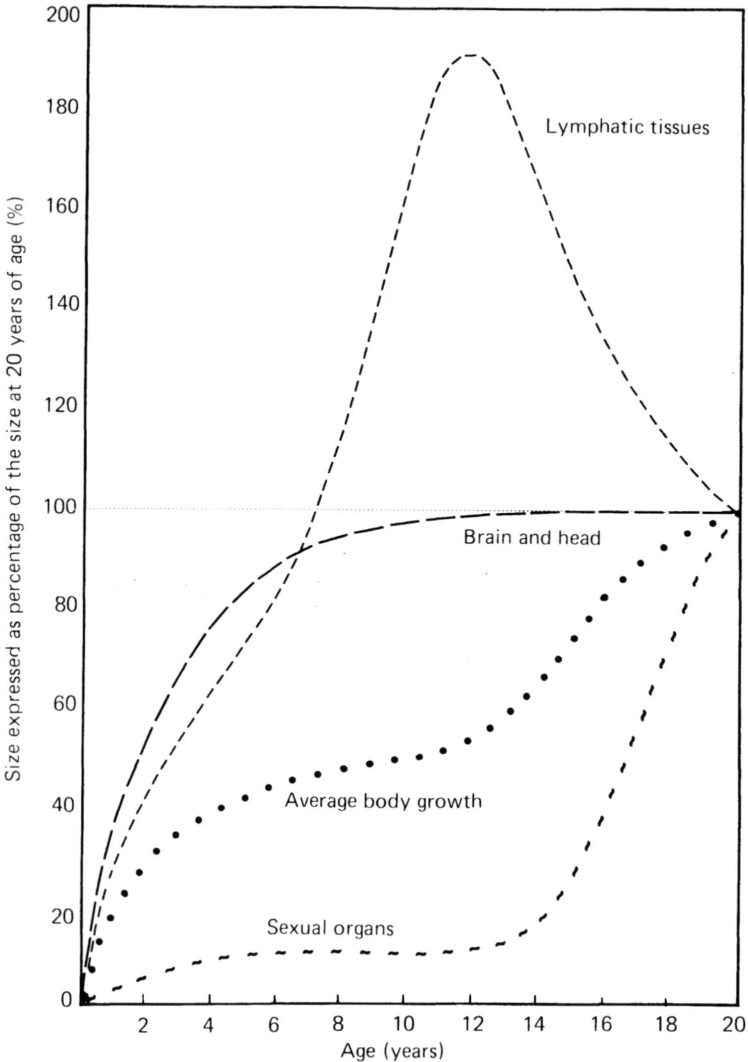


*Figure 1.9* Growth curves after birth for various tissues. The size of the tissue is expressed as a percentage of the size at 20 years of age. (After Solomon, 1971)

With increasing age a significant reduction of the central lymphoid organs will occur accompanied by a corresponding decrease in the production of new immunocompetent lymphocytes. Despite this it is generally agreed that even in old age the human being produces a significant number of new lymphocytes. The capacity to produce antibodies against new, not previously encountered, immunogens does, however, decline with certain exceptions. Relatively speaking it would also seem that the cell-mediated immune system decays with age at a more rapid rate than that of the humoral system. The function of the thymus has largely disappeared at around 40 years of age in the human. Parallel to this weakening of the cell-mediated immunity there is frequently an increase in the number of autoantibodies being made, i.e. antibodies which can react against 'self' components. 'Ageing' of the immune system is a likely reason for the increased incidence of infections known to affect elderly people. Furthermore, the frequency of many malignant diseases increases with increasing age but a possible connection to age-related immune defects should still be regarded as a hypothetical assumption for most types of tumours.

## Bibliography


COOPER, E. L. (1976). *Comparative Immunology*. Prentice-Hall Inc., Englewood Cliffs, NJ.
KATS, D. H. (1977). *Lymphocyte Differentiation, Recognition and Regulation*. Academic Press, New York.
METCALF, D. and MOORE, M. A. S. (1971). *Haemopoietic Cells*. North-Holland Publ. Co., Amsterdam, London.
MELLORS, R. C. and KORNGOLD, L. (1963). *Journal of Experimental Medicine*, **118**, 37.
SINGHAL, S. K. *et al.* (1979). *Aging and Immunity*. North-Holland Publ. Co., Amsterdam, London.
SOLOMON, J. B. (1971). *Neonatal Immunology*. North-Holland Publ. Co., Amsterdam, London.

# Chapter 2

# Immunoglobulins

**Hans Bennich**

Immunoglobulin is a common term for a complex group of proteins with antibody function. Immunoglobulin in blood or secretions is produced as a consequence of specific antigen-activated processes in the lymphoid organs. Every immunoglobulin with antibody activity (i.e. antibodies) can be characterized by its specific capacity to react with a defined antigen (*see* chapter 4).

Antibodies with different specificity must thus have different chemical structures, at least in that part of the molecule with binding affinity for the antigen. It has also been found empirically that immunoglobulins can be subdivided into classes and subclasses according to features which are independent of a particular antibody specificity.

## Common features

Circulating (humoral) antibodies can be shown to exist in body fluids and secretions such as serum, saliva, urine and milk. When serum is subjected to electrophoresis antibody activity is mainly recovered in the gamma region and the term gamma-globulin was commonly used for antibody-active proteins. Immunoglobulins (Ig) can be subdivided according to the different antigenic properties and, in serum from healthy human beings, it has so far been possible to identify five classes, namely IgG, IgA, IgM, IgD and IgE. As can be seen in *Table 2.1* the various classes differ with regard to physical and chemical features, localization and biological function.

## Basic structure

All immunoglobulins can be described starting with a common basic formula. As seen in *Figure 2.1A* the ground structure is composed of two kinds of polypeptide chains, light (L) and heavy (H) which are kept together as a symmetric four chain molecule ($H_2L_2$).

L chains have a molecular weight around 23 000 dalton and exist in two forms, kappa ($\kappa$) and lambda ($\lambda$). Both L types exist in all immunoglobulin classes but for every single antibody the rule is that it may contain either $\kappa$ or $\lambda$ chains, never both at the same time.

H chains (molecular weight 50 000–70 000 dalton) have antigenic features which are typical for each Ig class. The heavy chains of different Ig classes differ with regard to molecular weight and carbohydrate content. Furthermore there exist subclasses of

**TABLE 2.1. Common features of different immunoglobulin classes**

| | *IgG* | *IgA* | | *IgM* | *IgD* | *IgE* *serum* [a] |
| --- | --- | --- | --- | --- | --- | --- |
| | | *Serum* | *Secretion* | | | |
| *Molecular weight* | 150 000 | 150 000 | 370 000 [b] | 900 000 | 170 000 | 190 000 |
| Sedimentation $(S_w^{\circ})$ | 6.6–7S | 7–9S | 11S | 19S | 7S | 8S |
| Carbohydrate $(g\%)$ [c] | 3 | 9 | 12 | 12 | 12 | 12 |
| *Polypeptide chains* | | | | | | |
| Heavy: | | | | | | |
|    Molecular weight (incl. CHO) [i] | 50 000 | 54 000 | | 70 000 | 62 000 | 72 000 |
|    Molecular weight (excl. CHO) | 46 000 | 46 000 | | 60 000 | 52 000 | 60 000 |
|    Class | gamma $(\gamma)$ | alpha $(\alpha)$ | | mu $(\mu)$ | delta $(\delta)$ | epsilon $(\varepsilon)$ |
|    Isotypes (number) | 4 [d] | 2 | | ? | ? [e] | ? |
|    Allotypes (number) | Gm(25) | Am(2) | | ? | ? | ? |
| Light: | | | | | | |
| Molecular weight | 23 000 | 23 000 | | 23 000 | 23 000 | 23 000 |
| Types | $\kappa, \lambda$ | $\kappa, \lambda$ | | $\kappa, \lambda$ | $\kappa, \lambda$ | $\kappa, \lambda$ |
| Isotypes [f] | 9 | 9 | | 9 | 9 | 9 |
| Allotypes [g] | Km(3) | Km(3) | | Km(3) | Km(3) | Km(3) |
| *Biological features* | | | | | | |
| Serum levels (g/l) | 8–17 | 1–4 | | 0.5–2 | 0–0.5 | 0–0.0009 |
| Complement binding | | | | | | |
|    classical | Yes [h] | No | | Yes | No | No |
|    alternative | No | Yes | | No | No | No |
| Placental passage | Yes | No | | No | No | No |
| Secretion from serous membranes | No | No | Yes | No | No | Yes |
| Binding to homologous tissue | No | No | | No | No | Yes |
| Binding to heterologous tissue | Yes | No | | No | No | No |

[a] IgE in secretion is identical to IgE in serum.

[b] Dimer of IgA in serum kept together by two J (join) chains (mol wt 15 000) to which during secretion is added the secretion peptide (mol wt 50 000) from epithelial cells.

[c] Covalently bound to H-chains; the number of oligosaccharide moieties varies with the class, $\gamma$ chain has 1, $\mu$ chain 5 and $\varepsilon$ chain 6.

[d] *See Table 2.2* for IgG. $V_H$I–IV subgroups can be included in this.

[e] Membrane-bound IgD and serum IgD have been suggested to represent different subgroups.

[f] $V_L$ subgroups: 4 $V_k$ and 5 $V_L$.

[g] Is valid for $\kappa$ chains; for $\lambda$ chains no allotypes are known in the human.

[h] Complement binding features for $\gamma$ chains vary with subclass (isotype) (*see Table 2.2*).

[i] CHO, carbohydrate chains.

heavy chains. For example, the $\alpha$ chains exist in two forms, $\alpha$-1 and $\alpha$-2, which differ with regard to the way in which the light chain is combined with the $\alpha$ heavy chain. In the $\alpha$-1 molecule this is through a disulphide bridge, while in the $\alpha$-2 this binding occurs via non-covalent bonds. When discussing $\gamma$-chains there are four subclasses, $\gamma$-1, $\gamma$-2, $\gamma$-3 and $\gamma$-4, which differ with regard to the number of disulphide bridges that unite their heavy chains.

As all these antigenic variants exist in all individuals of the same species they are called isotypes. But, in addition, there may exist antigenic variants which are determined by a gene locus which, in the same species, may exist in two or more allelic forms; these are then called allotypes. *Table 2.2* shows various subclasses (isotypes) and allotypes of IgG which have different biological functions.

The polypeptide chains in Ig are kept together by covalent as well as by non-covalent bonds. The former consist of disulphide bridges that are sensitive to mercaptan (SH

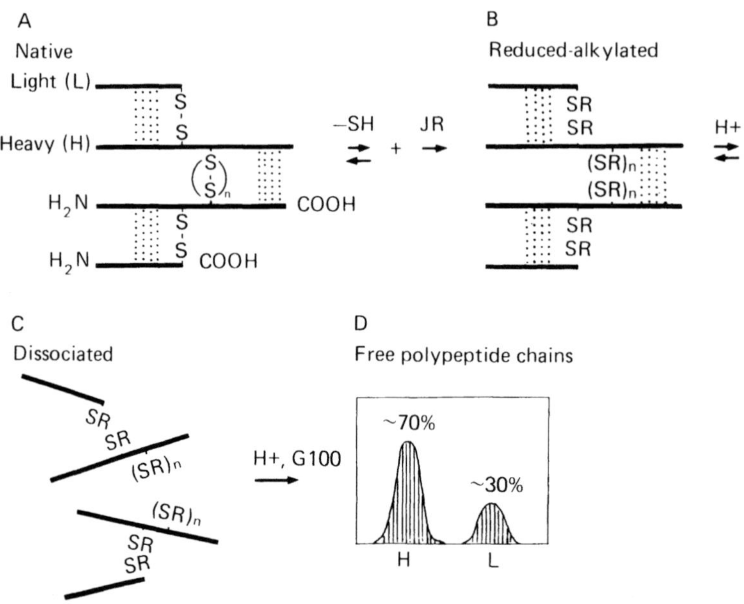


*Figure 2.1* A. The basic structure of immunoglobulin is constituted by a symmetrical four chain structure composed of two light (L) and two heavy (H) polypeptide chains kept together by disulphide bridges (—S—S—) and noncovalent bonds (dotted lines). B. Despite reduction and alkylation (SR) of the disulphide bridges the four chain structure will remain intact in a neutral environment through the influence of noncovalent bonds. C. Acid milieu or presence of dissociating substances (e.g. urea) will diminish the attractive forces between the chains making them into single chains. D. Isolation of heavy and light chains after reduction and alkylation is most easily carried out via filtration through a molecular sieving device in acid milieu separating the molecules according to size

**TABLE 2.2 Subclasses (isotypes) and allotypes of IgG in the human: Biological and chemical features**

|  | *IgG1* | *IgG2* | *IgG3* | *IgG4* |
|---|---|---|---|---|
| Heavy chain | $\gamma 1$ | $\gamma 2$ | $\gamma 3$ | $\gamma 4$ |
| Relative concentration (%) | 70 | 20 | 8 | 2 |
| Number of disulphide bridges ($\gamma$-SS$\gamma$) | 2 | 4 | 13 | 2 |
| Allotypes (Gm groups) | 1, 2, 4, 17, 22 | 24 | 3, 5, 6, 13, 14, 15, 16 | [a] |
| Placenta passage [b] | Yes | (Yes) | Yes | Yes |
| Complement binding (C 1) [c] | Yes | (Yes) | Yes | No [d] |
| Binding to heterologous tissue [e] | Yes | No | Yes | Yes |
| Binding to *Staphylococcus aureus* protein [b] | Yes | Yes | No | Yes |
| Binding to macrophages [f] | Yes | (Yes) | Yes | (No) |

[a] Allotype is not yet shown to exist.
[b] Domain: Both $C_H2$ and $C_H3$.
[c] Domain: $C_H2$.
[d] True for intact IgG4: Fc fragment of IgG4 does bind C1, which indicates that the Fab parts of the intact protein may block complement binding.
[e] Domain: $C_H3$.
[f] Domain: $C_H3$.

reagent) and can be split by reduction without affecting the individual structure of the chains (*Figure 2.1B*). This reaction is reversible and thus the resulting sulph-hydryl groups must be blocked, e.g. by alkylation using an iodoacetamide. Mild reduction and alkylation of an antibody does not normally affect its ability to bind antigen; nor are the physicochemical features changed. The explanation for this is that non-covalent bonds (e.g. hydrophobic forces, hydrogen and salt bonds) keep together the antibody molecules in a physiological state. If, however, the environment is changed, e.g. by lowering the pH or by increasing the ionic strength in the solution, one may observe that the non-covalent forces weaken in such a manner that the molecule dissociates into heavy and light chains (*Figure 2.1C*). The same results are obtained if the partially reduced and alkylated antibody is brought into contact with substances which have dissociating power, such as carbamide. In order to characterize the individual peptide chains of the immunoglobulin it is necessary to isolate and analyse them using dissociating conditions (*Figure 2.1D*). Isolated heavy and light chains have largely lost the antigen-binding capacity of the native antibody molecule. However this can be recovered if the chains are allowed to recombine as pairs using a weakly acid pH (5.5).

## Antibody activity and specific functions

An antibody can have several functions; besides binding to a specific antigen it can also participate in several different biologically important reactions (*see Tables 2.1 and 2.2*). Using partial enzymatic and reductive splitting of an antibody molecule it is possible to demonstrate that antibody activity and class-specific functions are localized to various compartments of the molecule (*Figure 2.2*). Splitting with proteolytic enzymes such as papain or trypsin gives rise to three fragments. Two are identical Fab fragments that retain antibody activity with regard to the antigen binding, while the third is the Fc fragment that consists of the carboxyterminal part of two heavy chains that are responsible for other biological functions (*see Figure 2.2 and Table 2.1*). The Fab fragments are composed of the aminoterminal portion of a heavy chain and a complete light chain held together by a disulphide bridge. Every antibody contains two such identical antigen binding areas, one per Fab fragment. This arrangement explains the secondary impact of a reaction between an antigen and an antibody, e.g. agglutination or precipitation (*see* chapter 4). The environment within the Fab-part of the antibody which is capable of binding to an antigen is formed through the creation of a cleft between defined structural areas within both the heavy and the light chains (see the variable regions).

## Monoclonal immunoglobulins

Antibodies which are synthesized as a response to stimulation with a chemically pure immunogen are normally composed of a mixture of molecules with different structures. Two major reasons exist for this, one being that most immunogenic compounds represent a mosaic of antigenic determinants (*see* chapter 3). The second is that a single antigenic determinant can be viewed in the fluid phase in several different ways and thus produce antibodies with varying specificities and binding capacities. For such reasons it is not possible to determine the structure of the antigen-binding areas because of the chemical heterogeneity of the antibodies.

The production of chemically quite homogeneous immunoglobulins is, however, a characteristic feature in patients with multiple myeloma (a disease which occurs in human and in certain rat strains; it can also be induced in some mouse strains), in

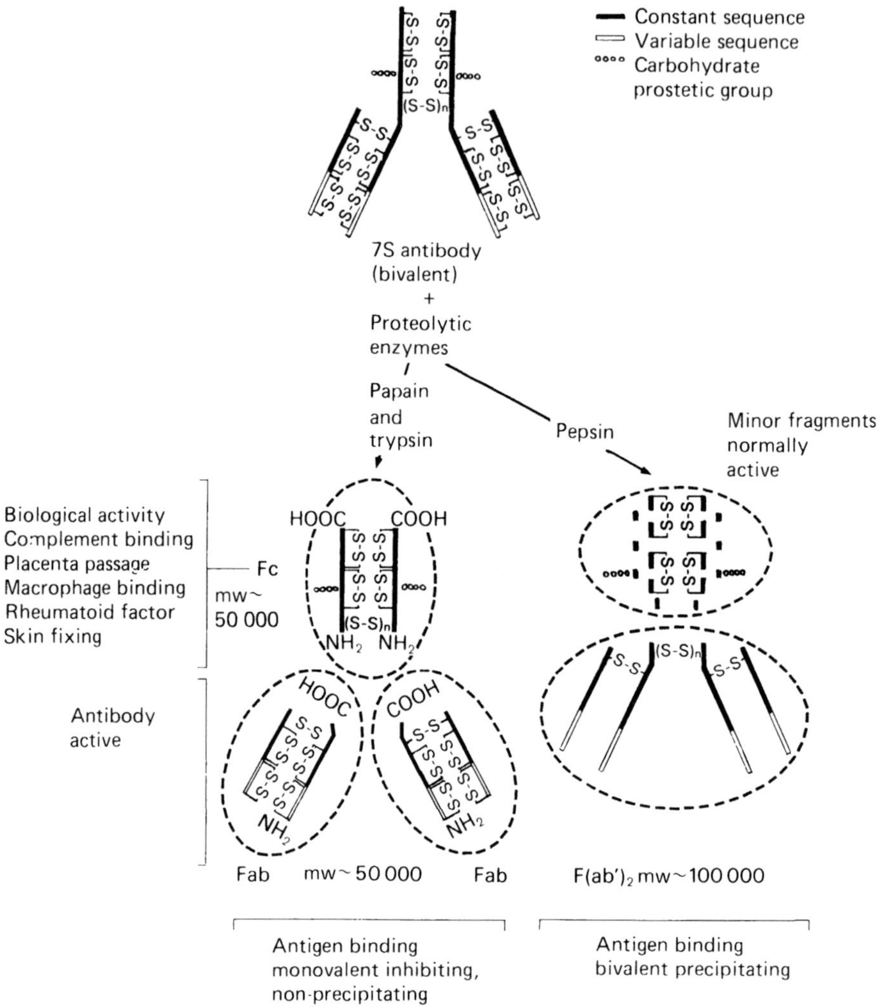


*Figure 2.2* Diagram of fragmentation of an IgG antibody using proteolytic enzymes like papain, trypsin or pepsin. Note the distribution of biological functions of different parts of the molecule

macroglobulinaemia and in certain other neoplastic conditions. Such immunoglobulins (myeloma proteins or M components) are produced due to the abnormal growth of single clones of plasma cells and the proteins are called monoclonal immunoglobulins. Most monoclonal immunoglobulins of such origin lack known antibody activity and it is not certain whether they have been synthesized by antigenic stimulation in the ordinary sense. There is nothing to indicate that such immunoglobulin molecules differ from normal antibodies with regard to biological, immunological or chemical structural features (*see Table 2.1*). In the human the distribution of M components with light chains of $\kappa$ or $\lambda$ isotype is normally 2 to 1, which corresponds to the distribution found in immunoglobulins from normal human beings. An exception is constituted by M components of the IgM class, where $\kappa$ chains are considerably more frequent than $\lambda$ chains. Certain patients with myelomatosis have characteristic proteins in the urine which are related to immunoglobulins. The Bence-Jones protein (BJP, discovered 1846) belongs to this group and consists of light chains of $\kappa$ or $\lambda$ isotype.

The secretion in urine of light chains of monoclonal origin suggests that the normal balance between the synthesis of heavy and light chains in the plasma cells has been shifted in such a way that considerably more light chains are synthesized than are needed in order to construct immunoglobulin molecules of intact type. About 10% of patients with myelomatosis also have in their urine amyloid substance which is a chemical structure homologous with the variable (V) part of the light chains (*see below*). Rare patients may also display the so-called heavy chain disease which means that they secrete isolated $\alpha$, $\gamma$, or $\mu$ chains in their urine. The reason why the plasma cells in the above mentioned patients sometimes produce only BJP or heavy chains is not known in detail. In this context one should also realize that in urine one normally detects $\beta$-2-microglobulin (molecular weight 12 000 dalton) which has a chemical structure which is homologous to the constant (C) regions of the $\gamma$ chain. The particular interest in $\beta$-2-microglobulin is due to the fact that it is one of the polypeptide chains of the major transplantation antigens (*see* chapter 9). An increased secretion of $\beta$-2-microglobulin in the urine occurs especially during certain chronic kidney diseases caused by, for example, cadmium poisoning.

It is now also possible to produce at will monoclonal immunoglobulins with known antigen-binding capacity. This will be discussed later in detail (*see* chapter 6).

## Structural areas with variable or constant amino acid sequences

Comparative investigations of H or L chains isolated from M components have shown that both polypeptide chains contain two distinct structural areas, one with a variable (V) and the other with a constant (C) amino acid sequence (*Figure 2.3A*).

The variable region of the human L chains ($V_L$) comprises the amino acids 1–106 or roughly half the L chain. From amino acid 107 to 214 the structure is constant for L chains of a particular isotype ($\kappa$ or $\lambda$). The only exception in the human is the amino acid in position 191, which, in the $\kappa$ chains, can be leucine or valine; this determines the allotype of this chain (Km factor). A corresponding change of amino acids in a specific position also occurs within the $\lambda$ chains (Oz factor), but here this represents isotypic variation and not allotype polymorphism.

The size of the H chains does vary with Ig class and they may consist of 450 to 570 amino acids. The variable region ($V_H$) is approximately of the same size as the $V_L$ and normally comprises the amino acids 1–120, which corresponds roughly to half of that part of the H chain which participates in the creation of one Fab fragment. This particular segment is called the Fd fragment (*see Figure 2.2*). The rest of the H chain has a constant structure ($C_H$), typical for that particular class or subclass. As for the L chains there are allotypic variants of H chains (*see* Am and Gm allotypes, *Tables 2.1* and *2.2*).

Analyses of a large number of L chains have shown that the $V_L$ region can be subdivided into subgroups which strictly follow the isotype. With regard to $\kappa$ chains in the human four such subgroups have been identified, and for $\lambda$ chains there are five $V_L$ subgroups (*Figure 2.3B*). Certain amino acids in defined positions are never interchanged. However, cysteine in position 23 and 88 and tryptophan in position 34, for example, constitute such amino acids while other amino acids which localize to a

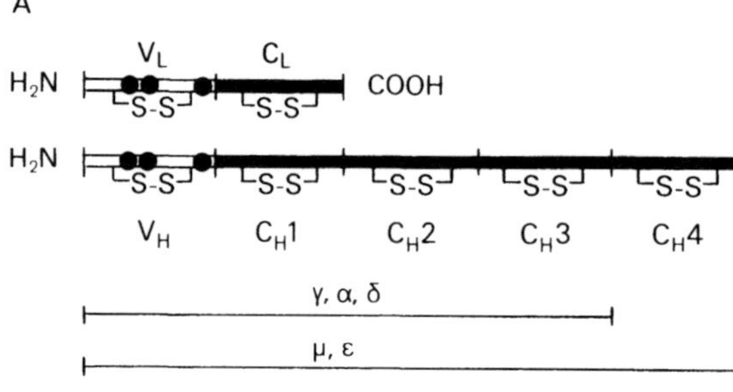



*Figure 2.3* A. Distribution of variable (V) and constant (C) sequence areas within light (L) and heavy (H) chains. The number of amino acids between the half cystinyl residues, which constitute the disulphide bridges (—S—S—) is around 60. Note that there is an extra C region in the $\varepsilon$ and $\mu$ chains. B. Subgroups of the variable region exist in both light and heavy chains. The $V_L$ subgroups are linked to the chain type ($\kappa$ or $\lambda$) while the $V_H$ subgroups can be combined with $C_H$ regions from all Ig classes

nearby structure segment may display what would seem to be, in principle, unlimited variability.

Both $\kappa$ and $\lambda$ chains contain three such hypervariable segments, which constitute the amino acids in position 24–34, 50–56 and 89–97. Investigation of a large number of $V_H$ regions has shown that their structure is similar to that of the $V_L$. So far four subgroups of $V_H$ have been identified. They are not coupled to any particular isotype but can be found combined with $C_H$ regions from all different classes and subclasses of Ig (*Figure 2.3B*). The hypervariable segments within $V_H$ are represented by amino acids in position 31–35, 50–65 and 95–102. The hypervariable segments (in structural context now called complementarity determined regions or CDR) are surrounded by preserved structural areas (framework regions or FR) which are characteristic for each V subgroup. The specificity of an antibody is thus determined by the structures of the CDR from both $V_H$ and $V_L$ (*see below*). When considering a single antibody this usually means that its antigen-binding areas have a unique structure which can serologically be identified and it is then called an idiotype.

### Structural and functional units: the concept of domains

When the primary structure of H chains was studied it was shown that the $C_H$ region consists of several segments of approximately equal size ($C_H 1, C_H 2$, etc., *see Figure 2.3A*) which are homologous to $C_L$ regions ($\kappa$ or $\lambda$). Each segment consists of approximately 110 amino acids and contains one disulphide bridge which is formed by two cysteines placed approximately 60 amino acids from each other.

The fact that the C and V segments from H and L chains are similar in structure and size, indicates that the peptide chains of immunoglobulins have probably been developed from a common primordial 'polypeptide'. The gene for such a peptide, which can be assumed to correspond to a modern C or V segment of approximately 110 amino acids has then segregated to create primitive C and V peptides. Subsequently these peptides have, through a series of duplications and point mutations at the DNA level, probably been developed into the C and V segments or domains, which together create present-day classes, subclasses and subgroups of immunoglobulins.

According to the domain hypothesis this development has led to the different biological activities which are localized to the Fab and Fc regions of the antibody molecules and allow the expression of specific features in different segments (domains) present in heavy and light chains. Experimental support for this domain hypothesis has come at the level of protein chemistry by testing various V and C segments isolated after brief enzymatic splitting of intact antibodies with different activities. The distribution of information for protein synthesis at the DNA level has also corresponded to the domain hypothesis.

As can be seen in *Figure 2.4* the immunoglobulin molecule is composed of a series of globular entities with compact structure and defined biological function (*Table 2.2*).

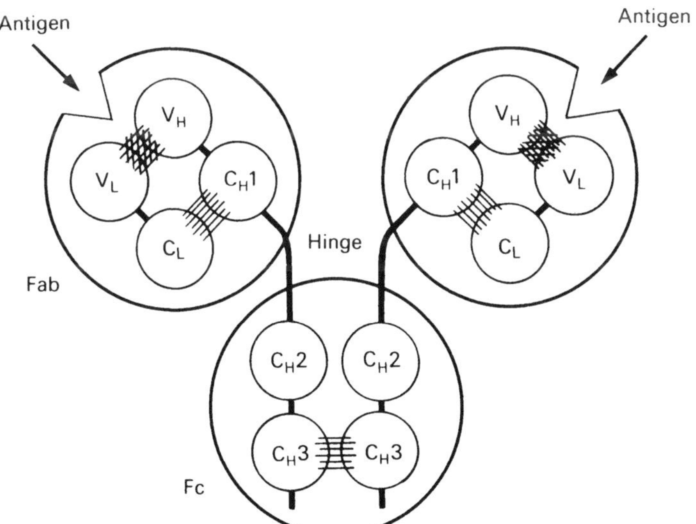


*Figure 2.4* Schematic model of an IgG antibody according to the domain hypothesis. Each domain constitutes a globular entity with compact structure and determined biological function, e.g. $V_H$–$V_L$ domains constitute the binding site for antigen. $CH_2$ binds complement (*see Table 2.2*). Areas involving non-covalent interactions are the $C_H1/C_L$ and the $C_H3/C_H3$. Disulphide bridges between H chains are placed in the hinge region. Areas between domains have a loose structure and are thus 'open' for enzymatic attack

These units are linked together by small peptide segments with a looser structure which allows a certain flexibility within the antibody molecule. In the same way that the V regions of the heavy and light chains are in close contact with each other, so are the $C_H1$ and the two $C_H3$ domains (*see Figure 2.4*). In contrast there is a lack of contact between the $C_H2$ domains which are united through disulphide bridges localized in the hinge region. The schematic picture of IgG as shown in *Figure 2.4* which summarizes the result of immunochemical, physicochemical and biological studies does in all essential parts agree with the model of the molecule constructed through the help of X-ray crystallography (*see Figure 2.5*). The new information gained through the crystallographic studies relates to three-dimensional construction of the specific antigen-binding area as well as to the influence of carbohydrate chains on the tertiary structure. Through the analysis of Fab crystals isolated from antibody active M components, it has been possible to localize the antigen binding area to the aminoterminal region of the Fab fragments, which creates a cleft fully exposed to the surrounding medium. The opening of the cleft normally measures roughly $10 \times 2.5$ nm and its depth is about 0.1 nm, which gives enough space for an antigen determinant of a size corresponding to four to six amino acids or a corresponding number of monosaccharide units. The floor and the walls of this cleft are formed exclusively by amino acids from the hypervariable

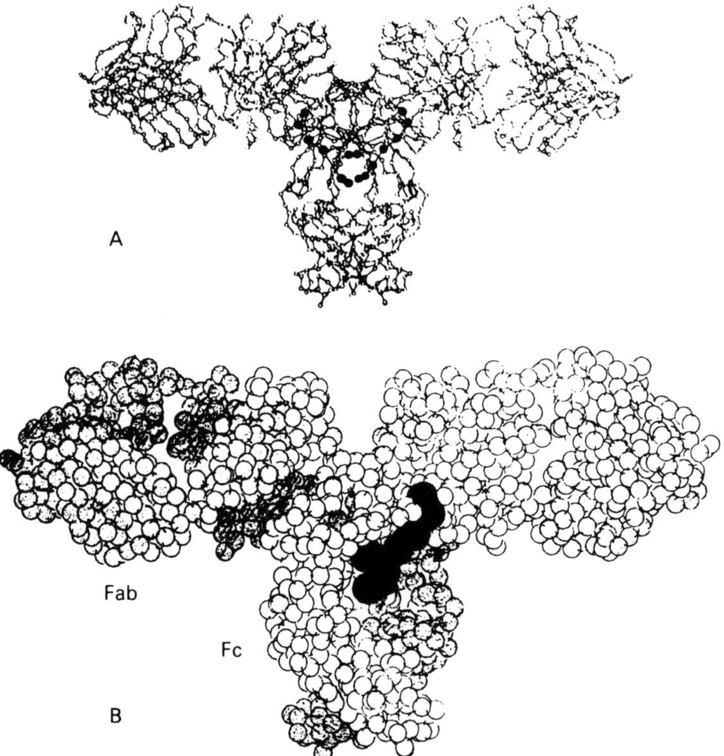


*Figure 2.5* A. The carbon skeleton for an IgG antibody determined by X-ray crystallography. Small circles, α carbon atom. Black circles, hexose units. B. A volume model of the structure in A. One H chain is marked with white balls, the second with dark grey balls, while light chains are light grey. Carbohydrate chains are marked in black. (After Silverton, E. W. *et al.* (1977). *Proc. Natl. Acad. Sci. (USA)*, **74**, 5140)

regions. The X-ray data have thus confirmed similar results using haptens binding irreversibly and affinity labelling techniques. The three hypervariable regions CDR 1, CDR 2 and CDR 3 from the heavy chain and CDR 1 and CDR 3 from the light chain are thus in contact with the binding site for the antigen. If one or more amino acids in one or more CDR are changed, both the dimension of the antigen binding area and single contactual points can be adapted to fit antigenic determinants of different sizes and chemical structures. Such modifications will not influence the conformation of the $V_H$ and $V_L$ domains as they are stabilized by structures within FR.

X-ray diffraction investigations have yielded unexpected results with regard to the localization of the carbohydrate chains within the Fc fragment of the IgG molecule. IgG contains only two carbohydrate chains which are localized to the $C_H2$ domains. Instead of being orientated out from the domains, towards the surrounding medium, as was previously assumed considering the hydrophilic features of carbohydrates, it turned out that the carbohydrate chains in IgG are localized inwards and orientated towards each other. As a result the two $C_H$ domains are kept apart creating a cavity filled with fluid. It also eliminates the possibility of contact between the $C_H1$ and the $C_H2$ domains. The exact function of the carbohydrate chains is not known but removal of them results in a significant reduction in the biological activities normally associated with the $C_H2$ domain. The oligosaccharide chains of the IgG molecules are of a complex nature and consist of hexoses (galactose, mannose), amino sugar (N-acetyl-glucosamine, fucose and sialic acid. Other Ig classes which contain 10–15% peptide bound carbohydrates have both simple and complex carbohydrate chains. Removal of sialic acid from the glycoprotein normally results in the binding of that protein to asialoreceptors on the surface of several cell types, i.e. liver cells. IgG is here an exception together with transferrin.

## Immunoglobulin classes and biological function

Five Ig classes have so far been isolated from the serum of adults as represented in *Table 2.1* and *Figure 2.6*. Immunoglobulins also normally exist in colostrum, milk, saliva, spinal fluid and urine, but the distribution and concentration in these fluids is very typical and distinct from that of the serum. This indicates that antibodies belonging to various classes have developed the ability to take over distinct immunobiological functions. The part played by the Fc region of the Ig molecule in several non-antigen related functions has already been touched upon. In the following section we will discuss the features which are typical for each Ig class.

IgG, which is the dominating Ig class in the serum, exists normally as a monomer with the basic structure $H_2L_2$. The molecular weight is around 150 000 dalton out of which 3% are carbohydrates bound to the $C_H2$ domain. IgG is characterized by a high degree of polymorphism: four isotypes and 25 allotypic variants have so far been identified in man. IgG antibodies that pass through the human placental membranes, can activate the complement system (*see* chapter 5), can be fixed to receptors on macrophages and be attached to mast (basophil) cells in heterologous tissue. These constitute some examples of biological reactions, that are due to structural features in various $C_H$ domains. As can be seen in *Table 2.2* various biological functions and genetic markers (Gm allotypes, *see* chapter 9) are distributed evenly on the four IgG isotypes. The majority of the IgG molecules are synthesized by plasma cells in the regional lymph nodes and the metabolism of IgG is demonstrated in *Table 2.3*.

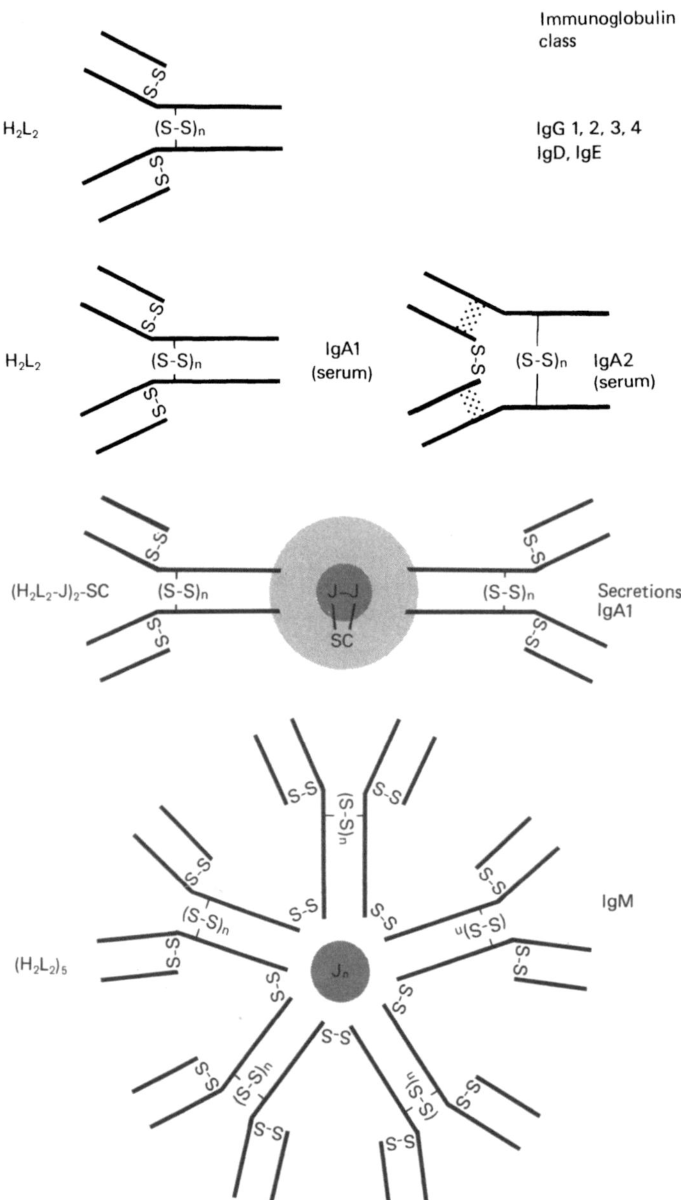


*Figure 2.6* The build-up of various immunoglobulin classes using as the basic element the four chain structural unit. Note that light chains in IgA2 exist in the form of disulphide linked dimers associated with the α chains through non-covalent bonds. The number of disulphide bridges between the heavy chains varies with class and subclass of immunoglobulin (*see Table 2.2*). SC, secretory component—a polypeptide of epithelial origin. J, joint chain—a polypeptide which is synthesized by B cells or plasma cells (mol wt 15 000)

**Table 2.3. Metabolic properties of immunoglobulins in healthy adult individuals**

| Ig class | Serum concentration (g/l) | % Intravascular (i.v.) | Total circulating pool (mg/kg) | Survival T 1/2 (days) | Catabolism. Fraction of the (i.v.) pool per 24 hours | Synthesis (mg/kg per 24 hours) |
|---|---|---|---|---|---|---|
| IgG | 12.1 | 45 | 494 | 22.9 | 0.067 | 34 |
| IgA | 2.5 | 42 | 95 | 5.8 | 0.252 | 24 |
| IgM | 0.93 | 80 | 37 | 10.1 | 0.088 | 3.3 |
| IgD | 0.023 | 75 | 1.1 | 2.8 | 0.37 | 0.4 |
| IgE | 0.0001 | 51 | 0.0035 | 2.3 | 0.71 | 0.0023 |

IgA in serum exists both as a monomer, of the type $H_2L_2$, and as a dimer $(H_2L_2)-J_2-(H_2L_2)$, where J (join) represents a special type of polypeptide chain (mol wt 15 000 dalton) which can be synthesized in plasma cells and bind not only to IgA but also to IgM. In milk, saliva and intestinal secretions IgA also exists as a complex of $(H_2L_2)_2-J_2$ and an additional protein, the secretory component (SC, mol wt 50 000 dalton), which is synthesized in epithelial cells. The function of these extra components is not entirely clear but it is assumed that the combination of J chains with IgA (which are both synthesized in the same cells) forms a secondary binding site for the secretory component. The presence of this is necessary for the transport of IgA antibodies through glandular epithelium to serous membranes. Active immunization results in the synthesis of IgA antibodies which causes an increased titre of IgA in secretions but not necessarily in serum.

Two isotypic forms of IgA exist which differ in the way in which the L chain is linked to the α chain (*see Figure 2.6*). One consequence of this type of variation is that IgA2 antibodies, functionally speaking, will have monovalent binding features.

Early transfer of IgA antibodies through the mother's milk will complement the supply of IgG antibodies that a newborn human being has received from the mother during the embryonic period. IgA antibodies are not resorbed however but offer local protection in the intestinal tract of the newborn.

The metabolism of IgA is shown in *Table 2.3*.

IgM antibodies are constructed in five identical ground structures, which are united through disulphide bridges to create a pentamer, $(H_2L_2)_5$.

The molecular weight of IgM is 900 000 dalton out of which roughly 12% are carbohydrates, which are linked to the CH1, CH2 and CH3 domains. IgM antibody has ten binding sites for antigen, but in reality IgM functions as an antibody with five binding sites, probably due to some steric blocking. The multivalent features, however, mean that IgM antibodies can react in a most efficient manner with polyvalent antigenic determinants on the cell surfaces (e.g. bacteria, viruses). IgM is also an efficient complement activator and the binding site has been localized to the $CH_2$ domains. IgM molecules bind a J chain through a disulphide bridge, which together with SC may allow for selected transport through glandular epithelium and secretion. On active immunization IgM antibodies rapidly appear in the serum but normally the amount decreases after about a week, which usually parallels a significant increase in the IgG response (*see* chapter 6).

IgD in serum exists as $H_2L_2$ monomers with a molecular weight around 170 000, out of which 12% are carbohydrates. It is present in quite a low concentration in the serum (*see Table 2.3*), and no specific functions have yet been ascribed to the serum IgD molecules. IgD exists, however, as a functional antigen binding receptor (together with IgM) on the majority of newly mature B lymphocytes in peripheral blood. The appearance of the IgD molecules on the B cells has been found to be linked with a more mature action of B lymphocytes, with the cells being more resistant to inactivation by antigen contact. More than 90% of human IgD myeloma proteins are of $\lambda$ type while the membrane-bound IgD-like normal immunoglobins are mainly of $\kappa$ type. This indicates that cells which secrete IgD may represent a small group of plasma cells selected for a particular purpose. Difficulty in demonstrating IgD-producing plasma cells in normal individuals also suggests that the low serum concentration may represent breakdown of shed membrane IgD rather than being a result of active secretion.

IgE has the form of a basic structure, $H_2L_2$, but with a molecular weight of 190 000 dalton. Like IgA, IgD and IgM, IgE contains several oligosaccharide chains, which together represent approximately 12% of its molecular weight. The size of the heavy chain of the IgE molecule ($\varepsilon$) is due to the fact that this chain like the $\mu$ chain contains one extra $C_H$ domain. It is localized at a place corresponding to the hinge region in $\alpha$, $\delta$ and $\mu$ chains, which suggests that this region may in fact represent the rest of a previous domain. The serum concentration of IgE in healthy individuals is well below 1 mg/l. Qualitative and quantitative determinations of IgE have accordingly been done using highly sensitive radioimmuno or enzyme-coupled techniques (*see* chapter 4). An increase in the IgE concentration in serum is normally related to allergic hyper-sensitivity reactions of type I (*see* chapter 17), i.e. hay fever, allergic asthma and atopic eczema. An increase in the IgE level (up to 50 mg/l) may also normally occur with certain parasite infections, such as *Ascaris lumbricoides.*

IgE antibody has a unique capacity to bind avidly to specific receptors on basophil blood leucocytes and tissue-bound mast cells using its Fc region. Contact with relevant antigens via the Fab part may thus lead to a release of histamine and other vasoactive amines, as well as chemotactive factors which, in turn, may regulate secondary reactions such as vasodilatation and bronchoconstriction depending on the local organ. Several of these reactions can be shown to have detrimental consequences for the parasites in question. The half-life of IgE, which is bound to mast cells is around two to three weeks in contrast to the very rapid turnover of freely circulating IgE molecules (*see Table 2.3*).

## Immunoglobulin levels and age

A normal newborn child has an IgG level in the serum which is about 150% compared to that of the mother. Transport of IgG through the human placental mambranes is an active process which is regulated in part by the $C_H2$ and/or $C_H3$ domains of the $\gamma$ chains (*see Table 2.2*). Active synthesis of IgG antibodies in a child will only start towards the end of the embryonic period. Thus a passive immunization via transferred IgG antibodies from the mother is important in providing protection against infections during the first few months after birth. Synthesis of IgM and IgA will start during the twentieth embryonic week and intrauterine infections may thus lead especially to increased levels of, above all, IgM antibodies. After birth the development of Ig levels varies for the different Ig classes (*see Figure 2.7*). During the first year of life there is, for instance, an initial rapid decay of maternal IgG relative to that of the synthesis of the child's own IgG antibodies.

Thus, at three to four months of age the level of IgG in the serum of the child will be comparatively low.

Adult levels of IgG through active synthesis will only be reached at about five to six years of age, IgM at one year of age, and for secretory IgA at around two to three months, whereas for serum IgA adult levels will not be reached until puberty. It is normally difficult to detect IgD during the first year of life. Adult levels are only reached around four to five years of age. In adults about 20% lack detectable IgD and between 0.1–0.3% lack IgA. The consequences of such presumably genetically determined defects with regard to infections are discussed in chapter 13.

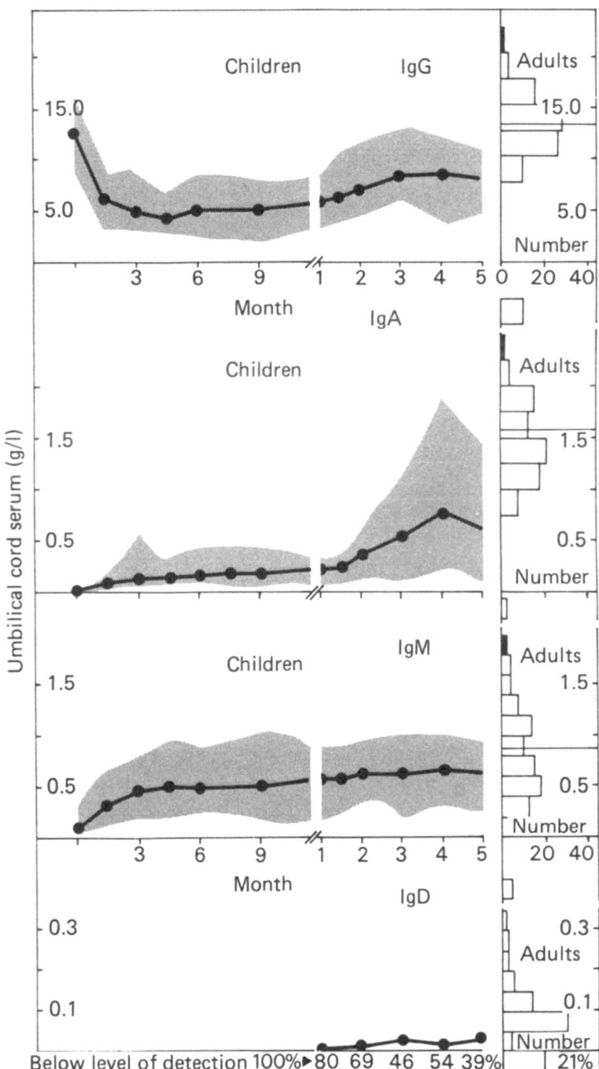


*Figure 2.7* Mean and normal range of immunoglobulin concentration in the sera from 188 healthy children varying in age from 0–5 years, compared to normal adults (S. G. O. Johansson and T. Berg (1967) *Acta. Paediat. Scand.* **56**, 572)

## Biosynthesis of immunoglobulins

Synthesis of H and L chains and their coming together as a disulphide-linked $H_2L_2$ molecule occurs within the same cell, i.e. an antibody-forming B lymphoblast or a plasma cell. The plasma cells represent one of the final stages in the differentiation process, which is initiated through contact between antigen and mature B lymphocytes (*see* chapter 6).

The synthesis of the two polypeptide chains is regulated by separate unlinked genes which are localized in different chromosomes and which are transcribed to separate H and L mRNA molecules.

Active protein synthesis occurs on the polysome—a complex between an mRNA chain and several ribosomes—which is linked to the granular membrane of the endoplasmic reticulum. The number of ribosomes varies with the length of the mRNA, which is proportional to the length of the polypeptide chain for which it is coded. Newly synthesized H and L chains contain an aminoterminal presequence of 18 amino acids, which is split before the chains are brought together into one Ig molecule. The existence of such presequences in other proteins as well indicates that the extra peptide segment has a regulatory function in protein synthesis. It has been suggested that it may constitute a sequence for binding of the ribosome to the endoplasmic reticulum. Isolated L mRNA contains around 1200 nucleotides, which is approximately twice as many as will be needed for the coding of the L chain. The explanation is that between 200–300 nucleotides in the 5′ and 3′ end respectively are not translated. In normal cells the synthesis of H and L chains is balanced with a slight excess of L chains. The time required for synthesis of a single L chain is around 30 seconds and for an H chain 60–70 seconds. The combination of the chains to a four chain structure occurs at the time of or closely after the chains have left their polysomes. If the Ig molecule is to be secreted it will take approximately 30 minutes after synthesis until secretion does occur. During the transport of the polypeptide chains from the site of synthesis via the Golgi apparatus to the cell surface, there is normally a successive build-up of the oligosaccharide chains of the H chain, through membrane-bound glucosyl transferases. The composition of the saccharide side chains with regard to hexosamine, mannose, galactose, fucose and sialic acid varies as does the number of chains according to the type of H chain. A general rule exists that the single plasma cell can at any given moment normally only synthesize one particular class of antibody.

The selection of specificity (V regions) and the coupling of V regions with C regions is described at the DNA level in chapter 6.

# Chapter 3

# Antigens

Sten Hammarström and Peter Perlmann

## Antigenicity and immunogenicity

In order to induce an immune response the substance must be perceived as foreign to the body by the immune mechanism of the reacting organism. The meaning of the concept foreign ('non-self') is a basic problem of immunology. According to accepted terminology the substance is called an immunogen when it provokes a specific immune response. The words antigen and antigenicity are frequently used to describe the capacity of the substance to react in a specific manner with the effect or mechanisms of the immune response, i.e. the antibodies or the antigen-reactive cells. Antibodies are directed against small structures on the surface of the antigen (determinants). Exactly which fine structures will be perceived as foreign and thus give rise to antibody production is genetically determined and can vary between various species and between individuals of the same species. The immune apparatus displays a significant disinclination to produce antibodies against the body's own substances (natural immunological tolerance). A substance does not, however, necessarily have to come from the outer environment in order to be perceived as foreign. Natural tolerance can be lost in various ways. 'Self' substances can then start to function as immunogens. This gives rise to autoimmunity and autoantigens. Autoantigens can also be 'self' substances which have been changed, where, for example, such a change has been induced through a virus infection or a malignant cell transformation. Under certain conditions it is also possible for a native cell substance to behave like an autoimmunogen.

An immune response registering genetic differences in macromolecules from different individuals within the same species is called alloimmunity and the immunogens are called alloantigens. The antigens derived from other species are called heteroantigens or xenoantigens.

To be foreign is in itself not enough to be immunogenic. The molecules must also express certain physicochemical and biochemical features in order to be able to provoke an immune response. The substance should be of high molecular weight but an exact lower limit cannot be given as this varies from substance to substance. The state of aggregation of the molecule is also of great importance. A substance which is brought into the organism in an aggregated state is thus often an efficieint immunogen which can give rise to a strong immune response. If the same substance is brought into the organism in a solution deprived of aggregates, e.g. through ultracentrifugation this may weaken or sometimes completely eliminate the immune response. In fact such administration of a substance may provoke the immune system in a negative way and induce a more or less complete absence of reactivity (tolerance) against the substance in question. Under such conditions the substance can be called a tolerogen.

Immune responses can also be directed against low molecular weight substances. Many allergic responses constitute examples of such a situation (*see* chapter 17). Low molecular weight substances which are able to react specifically with antibodies, even when they are not immunogenic, are called haptens. An immune response against a hapten can be easily provoked experimentally by immunizing an animal with a hapten coupled to a high molecular weight carrier substance. It is assumed that immune responses against low molecular weight compounds, for example in certain allergies, depend on the fact that such molecules may become coupled to high molecular weight carrier 'self' substances. Alternatively, they may have such a strong aggregating tendency that they will become functionally polyvalent in the organism.

There is also a minimum time requirement for the immunogen to remain in the body in order for an immune response to be initiated. Substances which are rapidly cleared from the blood or are catabolized through enzymatic breakdown are thus often weak immunogens. The parenteral way of introducing an immunogen is normally the safest way to assure that an immune response will be initiated. Administration of foreign substances via the food intake is, in normal situations, a less efficient manner of inducing a systematic immune response. A particular route of administration of antigen, however, can sometimes give rise to strong local immune reactions. The functional state of the immune apparatus is, of course, of great importance.

Genetic factors not necessarily related to the antigenicity of the foreign substance may also play a role in the immunogenicity. This is due to the fact that the immune response is a complicated chain of reactions with many steps where genetic or physiological blocks may exist at different levels.

## Antigenic determinants

Our knowledge of the size and chemical features of the antigenic determinants, as well as their numbers and localization in macromolecules, is mainly derived from *in vitro* experiments using antisera (i.e. sera containing antibodies), isolated antibody fractions or from experiments using monoclonal antibodies (*see* chapter 6).

As previously mentioned, an antibody does not recognize an antigenic molecule *in toto*, but only discrete minor reactive areas, antigenic determinants or epitopes. Most immunogens are polyvalent, i.e. they have several determinants which may be identical or different depending on the chemical nature of the antigen. Every single determinant normally gives rise to a population of antibodies which fit to varying extents to the determinant. Antibodies can also react with determinants which are similar but not identical with those which have been used for the production of antibodies. Such reactions are called immunological cross-reactions. Cross-reactions can, however, also exist due to the fact that the same determinant may exist on different macromolecules.

The structure of the antigen-binding area in an antibody molecule determines the size of the antigenic determinant. In polysaccharide antigens the determinant can comprise three to six monosaccharides, while, with regard to protein, it may at the most involve six to seven amino acids.

The number of determinants on macromolecular antigens may also vary depending in part on the genetic relationship between the responding organism and the donor of the antigen and also on the size and chemical complexity of the antigen itself. Immunization of rabbits using human serum albumin (HSA, molecular weight 67 000 dalton), thus gives rise to antibodies against HSA. A maximal number of six antibody molecules can be bound to each HSA molecule using antibody saturation levels. The minimum number of antigenic determinants on HSA is six. The ten times heavier thyroid protein, thyroglobulin, can bind up to 40 antibody molecules.

## Haptens

Fundamental knowledge about the capacity of antibodies to distinguish between different chemical structures was obtained in the 1930s and 1940s, predominantly through the studies of Landsteiner and co-workers with regard to haptens. In these experiments simple organic compounds (haptens) were coupled to proteins using covalent bonds. The artificial antigen was then inoculated into animals, e.g. rabbits, and antiserum was collected. Such antisera contain antibodies against the hapten, against the protein and also against the linkage between the protein and the hapten. The specificity of the antibodies directed against the hapten were studied, e.g. by exploring their ability to precipitate related hapten–protein conjugates (the precipitin reaction, *see* chapter 4). During such analysis the haptens were coupled to another protein than the one used during immunization in order to eliminate the reaction of antibodies against the protein component. The specificity of the antibodies was also investigated by making use of the capacity of different free haptens to inhibit the reaction between the antibody and the hapten–protein conjugate. The hapten, because of its low molecular weight, is normally monovalent, which means that it can only react with one combining site of the antibody. It is thus unable to form a lattice with the antibody, which is required in order for a precipitate to develop.

*Table 3.1* shows the result of a classical experimental series in which the immunizing

**TABLE 3.1. Precipitation of different protein–hapten conjugates using antisera against the haptens *m*-aminobensoic acid and *m*-aminobensulphonic acid**

| Antiserum produced against | Antiserum tested against | | | | | |
| --- | --- | --- | --- | --- | --- | --- |
| | azobenzene | azobenzoic acid (COOH) | azobenzoic acid (COOH) | Cl-azobenzoic acid (COOH) | H₃C-azobenzoic acid (COOH) | azobenzenesulphonic acid (SO₃H) |
| $m$-aminobenzoic acid (COOH) | 0 | +++ | 0 | ++++ | +++ | + |
| $m$-aminobenzenesulphonic acid (SO₃H) | 0 | 0 | 0 | | 0 | ++++ |

0 = no reaction: + to + + + + = positive precipitin reactions of various strengths. (After L. Landsteiner, from W.C. Boyd, *Fundamentals of Immunology*, 1956).

hapten was made up of two different aromatic acids. The amino groups were used to couple this hapten to a carrier protein. As seen, the antibodies can distinguish very well between carboxyl and sulphonic acid groups, but the occurrence of cross-reactions at the same time proves that the discriminatory power of the antibodies has certain limitations. The antibodies do not react with test antigens, where the non-substituted benzene ring serves as a hapten or where the acid group is in the *p* position. On the other hand the introduction of a Cl- or $CH_3$-group in the *o* position does not seem to change the reactivity of the hapten significantly. Hapten studies similar to this experiment have provided important information of general validity. Thus, the presence of a charged group is of relevance for the specificity. Presence of groups that can be ionized is, however, not a compulsory requirement. It is possible to produce antibodies against neutral antigens, e.g. dextran (a homopolymer of $\alpha$-1.6-linked glucose).

The steric configuration of the haptens is of the greatest importance. Antibodies can clearly distinguish between mirror image isomers (L and D forms of molecules with asymmetric carbon atoms). When the hapten consists of several elementary components, such as amino acids or simple sugars, antibodies are able to register the sequence order between the single components. The component which is situated furthest out in such a hapten chain is normally the most relevant for specificity; it is immunodominant.


# Natural antigens

All classes of biological macromolecules, i.e. polysaccharides, proteins, glycoproteins, lipoproteins, nucleic acids, glycolipids, phospholipids and lipopolysaccharides can serve as antigens. Although normally able to induce an immune response their relative efficiency may vary considerably due to such parameters as genetic relationship between the antigen donor and the responding individual, the chemical complexity of the molecule, its size, etc. (*see below* for some examples of antigen determinants of carbohydrate and protein nature). As for nucleic acids the rules are very similar to those for carbohydrate antigens.

### Polysaccharides

Determinants of a carbohydrate nature are normally easier to study than peptide determinants. The reason for this is that the former are less conformation dependent than the latter. Immunologically active carbohydrate fragments can be obtained by treating the polysaccharide or glycoconjugate with dilute acid or enzymes. After purification the ability of various fragments to inhibit the precipitin reaction between antibody and the intact antigen is determined.

Kabat and co-workers have studied the simple polysaccharide antigen dextran and antibodies against this substance. Dextran is a homopolymer of glucose and the predominant linkage is $\alpha(1\rightarrow6)$. The results can be summarized as follows:

(1)   Antidextran antibodies of two different types exist, i.e. those which react at the terminal non-reducing ends of $\alpha(1\rightarrow6)$-linked dextran chains and those which react at non-terminal locations along $\alpha(1\rightarrow6)$-linked dextran chains. Normally an antiserum contains a mixture of these types of antibodies in varying proportions.

(2)   For certain antibodies with terminal specificity as much as half of the total binding energy is directed against the terminal non-reducing monosaccharide unit, i.e. it is clearly immunodominant.

(3)   The size of the antigenic determinants normally comprises three to six mono-saccharide residues.

(4)   The strength of the interaction was dependent upon the way the monosaccharide units were linked to each other [$\alpha$ or $\beta$ glycosidic linkage; (1→2), (1→3) etc.]. When structural analogues to the isomaltose series of oligosaccharides were studied as inhibitors they were generally found to react weakly or not at all with the antibodies.

Complex carbohydrates can contain several different antigenic determinants. One example is the lipopolysaccharide (LPS) derived from Gram-negative bacteria. LPS is a component of endotoxin which exists in the cell wall of certain bacteria, for example from the family Enterobacteriaceae. LPS is a carrier of the O antigens, which serves as a basis for serological classification of Enterobacteriaceae. LPS consists of three regions—one O specific side chain which is different from serotype to serotype, one common 'core' polysaccharide and one lipid part (lipid A). The schematic structure of the LPS of *Salmonella typhimurium* with the immunodominant sugars for the three O factors marked is shown in *Figure 3.1*.

Human and animal erythrocytes carry surface antigens which differ between individuals within the species. A number of human blood group systems are known of which the ABO system is the most important (chapter 9). The ABO antigens are not only found on the surface of erythrocytes but also on many other cells. In about 80% of all individuals they are also present in secretions such as saliva and gastric juices. The secreted substances are water-soluble molecules with molecular weights ranging from 200 000–1 000 000. The chemical composition is approximately 75% carbohydrate and 25% polypeptide. The polypeptide constitutes a sort of 'backbone' onto which oligosaccharide chains of various lengths are attached. The blood group specificities (A, B, O, Le$^a$, etc.) are linked to the outer parts (the non-reducing ends) of these chains. In the erythrocyte membrane the antigens occur as glycolipids of varying complexity. The structures of the determinants of the ABO, Le system are shown in *Table 3.2*. The A, B, O(H) determinants occur both on type I and type II chains, while the Le$^a$ and Le$^b$ determinants only occur on type I chains. Antibodies against pneumococcal polysaccharide type 14 cross-react with type II chains lacking terminal N-acetyl-D-galactosamine (A) or D-galactose (B) as well as L-fucose. The ABO, Le specificities arise through the action of different sugar transferases on type I and type II chains. Several independent pairs of genes control the different transferases. For example the co-dominant alleles A and B control, $\alpha$-N-acetyl-D-galactosaminoyl transferase and on $\alpha$-D-galactosyl transferase respectively which act on the H-active oligosaccharide chain.

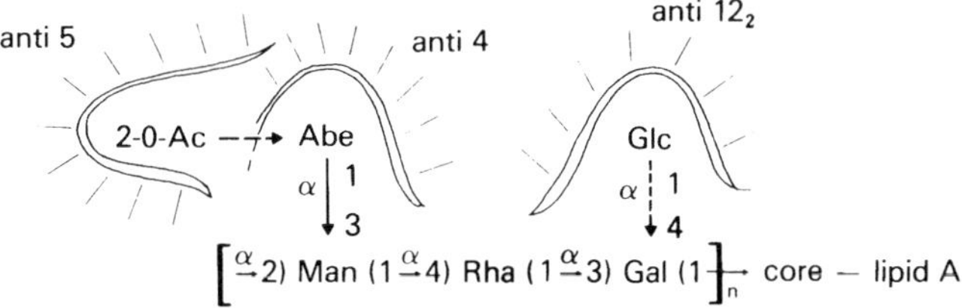


*Figure 3.1 Salmonella typhimurium* lipopolysaccharide where the immuno-dominant sugars for the O-factor 4, 5 and 12$_2$ (Kauffmann–White) have been indicated. ——→ indicates partial substitution. Abe, D-abequose, Rha, L-rhamnose; Man, D-mannose; Gal, D-galactose; Glc, D-glucose. $n = 10$–20. (After A. A. Lindberg, 1983)

**TABLE 3.2. Blood group determinants in the ABO, Le system**

| *Specificity* | *Determinant* |
|---|---|
| A | α-L-Fuc<br>↓1<br>↓2<br>α-D-GalNAc-(1 → 3)-β-D-Gal(1→3 or 4)-β-D-GNAc-(1 ... |
| B | α-L-Fuc<br>↓1<br>↓2<br>α-D-Gal-(1 → 3)- β-D-Gal(1→3 or 4)-β-D-GNAc-(1 ... |
| H(O) | α-L-Fuc<br>↓1<br>↓2<br>β-D-Gal(1→3 or 4)-β-D-GNAc-(1 ... |
| Le$^a$ | α-L-Fuc<br>↓1<br>↓4<br>β-D-Gal(1→3)-β-D-GNAc-(1 ... |
| Le$^b$ | α-L-Fuc    α-L-Fuc<br>↓1      ↓1<br>↓2      ↓4<br>β-D-Gal(1 → 3)-β-D-GNAc-(1 ... |
| type II chain  pn type XIV | β-D-Gal(1 → 4)-β-D-GNAc-(1 ... |
| type I chain | β-D-Gal(1 → 3)-β-D-GNAc-(1 ... |

(After Watkins, 1967.)
D-Gal, D-galactose; D-GalNAc, N-acetyl-D-galactosamine; D-GNAc, N-acetylD-glucosamine; L-Fuc, L-fucose; pn type XIV, specificity of the capsule polysaccharide from pneumococci type XIV.

example, α-N-acetyl-D-galactosaminoyl transferase and α-D-galactosyl transferase respectively and can then act on the H-active oligosaccharide chain.

## Proteins

Proteins are made up of 20 different amino acids which are linked together through covalent bonds to form polypeptides of varying lengths. Since many of the bonds in the polypeptide chain allow free rotation of the joining atoms a protein molecule can, in principle, adopt a very large number of different shapes or *conformations*. However, due to the interactions of different amino acids with each other and with water to form non-covalent bonds the peptide folds in only one particular conformation under physiological conditions. The particular folding adopted by a given protein is mainly determined by the distribution of its polar and non-polar side chains. Many proteins often form additional covalent intrachain bonds such as disulphide bonds between cysteine-SH groups in the folded peptide chain.

Antigenicity of proteins are in most cases strongly dependent on protein conformation. Information about protein determinants is acquired through methods which by various means modify the protein through chemical derivation of different types of amino acids, followed by the investigation of the capacity of the modified protein to react with antibody. If the antigenicity of the protein is significantly decreased this may be due to the fact that one or several of the modified amino acids is (are) part of antigenic determinant(s). Alternatively, the conformation of the protein is changed, which will usually lead to a decreased immune reactivity. Thus it is necessary to investigate to what degree the modified product has retained its native conformation. This can be determined using optical or other methods. Further information may be obtained by studies of large fragments which, because of their size, may be expected to retain a large part of their native conformation. In proteins containing disulphide bridges it has been shown that these must be intact in order for the antigenicity to be retained. Immunologically active fragments can be produced from such proteins through tryptic hydrolysis after blocking of the lysines in the protein by citraconylic groups. The citraconylic groups may then be removed by treatment with weak acid. In the final detailed analysis of the limits of the determinants peptide synthesis will become an important aid.

Myoglobin from sperm whale was the first protein in which antigenic features were determined in detail. The protein consists of a single 153-amino-acid-long polypeptide chain containing many regions of $\alpha$-helices. The amino acid sequence and the three-dimensional structure of the molecule has been known since the 1960s. Early antisera

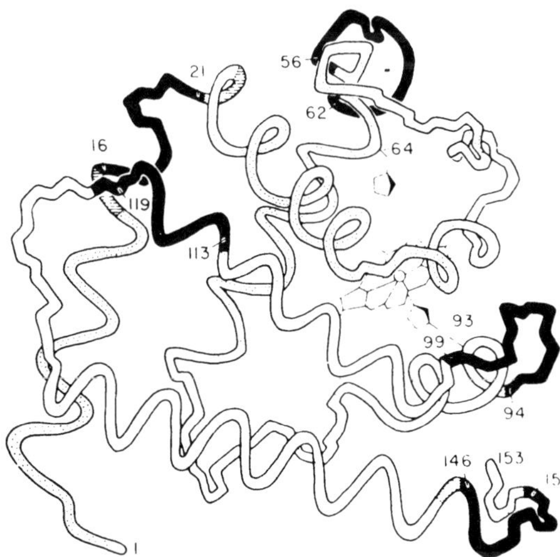


*Figure 3.2* Diagram of myoglobin displaying polypeptide folding and antigenic determinants. The black segment indicates the exact localization and size of the five antigenic determinants. The three striped segments are single amino acids which may participate in the relevant determinant as suggested by certain antisera. The dotted segments are antigenically inactive. (After M. Z. Atassi, 1975)

obtained from individual rabbits or goats were used for the immunochemical analysis. Myoglobin was found to have five antigenic determinants which were all different from each other. The positions of the determinants are depicted in *Figure 3.2*. As seen the determinants comprise five well-defined amino acid sequences located in 'corners' of the molecule often between two α-helix regions. Each determinant is comprised of six to seven amino acids. The superficial positions in the molecule of the determinants make them easily accessible for the reaction with antibodies. The amino acid composition of the determinants shows that basic and acid amino acids often are present, which means that polar bonds play an important role in the interaction with the combining site of antibodies. Hydrogen bonds and hydrophobic interactions, however, add an important stabilizing factor to the reaction. The determinants are normally strongly conformation dependent. Thus, isolated determinant peptides only react weakly or not at all with the antibodies against the native protein. This reactivity can, however, be improved if an isolated peptide is comprised of several neighbouring amino acids as well, which could then help to fix the determinant in its native spatial form.

The five determinants of myoglobin in all cases comprise limited amino acid sequences where the amino acids are directly linked to each other. This is, however, not a common rule. In protein with disulphide bridges, amino acids, which are far apart in the sequence, may be very close to one another when the thread is folded, and therefore be contained in the same antigenic determinant. One example is the carbohydrate-splitting enzyme lysozyme from the egg white of chicken, whose primary and tertiary structure has been known about as long as that of myoglobin. This protein consists of a single polypeptide chain (129 amino acids) whose three-dimensional structure is stabilized via four disulphide bridges. Analysis using goat or rabbit antisera has demonstrated that the protein has three superficially positioned antigenic determinants, each one comprising six to seven amino acids. However, in contrast to myoglobin, each determinant is composed of amino acids which are far apart in the primary sequence. The integrity of the S—S bonds is necessary to retain the reactivity of the determinants with the antibodies. Thus reversible denaturation of the protein through reduction of the S—S bridges will lead to the elimination of antigenicity without changing the primary structure. Removal of small peptides, although they may be immunologically inert, can also lead to a loss of immunological activity of the residual large fragment because the small fragments are necessary for the maintenance of the native configuration of the molecule.

Many proteins are composed of several more or less equal segments (homology regions), which have arisen through duplication of a primordial gene. The different segments display a varying degree of relatedness to each other. Albumin consists of three compact domains; each comprising approximately 190 amino acids. The degree of homology is 18–25%. Preliminary immunochemical analysis of bovine serum albumin using rabbit antisera has shown that each domain has two different determinants and that both are present in a more or less identical form in the three domains (i.e. A', A", A''' and B', B", B''').

The haemagglutinin of the influenza virus, which is a complicated membrane protein, has recently been analysed with regard to antigenic determinants. The haemagglutinins are present in the spherical membrane of the virus where they protrude like clubs. Their function is to attach the virus to the host cell and probably also to allow the penetration of the virus through the plasma membrane of the host cell. The haemagglutinin consists of two peptides (HA-1 and HA-2) kept together through non-covalent bonds plus one disulphide bridge. The native haemagglutinin is a trimer of these peptides (*Figure 3.3a*). Studies of amino acid substitutions in the haemag-

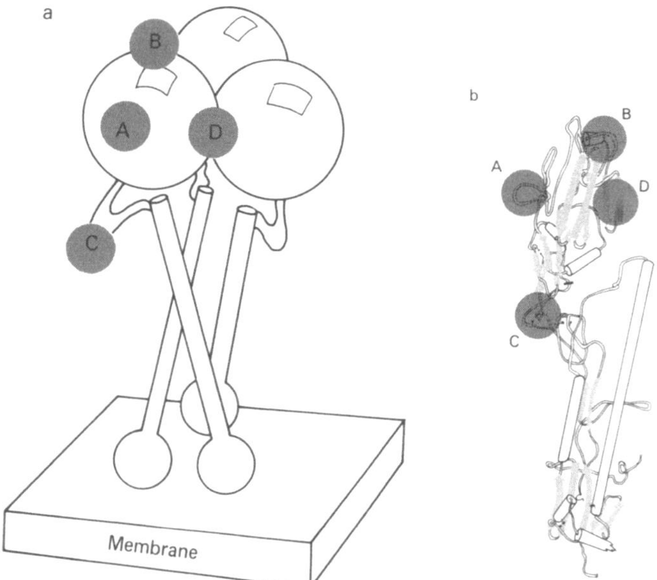

*Figure 3.3* Schematic model of the influenza virus haemagglutinin. (a) Trimer, (b) monomer. Encircled areas show the position of the four antigenic determinants (A–D). Shaded areas in (a) = host cell binding surface. Carbohydrate residues are not indicated. Flat twisted arrows and cylinders in (b) indicate $\beta$-structure and $\alpha$-helix respectively. (Modified from Wilson *et al.*, 1981)

glutinin from different epidemic strains of influenza virus show that it contains four antigenic determinants. Their position in the three-dimensional structure of the haemagglutinin can be seen in *Figure 3.3b*. The determinants A, B and D are situated close to the host cell binding region of the haemagglutinin and this probably explains why antiviral antibodies, which are predominantly directed against the haemagglutinin, have such a good neutralizing capacity. It is most interesting that at least one amino acid substitution in each of the determinants A–D is required in order to create a new epidemic strain of virus. It is somewhat surprising that normally antibodies are not formed against other, more constant areas also present at the surface of the haemagglutinin.

In this context the studies of Lerner and others on synthetic virus vaccines are of great importance. He synthesized peptides corresponding to various parts of HA-1 and HA-2. They were comprised of about 15 amino acids each and were then chemically coupled to macromolecular carriers and inoculated into rabbits. Many antipeptide antibodies did react with the native haemagglutinin and were able to neutralize the virus. Of particular interest was the finding that it was possible to produce virus neutralizing antipeptide antibodies against areas of constant amino acid sequence. In the native protein these areas do not normally trigger production of antibodies. It is obvious that peptide vaccines of this type may have an enormous practical importance in the future.

Many proteins consist of several equal or unequal polypeotide chains. When such peptides are brought together to construct the native molecule, this will add a further dimension to their immunological properties. An example of this is haemoglobin which is constructed of two pairs of a similar polypeptide chain ($2\alpha$ and $2\beta$ chains in human haemoglobin A). Antibodies against isolated chains are specific for the corresponding polypeptide chains but they also react in part with the native haemoglobin. The reactivity is however not the same as with isolated chains because the assembly of the peptides influences the conformation of the chains. Correspondingly the native tetrameric molecule contains determinants which are not found in the isolated chains.

# Chapter 4

# Antigen–antibody reactions

Peter Perlmann and Sten Hammarström

Our knowledge about antigen–antibody reactions is derived from studies of the reaction patterns of humoral antibodies. Immunological reactions can, however, also be produced by cells equipped with specific antigen-binding receptors (chapter 7). In this chapter we will only describe the reaction of humoral antibodies with antigen.

Antibodies are glycoproteins. The chemical and physical laws which govern the properties of proteins are also valid for antigen–antibody reactions. Such reactions exhibit specificity, which is however not unique since specific receptor structures with a similar discriminating power regulate much of the physiology of the cells in a multicellular organism. In fact certain enzyme reactions display great similarities with antigen–antibody reactions as far as specificity requirements are concerned. Differences between enzymes and antibodies mostly occur in the way they react to contact with a specific substrate. While the substrate of enzymes is decomposed or changed, the 'antibody substrate', the antigen, is more or less firmly bound to the antibody without being degraded.

The uniqueness of the antibodies does not lie in the level of specificity but rather in the heterogeneity and variability of antibody molecules. If certain biological and chemical basic requirements are fulfilled, the adult mammal can produce antibody-active immunoglobulins against virtually any chemical structure. Regardless of their specificity the antibodies are principally constructed in the same way by closely related polypeptide chains (chapter 2).

When trying to understand the kinetics and features of the antigen–antibody reactions it is advantageous to distinguish between primary reaction and secondary phenomena. The primary reaction is defined here as the specific binding reaction between the antigen determinants (chapter 3) and the antigen-binding area or combining site of the antibody molecule (chapter 2). It is this reaction which constitutes the basic specific immunological reaction. However, when observing an antigen–antibody reaction, it is normally not the primary reaction which is studied or seen. What is normally registered is a secondary manifestation, such as precipitation of antigen–antibody complexes, agglutination or lysis of cells. These complicated late reactions will be dealt with in the following sections.

## The primary reaction

### Reversibility and kinetics

The primary reaction between an antigenic determinant and its corresponding antibody is a reversible reaction where the reactants are bound to each other by non-covalent bonds.

The reactions follow common laws of equilibrium and can, in principle, be defined by the conventional thermodynamic units. The strength of the binding is defined by the association constant of the antibodies. When the equilibrium is shifted a long way towards the product side (the association constant is high), the antibodies are called high-affinity antibodies. Affinity is normally used to denote the binding strength between a single combining site and a hapten. The term avidity is used to denote the total sum of bindings between multivalent antibodies and antigens. As natural antigens frequently are polyvalent, i.e. have many antigenic determinants, and the antibodies are at least bivalent, i.e. have two antigen-combining sites directed against the same antigenic determinant, it will follow that the total reaction is a complicated function of the various binding equilibria. The forward reaction between hapten and antibody is extremely fast and constitutes one of the fastest known bimolecular biochemical reactions. One can draw the conclusion from the relatively sparse data available that the rate limiting step is the diffusion of the hapten from the solution into the antigen-binding site of the antibody molecule.

**Hapten binding and equilibrium dialysis**

Most methods available for the analysis of the binding reactions are of a physico-chemical nature. Spectroscopic methods using fluorescent haptens exploit the decrease or quenching in fluorescence of the hapten as the binding reaction occurs. Other methods take advantage of fluorescence polarizations, change in the optical qualities of the solution due to complex formation, labelling of the reactants with radioactive isotopes. One simple and very useful way to study reactions between antibodies and low molecular weight haptens is to use equilibrium dialysis. In such studies hapten and purified anti-hapten antibodies (presence of other serum proteins can influence the reaction) are placed on either side of a semipermeable membrane through which the hapten, but not the antibodies, can pass. After dialysis to equilibrium at a constant temperature, the concentration of the hapten is determined on both sides of the membrane and the concentration of bound hapten can then be easily obtained by subtraction of the concentration in the antibody-free part from that in the antibody-containing part of the reaction mixture.

Reaction between the binding structure of the antibody B and hapten H can be formulated $B + H = BH$ with the association constant $K = (BH)/(B) \times (H)$. If all binding structures have the same equilibrium constant and do not affect each other, the relationship is obtained $r/c = nK - rK$, where $r = $ mol hapten bound/mol antibody, $c$ = concentration of the hapten in the protein-free solution in mol/l and $n = $ the valency of the antibodies. If the expression $r/c$ is plotted as a function of $r$ a straight line is obtained, where the intercept of the abscissa at $r/c = 0$ is equal to $n$ and where the intercept at the ordinate is equal to $nK$. With polyclonal antibodies however in practice a curved line is obtained (*Figure 4.1*).

In *Figure 4.1* the results of equilibrium dialysis at two different temperatures are shown with purified but polyclonal antibodies produced in rabbits against the hapten *p*-azophenyllactoside. As seen a straight line was not obtained in either case. Extrapolation to the abscissa gives the expected value 2 for the valency of the antibodies as they are in this instance of IgG class. When $r = 1$, $K = 1/c$ which gives a mean value of the association constant ($K_0$). It is then possible to calculate the other thermodynamic entities such as changes in the free energy of the system $\Delta F^0$, enthalpy, $\Delta H^0$ and entropy, $\Delta S^0$.

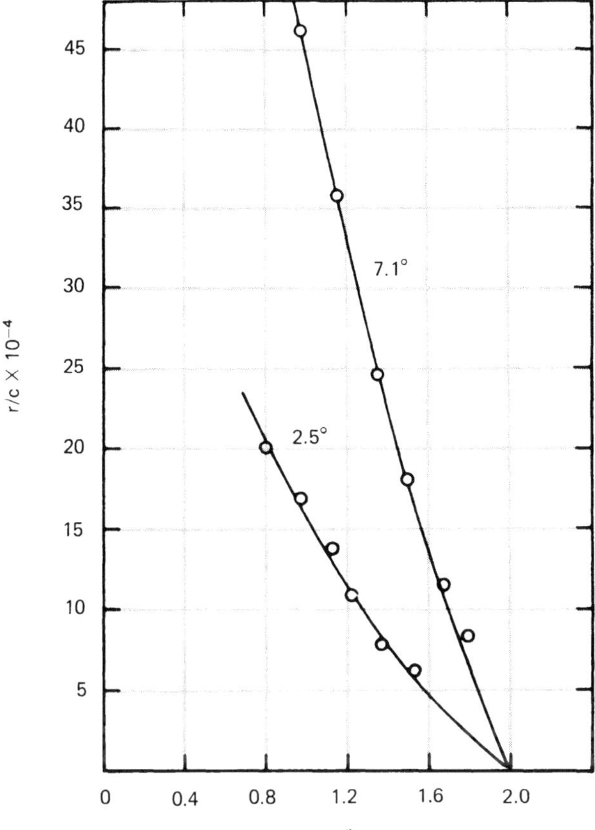



*Figure 4.1* Equilibrium dialysis. The reaction is measured between the coloured hapten phenyl-$\beta$-lactoside (Lac) and purified anti-Lac-antibodies using two different temperatures 25 and 7.1 C. The points are experimentally derived and the curve is theoretical. (After F. Karush, *Advances in Immunology*, **2**, 25, 1962)

The association constants provide information as to the affinity of the antibodies for the hapten in question. In many hapten/antibody systems $K_0$ will be around $1 \times 10^4$–$5 \times 10^5$ (l/mol). This corresponds to a $\Delta F^0$ of $-5$ to $-8$ kcal/mol and means that the average binding is comparatively weak. In other systems it is higher, for instance, $10^9$ l/mol. It should also be noted that these association constants refer to the binding between hapten and a single antigen-binding site. Using polyvalent antigen and bivalent antibodies a much higher binding constant is observed. This means that the equilibrium between native antigen and antibody may be driven towards the product side even though the association constants for the single discrete reactions are relatively low.

Studies using hapten binding and equilibrium dialysis or similar methods show that the antibody response is very seldom homogeneous even if the hapten is homogeneous itself and structurally quite simple. The heterogeneity of the binding features of antibodies, which is considered here, has nothing to do with immunoglobulin class (IgG, IgA, IgM, etc., *see* chapter 2). It exists even within the class, for instance within a population of IgG antibodies and is a reflection of the polyclonality of the normal antibody response. This means in other words that each hapten will give rise to the production of antibody molecules with different association constants. If instead monoclonal antibodies had been used in equilibrium dialysis as in *Figure 4.1*, a straight line would have been observed instead of the curved lines obtained.

## Specificity and binding forces

Chemical structures which can serve as antigenic determinants have been exemplified in chapter 3. Studies of haptens as well as of natural antigens have clearly shown that such determinants are small and can be charged or non-charged and that stereo-chemical relationships play a major part in determining specificity. As the antigen–antibody reaction is specific, it follows that antibodies must have binding structures which are complementary for single antigenic determinants. The interaction is created by relatively weak binding forces between determinants and binding sites of the antibody molecules. In order to allow such forces to act, a close contact has to be established between the reactant surfaces. This means that the binding surface must have a certain spatial configuration making it fit that of the determinant. An analogy which is frequently used is that of the antigen determinant fitting the binding structure of the antibody like a key fitting into a lock.

A steric fit is however not enough to ensure the specificity of the binding. Reactive atom groups in both the determinant and in the antibody molecule must be arranged in a complementary manner in such a way that the interatomic forces which give rise to the binding can become expressed. This, for instance, means that antibodies against a positively charged hapten may fail to react with a negatively charged hapten even if the spatial structure of the latter is related to the former.

Comparatively weak intermolecular forces of various kinds collaborate in the primary antigen–antibody reaction and through this cooperation they make the binding between the reactants quite stable. One such force is electrostatic attraction which can be induced by charge transfer or by mere attraction between positively and negatively charged side groups. Formation of hydrogen bonds between hydrophilic groups as well as van der Waal's forces, i.e. interaction between oscillating electrons in the outer surface of the molecules, also play an important role. Hydrophobic interactions, i.e. attraction between non-charged hydrophobic side groups (e.g. leucine, valine or phenylalanine residues in the proteins) are also of significant importance in stabilizing the antigen–antibody reaction.

## Secondary manifestations

### The quantitative precipitin reaction

The precipitin reaction is the best studied secondary manifestation of immunological reactions. It means that antigen and antibody after the primary reaction in solution will form larger aggregates, which may then make the solution cloudy in the form of visible precipitates. A necessary requirement is here that both reactants are at least bivalent.

The precipitin reaction between a homogeneous antigen and antibodies against such an antigen can be carried out in a quantitative manner and will then provide important information about the laws valid for such a reaction. It may be carried out using a series of tubes containing a constant volume of antiserum to which are added a dilution series of antigen. The tubes are allowed to stand in the cold for a few days in order to

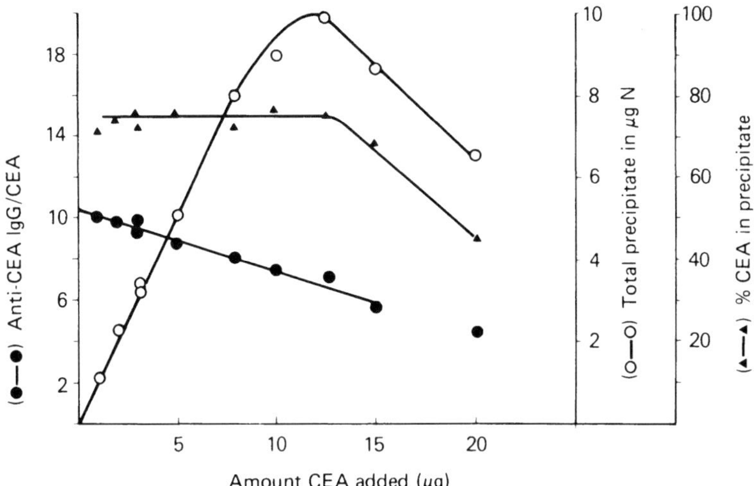

*Figure 4.2* Precipitation of carcinoembryonic antigen (CEA) using a rabbit anti-CEA IgG. CEA is labelled with $^{125}$I. The molar ratio between anti-CEA and CEA was determined by first measuring the radioactivity in the precipitate (i.e. the CEA present in the precipitate) followed by a calculation of the molar ratios from the total amount of N in the precipitate and the molecular weights and N content of both reactants

ensure complete precipitation of insoluble antigen–antibody aggregates. The precipitates are then centrifuged away and analysed for total amount of protein by, e.g. nitrogen determination. A typical example of such a reaction is that depicted in *Figure 4.2*.

The precipitation curve can be subdivided into three different areas:

(1)   Area of antibody excess where the precipitin curve rises rapidly. All added antigens will be found in such a precipitate. With certain antisera a prozone phenomenon will be obtained which means that the complexes formed in antibody excess are soluble due to the solubility of the reacting antibodies.

(2)   The equivalence zone where the precipitin curve has a maximum and where all antigens as well as antibodies have precipitated out. In this zone the reactants have been mixed in optimal proportions and this gives the most rapid precipitation, which frequently occurs within a few minutes after mixing.

(3)   Area of antigen excess where no free antibodies but free antigen will be found in the supernatant. In this area the amount of precipitate will decrease more or less rapidly with increasing dose of added antigen. With extreme antigen excess, a complete inhibition of precipitation may occur. This does not, of course, mean that antigen and antibody have failed to react with each other. If such a mixture is studied by ultracentrifugation, it is easy to demonstrate the presence of antigen–antibody complexes of various sizes. These experimental findings fit with a theory that postulates that precipitates are constructed of large insoluble molecular complexes created by polyvalent reactions, the lattice theory. The results also indicate that the composition of the aggregates changes according to the proportion of antigen in the mixture in relation to antibody. If the ratio

antibody to antigen in the precipitate is plotted against the amount of added antigen a straight line is obtained (*Figure 4.2*). The number of antibody molecules which can maximally bind per antigen molecule will be obtained if the line is extrapolated to the Y-axis (infinite antibody excess). The value obtained here indicates the minimal number of antigen determinants per molecule.

## Immunological methods

Antigen–antibody reactions constitute the basis of a large number of methods. Because of their specificity and sensitivity they have widespread applications in immunology, chemistry, biology and medicine. Here they are used for structural determination of biochemically active substances, classification of micro-organisms, studies of genetic relationships, blood analysis, etc. Biological extracts often contain a mixture of macromolecules, many of which will provoke an antibody response, particularly if inoculated into individuals of a foreign species. The antibody response observed when injecting an antigen mixture is not proportional to the amount of the various inoculated antigens but is to a high degree dependent on the inherent immunogenicity of the various molecules. This means that sometimes tiny contaminants, for instance in a purified protein preparation, may induce a stronger immune response than the 'pure' protein itself. Another factor of importance, is the possible presence of the same or similar determinants on several unrelated macromolecules. This is particularly common in polysaccharide antigens and gives rise to cross-reactions which complicate the analysis.

The polyclonality of the immune response means that immunization with a highly purified antigen virtually always results in the production of immune sera, which contain a mixture of antibodies of separate specificities. The proportion of antibodies against the same determinants but of different isotypes (immunoglobulin class and subclass) varies from serum to serum. It is, among other things, a consequence of the method of immunization, the time and the individual response patterns of the immunized hosts. Isotypes differ significantly in their capacity to give rise to various secondary manifestations such as precipitation, agglutination, complement activation and so on. They may also vary considerably with regard to avidity for the antigen. But differences in avidity also occur within the class or subclass. The association constant for polyclonal IgG antibodies from individual animals against well-defined haptens will thus rise more than a thousandfold in a couple of weeks during a primary immune response.

Methodological problems which are caused by the heterogeneity of antibodies can be avoided using monoclonal antibodies selected with regard to specificity and avidity. It is also possible to make polyclonal antisera more homogeneous through absorption procedures. If an antiserum contains antibodies against, for example, two antigens A and B, and there is an extract of A available which is free from B it is possible, through the use of that extract, to neutralize anti-A antibodies before the antiserum is used for the analysis of B in an unknown mixture. In order to make this removal of antibodies efficient against soluble antigens it is frequently advantageous to make such antigens insoluble before the absorption step.

Immunological methods vary widely with regard to sensitivity and may differ by as much as three to four logs. Using the relatively insensitive precipitation methods, it is possible to detect between 1–10 μg/ml of antigen or antibody whilst the sensitive radio- or enzyme immunological methods may detect 1–10 ng/ml or even less.

The sensitivity of other methods such as agglutination, immunofluorescence, etc., are normally placed between these borders.

In the following section the principles for some frequently used *in vitro* procedures are described. Only such procedures which use humoral antibodies will be dealt with. Methods used in cellular immunology are discussed in chapters 7 and 9.

## Principles of representative methods

### Affinity chromatography

Antigen or antibody which have been made insoluble while their immune reactivity has been maintained are called immunosorbents. Such immunosorbents are frequently used for many different purposes, e.g. for the isolation or purification of antibodies or antigens through affinity chromatography.

The ways of making a soluble antigen or antibody molecule insoluble include the covalent binding of the antigen or antibody to a solid phase (e.g. agarose beads), cross-conjugation, incorporation into polyacrylamide gels or physical adsorption to active carbon, glass or plastic surfaces (e.g. to the walls of test-tubes made of polystyrene). Covalent coupling of antibodies or protein antigens to an agarose gel like Sepharose is done by first activating the Sepharose gel with cyanogen bromide under alkaline conditions; thereafter the protein is added to the activated particles. Cross-conjugation of proteins, so that they form an insoluble gel can be induced through bisdiazotized benzidine or glutardialdehyde.

When attempts are made to purify antigen or antibodies, they are normally mixed with the immunosorbent in a chromatography column where the immunologically active components will be bound while other soluble components of the solution will remain free and thus can be easily washed away. Alternatively the whole procedure may be carried out in a beaker and insoluble complexes removed by centrifugation or filtration.

When an immunosorbent is used for preparative production of antigen or antibody the elution step may constitute the largest problem. Non-specific methods used to dissociate antigen–antibody binding are lowering of the pH (pH 2–4), high salt concentration or the addition of substances which will break the bond, e.g. guanidine-HCl, urea, KSCN, etc. One problem is that some antigens (antibodies) may be denatured. The most satisfactory method is elution using free antigenic determinants in solution, e.g. a low molecular weight hapten or an oligosaccharide if the original immunogen is a polysaccharide. The hapten should be relatively weakly binding so it can later be removed from the antibody using gelfiltration or dialysis.

### Radio-immunological and enzyme immunological methods

The primary interaction between antigen and antibody constitutes the basis for some extraordinary sensitive, quantitative analytical methods with wide application in many areas, such as the determination of hormones, drugs, antigen in blood, antibodies, etc. The RIA methods (radioimmunoassay) use a radioactive marker on the antigen and allow the determination of free and antibody-bound antigen after interaction at low concentration in antigen excess. In the radiometric methods (IRMA) antibodies are radiolabelled using antibodies as the excess reagents. Radioactive iodine ($^{125}$I or $^{131}$I) is normally used to label protein antigens or antibodies forming radioactive reactants causing relatively little denaturation. Separation of free reactants from bound ones can be carried out in many different ways. In the Farr assay for determination of antibodies in an unknown serum, antigen–antibody complexes are precipitated using $(NH_4)_2SO_4$ or an excess of anti-immunoglobulin from another species. However, it is more common to use the immunosorbent principle, i.e. using antigen or antibody in a solid phase, e.g. bound to the walls of a plastic test-tube or agarose beads.

One commonly used method where the immunosorbent principle is applied in a competitive binding analysis for antigen is *RIST* (radioimmunosorbent test). In this test a fixed amount of radioactive antigen is mixed with varying amounts of standard antigen at a known concentration using a limited quantity of antibodies in the solid phase. The binding of labelled antigen to antibody will be inhibited in a quantitative manner through the competition with the unlabelled antigen. The amount of bound radioactive antigen in such a test is thus inversely proportional to the amount of unlabelled antigen. Using a standard curve created by known dilutions of the reference antigen the antigen concentration in single unknown samples can be determined. This method requires access to pure antigen for radioactive labelling. In a corresponding manner antibodies in unknown samples can be determined via competition, e.g. by mixing unlabelled antibodies with labelled antigen and using antibody in the solid phase. The reverse principle using antigen in a solid phase also creates the possibility for determining unknown antibody concentrations relative to a known standard. Antibody in solid phase can also be used for the analysis of antigen in a *sandwich-analysis* where the labelled antibody is added after the binding of the antigen to an antibody sorbent. The reverse principle is used in antibody determinations. One example of such is the *RAST* (radioallergosorbent test) method for the quantitative determination of specific IgE antibodies, i.e. reaginic antibodies. These tests normally require access to purified antibodies. Several other RIA variants are now available.

Lately, labelling of the reactants using certain enzymes instead of radioactive isotopes has found widespread application. *ELISA* (enzyme-linked immunosorbent assay) can be used following the same guidelines as for RIA or IRMA. The antibody or antigen is here conjugated in a covalent manner with a suitable enzyme such as alkaline phosphatase, peroxidase or beta-galactosidase. The enzymatic activity is measured through a colorimetric or fluorimetric test adding the substrate after completion of the antigen–antibody interactions. A schematic picture of a competitive ELISA for determination of antigen is shown in *Figure 4.3*. These enzyme methods are extremely sensitive allowing the determination of antigen or antibody at very low concentrations and are fully comparable with those that can be determined using RIA. ELISA has certain advantages in comparison with radioisotope techniques. While $^{125}I$ or $^{131}I$ labelled reagents have a relatively short life-span due to the comparatively short half-life of the isotopes, enzyme-labelled reagents can be used over a prolonged period. The dangers linked with isotope work are avoided and the measuring equipment is considerably cheaper. ELISA, like RIA, is suitable for automatic analysis allowing the performance of routine tests in large numbers every day.

Through the availability of monoclonal antibodies as analytical reagents it has been possible to further refine radioimmunological and enzyme immunological methods. It is now possible to perform two site assays in which monoclonal antibodies against different epitopes on the same antigen can be used. *Figure 4.4* shows one application of this principle using an enzyme conjugated second antibody to demonstrate the binding of antigen to the first antibody. An important advantage of using monoclonal antibodies is that they offer the chance of the most suitable reagents, e.g. antibodies against epitopes which are unique for the substance being assayed.

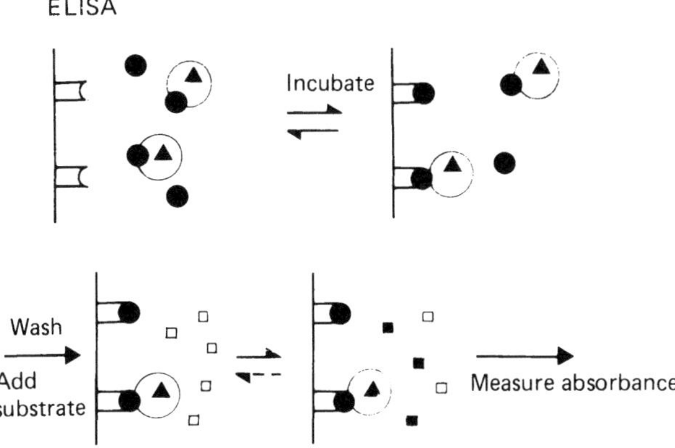



*Figure 4.3* Competitive ELISA used for the quantitation of antigen. (From Engvall and Carlsson (1976), *Immunoenzymatic Tehniques*, ed. by Feldman *et al.* North Holland Publ. Corp., Amsterdam)

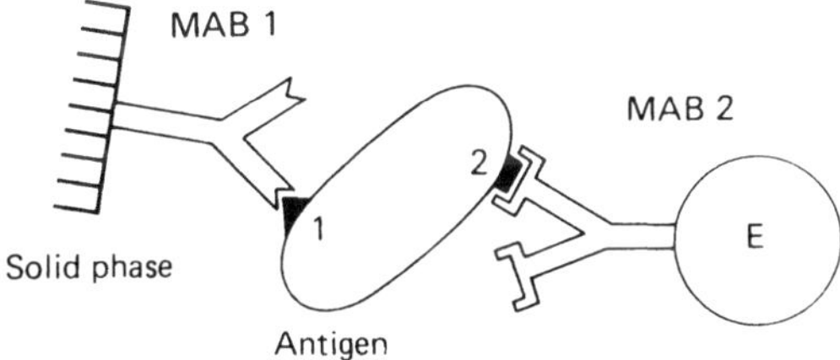



*Figure 4.4* Principle of a two site enzyme immunoassay, MAB 1 and 2 are monoclonal antibodies directed against two different epitopes (1 and 2) present on the same antigen. E = enzyme

## Immunodiffusion methods

A quantitative precipitation method has already been described (*see above*). Such precipitin reactions also serve as the basis for many other frequently used immunological methods. The most commonly used are assays where solutions of antigens and antibodies are placed in a thin layer of agar(ose) gel on a glass surface. In methods which use simple diffusion one reagent, e.g. the antibodies, may be mixed in a suitable concentration beforehand into the agar(ose). The test fluid containing antigen is then allowed to diffuse away from small reservoirs punched out in the antibody-containing gel. The diameter of the precipitin zones will provide a measure of the antigen concentration (*Figure 4.5*). Somewhat similar principles serve as the basis for the rocket electrophoresis (electroimmunoassay) according to Laurell. In this assay

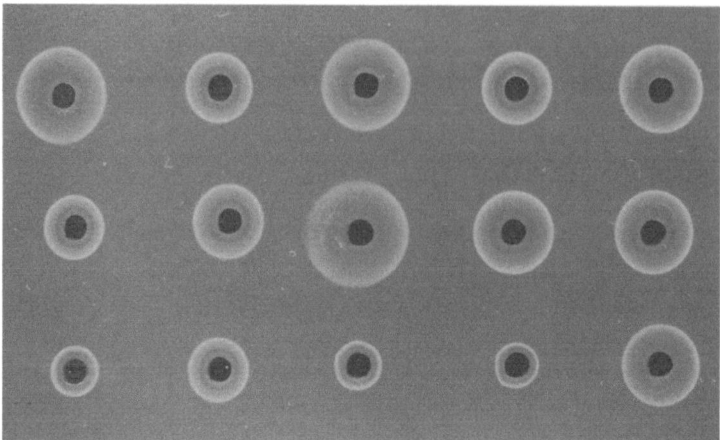

*Figure 4.5* Quantitative determination of antigen concentrations using simple diffusion in agar according to Mancini *et al*. In the present test a solution containing various concentrations of human immunoglobulin A (IgA) was added to the different holes (human IgA was used here as antigen). The agar layer contained rabbit antiserum against human IgA. The diameters of the precipitin zones constitute a measure of the antigen concentration and can be calibrated and quantitated using a standard reference curve

antibodies are incorporated beforehand in a buffered (pH 8.6) agarose gel after which antigen is added to small wells punched out in the gel. Using electrophoresis the antigen enters the gel (this is assuming that the isoelectric point of the antigen differs from the pH of the gel) while at the preferred pH (pH 8.6) the antibody will remain stationary during electrophoresis. If such an electrophoresis is allowed to run for long enough it will, in cases of specific antigen–antibody reaction, generate an immunoprecipitate which does not migrate any further. The concentration of antigen in an unknown sample can be determined using the height of the precipitin peak and relating it to a standard (*Figure 4.6*).

The immunodiffusion methods are relatively insensitive. Their strength is in the very high qualitative, discriminatory power. For instance, in the double-diffusion method according to Ouchterlony, both the antigen solution and antiserum are placed in punched holes in agarose gel at suitable distances from each other. Antigen and antibody will then diffuse against each other and precipitin zones (lines) will develop where the reactants meet in optimal proportions for the formation of precipitates. If several non-cross-reacting antigen–antibody systems exist in the same mixture each precipitate will, in principle, be localized at different positions as the position is determined by the relative concentrations of the reactants and their diffusion properties. If different solutions are allowed to diffuse from suitably placed wells on the same plate it is also possible, on the basis of the interference patterns of the precipitin lines as well as their features, to draw conclusions about the specificities of the antigens and antibodies. Precipitin lines which are formed by non-cross-reacting systems will cross each other (meaning no interference) while cross-reacting antigen–antibody systems will form lines which, to a greater or lesser extent, merge into one another (*Figure 4.7*).

The Ouchterlony technique is suitable as a qualitative analytical method when precipitating systems are available. It is frequently used in the analysis of body fluids

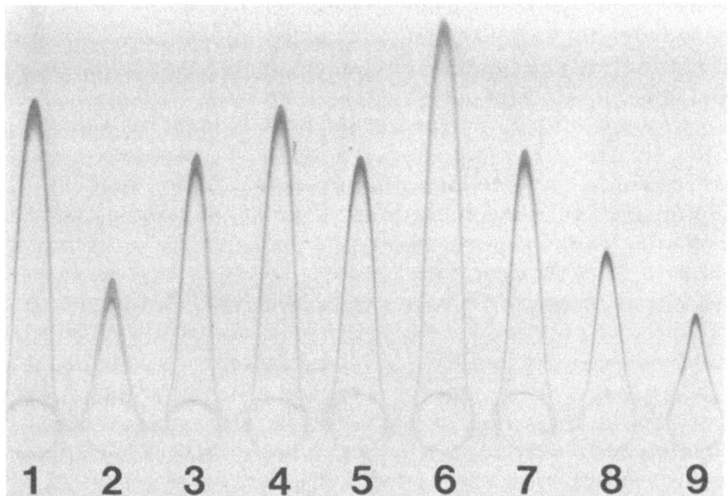

*Figure 4.6* Rocket electrophoresis of C3 in serum (C3 = third complement factor). In holes six to nine a normal reference serum has been added in dilutions 1/50, 1/100, 1/200 or 1/400. In the holes one to five different patient sera have been added all at a dilution 1/100. For further information, *see* the text. (Photo: A. B. Laurell)

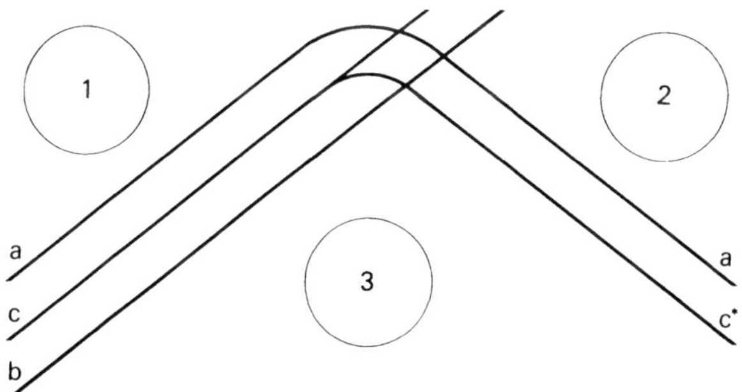


*Figure 4.7* Precipitin reaction in agarose gel according to Ouchterlony. 1. Pool containing a mixture of the antigens A, B and C. 2. Like for A, but containing the antigens A and C*. 3. Pool where antiserum has been added. Antiserum contains antibodies against antigens A, B and C. The precipitin pattern shows that pool 1 and 2 contain one common component (a) which has been precipitated by the antibodies against A (reaction of identity). Pool 1 does in addition contain one non-cross-reacting antigen (b) which is absent in pool 2. The antibodies against antigen C do not only precipitate this antigen but also the antigen C* (present in pool 2). The precipitin pattern indicates that C and C* are cross-reacting antigens where C* is lacking certain antigenic determinants present on C (reaction of partial identity). Alternatively C can consist of two non-cross-reacting antigens which happen to precipitate out in the same area

and tissue extract in parallel with biochemical methods, e.g. when following a purification procedure or when trying to analyse protein structure. The discriminatory power of this method can be further increased by a combination with electrophoresis in the same gel medium (immunoelectrophoresis). Here the antigens are first separated through migration in an electric field. Subsequently antibody is added via a slit cut in the gel parallel to the direction of electrophoretic migration. Precipitates are then subsequently formed according to the same principles which are valid for the ordinary double diffusion method. The combination of electrophoretic separation and immunoprecipitation will give the method a high discriminatory power. There are many different methods to define the identities of the components, e.g. by staining of the precipitates with histochemical reagents. This can define whether the antigens display certain enzymatic capacity. It is possible to increase the sensitivity and thus discriminatory power by the use of radioactive reactants followed by autoradiography of the agar plate.

An assay with a very high discriminatory capacity is the socalled two-dimensional or crossed immunoelectrophoresis. Here an ordinary gel electrophoresis in one direction is followed by a second electrophoresis into an antibody containing gel run at a 90 degree angle towards the first electrophoresis. In the precipitation pattern which will then be formed the antigen mixture can be analysed in great detail both with regard to the charge of the components and their immunological identities (*Figure 4.8*). The relative concentrations of the antigens can also be determined as described above.

Precipitin reactions of an immunological nature can also be used when analysing cell membrane proteins. The surface proteins of the cell are labelled using lactoperoxidase catalysed iodination with radioactive iodine or via the metabolic labelling of cellular proteins with radioactive precursors. After solubilization of the cells with non-ionic detergents the cell lysis is allowed to react with antibody followed by an anti-antibody or protein A from *Staphylococcus aureus* (coprecipitation) The precipitate can

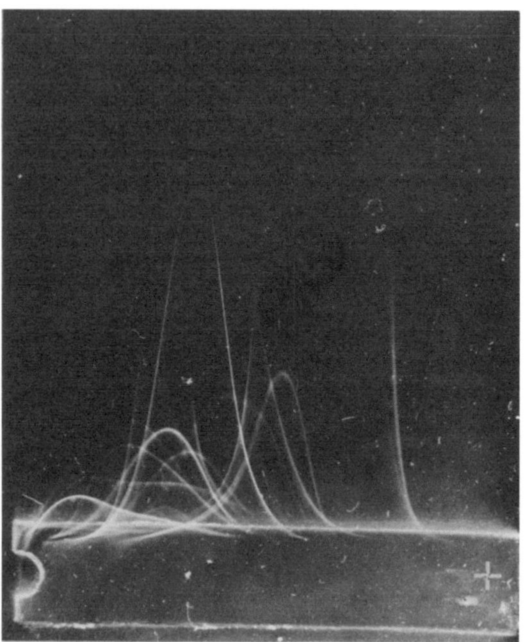

*Figure 4.8* Crossed immunoelectrophoresis. Lysosomal components from rat liver cells have been separated in the first dimension using electrophoresis (→), whereafter electrophoresis in a second dimension (↑) has been carried out into an agarose gel containing rabbit antiserum against lysosomes. Single precipitates formed after electrophoresis in the first dimension are resolved into several distinct precipitates after electrophoresis in the second dimension (about 15 different immunoprecipitates can be visualized on the picture). Using zymogram staining it was subsequently possible to demonstrate lysosomal enzyme activities in several of these in antigens (K. Berzins, unpublished data)

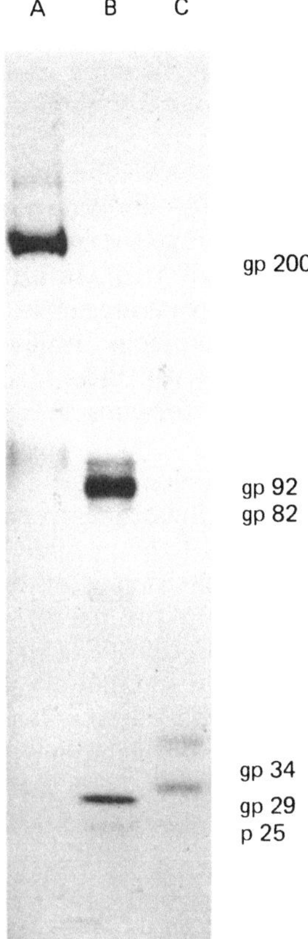



*Figure 4.9* Autoradiography of [125]I-labelled proteins separated on SDS–PAGE (sodium dodecylesulphate–polyacrylamide gel electrophoresis). B cells from a lymphoma patient were surface labelled using lactoperoxidase and radioactive iodine. The cells were lysed and incubated together with lectin or antibody conjugated Sepharose gel. Proteins which have bound specifically to the gels were then diluted with SDS and analysed in SDS–PAGE. A. Eluate from lectin–Sepharose containing a predominating glycoprotein of a molecular weight around 200 000 dalton (gp 200); B. Eluate from Sepharose conjugated with antibodies against human immunoglobulin (Fab′)$_2$-fragment. The eluated B cell components are immunoglobulin chains ($\mu$ chains, gp 92; delta chains, gp 82; and light chains gp 25); C. eluate from anti HLA–DR Sepharose containing the DR chains (gp 29 and gp 34) (B. Axelsson, unpublished data)

then be centrifuged down and solubilized in sodium dodecylsulphate (SDS) followed by analysis in polyacrylamide gel electrophoresis. The peptides in the precipitate will then be separated mainly according to molecular weight. Radioactively-labelled membrane proteins in the precipitate can subsequently be identified using autoradiography (*Figure 4.9*).

A new important technique is immunoblotting. In this technique the antigen mixture is separated via electrophoresis, isoelectric focusing or by other means, whereafter the antigens are transferred or blotted onto a nitrocellulose membrane using electrophoresis or by direct contact using pressure. The nitrocellulose membrane is subsequently incubated with an excess of irrelevant protein in order to block free binding sites whereafter specific antibody is added. After washing anti-antibody labelled with enzyme or with a radioactive isotope is added.

### Agglutination methods

Cells in suspension, which carry antigenic determinants on their surface, can be agglutinated using antibodies. Antibodies of IgM nature which have many binding sites (ten) are among the most powerful agglutinins but IgG antibodies can also be quite effective. The methods frequently require that complement is not present as this may change agglutination to a lytic reaction. Socalled direct agglutination methods are used in the classification of bacteria, blood group determinations. In the latter case the reaction is called haemagglutination. In certain situations haemagglutination of erythrocytes will only occur subsequent to enzymatic treatment of the red blood cells. The sensitivity of agglutination tests can frequently be increased using as a second layer anti-immunoglobulin antibodies from another species. This will then normally create agglutination even in situations where the first antibodies directed against the cellular antigens may exist in suboptimal concentrations or are insufficient on their own to cause agglutination. The concentration of antibodies in the serum is frequently defined by a determination at the highest dilution which will still give rise to visible agglutination under standardized conditions. This dilution is called a titre. The titre method is very simple but carries one significant disadvantage in that it depends on the varying agglutinability of the cellular material.

In agglutination inhibition different dilutions of antigen containing material are added to a series of tests containing a constant amount of antiserum. Subsequently to this agglutinable cells are added and the agglutination titre is recorded. If the added material did contain similar antigens as those involved in the agglutination reaction this will result in an inhibition of the latter. A requirement for this method to function is that the antibody concentration must not be too high. This method is very sensitive and allows for the determination of the relative antigen concentration in the inhibiting material, the specificity relationships, etc.

It is also possible to attach soluble antigens to cells which can then be agglutinated by antibody-containing serum (indirect agglutination). Red blood cells fixed with formaldehyde are frequently used as carrier cells for such soluble antigens. Certain complex polysaccharides, e.g. bacterial lipopolysaccharides, can be adsorbed to erythrocytes without having to use special chemical procedures. However, if protein antigens are to be linked to red blood cells, they have to be treated in various ways e.g. to form covalent bonds between the proteins or the haptens and the surface of the cells. Instead of red blood cells inert carrier particles can be used, e.g. latex or acrylic plastic particles. Such methods are frequently used in the determination of rheumatoid factor. The indirect agglutination methods are highly sensitive.

Antibodies against surface antigens present on tissue culture cells can also be used in very low concentrations through a socalled mixed haemadsorption test. Here the cells, growing on the bottom of a tissue culture dish, are first treated with a test serum. Subsequently the indicator system is added which consists of erythrocytes which have previously reacted with antibodies from the same species as the test serum followed by antibodies directed against immunoglobulins of the test serum. Such treated erythrocytes will then be able to stick to those cells which have reacted with antibodies in the initial test serum.


*Immunofluorescence and related methods*

Antibodies can be conjugated with dyes without losing their reactivity with antigen. They can then be used as specific histochemical reagents. A common method is to conjugate the immunoglobulin with fluorescein or rhodamines through isothiocyanate conjugation (immunofluorescence). In the direct technique such conjugates are added to the antigen-containing cellular material (bacteria, virus infected cells, smears, histological sections). Subsequently, the preparations are examined in a fluorescence microscope. Antibodies bound to antigenic structures will give rise to a staining

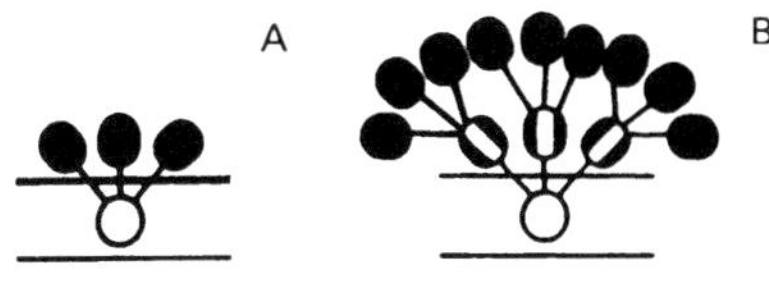

*Figure 4.10* Various modifications of immunofluorescence technique. A. Direct method for the demonstration of antigen using fluorescein conjugated antibodies. B. Indirect method. Unlabelled antibodies are used at the first step whereafter fluorescein conjugated antibodies directed against the first immunoglobulin type is added. ● Fluorescein labelled antibodies; ◑ Unlabelled antibodies; ○ Antigen. (After J. H. Humphrey and R. C. White (1970), *Immunology for Students of Medicine*)

characteristic for the conjugate which has been used (e.g. green in the case of fluorescein).

In the indirect method the test material is first treated using unconjugated antibodies whereafter a second layer of conjugated antibodies directed against the first immunoglobulins is added (*Figure 4.10*). The use of the indirect technique is increasing the sensitivity and areas of application of immunofluorescence. Another way of increasing fluorescence can be achieved if the low molecular weight vitamin biotin is coupled to the antibody molecules. Biotin has a very specific and high affinity for avidin, a protein from chicken egg white. Avidin can be conjugated with fluorescein or rhodamine to provide the fluorescence. It it is also possible to increase the discriminatory power of immunofluorescence by double staining, e.g. by using

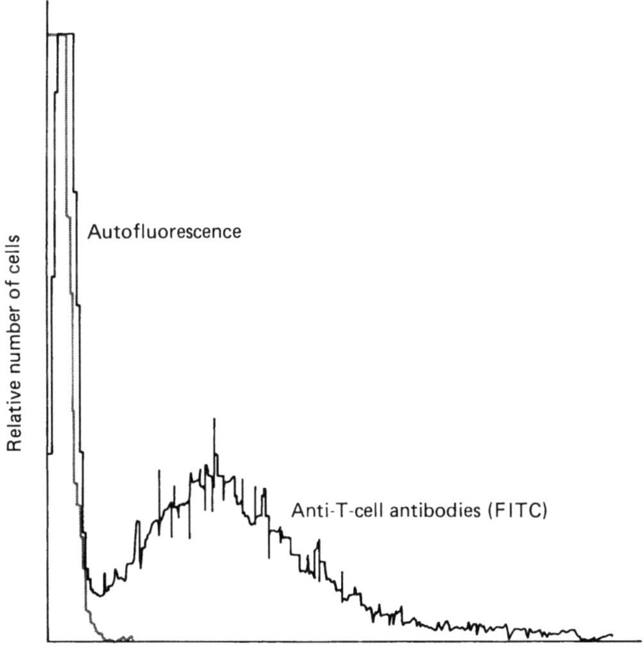


*Figure 4.11* FACS analysis of human peripheral blood lymphocytes treated with fluorescein conjugated monoclonal mouse antibodies which will only stain the surface of T cells. From the diagram it can be seen that around 70% of the added lymphocytes have been stained using these antibodies. It can furthermore be seen that the reactive cell population is heterogeneous with regard to surface fluorescence, i.e. density of the antigens in the T-cell surface

antibodies against different antigens conjugated with different fluorescent dyes and added to the very same test material.

Immunofluorescence techniques are highly sensitive. As qualitative histochemical methods of analysis they have no comparison. As antibody molecules normally are unable to penetrate living unfixed cells they do also constitute highly specific cell surface reagents in the analysis of heterogeneous cell populations, e.g. lymphocyte subsets. The staining of a lymphocyte preparation with antibodies specific for surface antigens present on only a certain subpopulation (e.g. certain T-cells, *see* chapter 7), provides a technique allowing the determination of the size of such a subpopulation. This can be done using the naked eye in fluorescence microscopy or by flow cytofluorometry. In the socalled FACS system (fluorescence activated cell sorter) the cells are allowed to pass one by one through a laser beam whereby each cell is characterized by light scattering, colour and fluorescence intensity. Here the results are obtained in the form of a histogram (*Figure 4.11*). Through the use of the FACS machine it is possible to separate cells differing in fluorescence intensity into antigen-positive and antigen-negative subpopulations.

Similar principles as are used in fluorescence immunology can also be used in the analysis of the ultrastructural localization of antigens using electron microscopy. Here antibodies conjugated with a protein ferritin in a molar ratio of 1:1 can be used as a stain. The ferritin molecule contains iron in characteristic micelles making the conjugate visible in the electron microscope.

Antibodies can also be conjugated with enzymes such as lactoperoxidase, whereafter the localization of the enzyme via the binding of the antibodies to the cellular material can be demonstrated in a light microscope using histochemical techniques. Enzyme conjugated reagents can here be used both for light and electron microscopical studies.


## Bibliography

AXELSEN, N. H. (ed.) (1983). *Handbook of Immunoprecipitation in Gel Techniques. Scand. J. Immunol.*, suppl. 10. Blackwell, Oxford.

BULLOCK, G. R. and PETRUSZ, P. (ed.) (1982). *Techniques in Immunocytochemistry*, vol. 1. Academic Press, New York.

EISEN, H. N. (1981). *Immunology*, 2nd edn. Harper & Brown, Hagerstown.

LANGONE, J. J. and VAN VUNAKIS (eds.) (1981–83). *Methods in Enzymology*, vol. 70, 73, 74 (1981): *Immunochemical Techniques;* vol. 84 (1982): *Selected Immunoassays;* vol. 92 (1983): Monoclonal Antibodies and General Immunoassays Methods; vol. 93 (1983): *Conventional Antibodies, Fd-receptors and Cytotoxicity.* Academic Press, New York.

# Chapter 5

# The complement system

**Anna-Brita Laurell**

Bordet notices in 1898 that the antigen–antibody reaction was only the first step in a chain of reactions which help to eliminate foreign cells and substances from the body. He demonstrated that lysis of foreign red blood cells or bacteria required, in addition to antibody, a thermolabile factor present in normal sera. This component was later named by Ehrlich as complement (C).

It was soon discovered that C is not a single homogeneous entity but is composed of a number of components which under certain conditions may be changed—activated—thus making them able to react with each other in a defined sequence. If activation occurs on the surface of a cell or a bacterium this may lead to the lysis of the cell.

C activation may, in addition to lysis of antibody-coated cells, also lead to a series of biologically important reactions which play a part, for example in the defence against infections, in creating inflammation and in the interplay between the coagulation and the kinin systems. It is also relevant for certain functions in monocytes, granulocytes, thrombocytes and possibly B lymphocytes.

The C system consists of 16 plasma proteins and at least six different controlling proteins which interact and inhibit certain defined steps in the cascade reaction which is initiated upon C activation. C components are normally present in serum as inactive proteins, zymogens. On activation specific proteolytic reactions occur, which convert zymogens to active components. Protein–protein complexes between the factors are created and these have important biological reactivities. C activation means that the individual C components are acted upon and will subsequently take part in an integrated biologically active system.

The activation of the C system occurs principally via two pathways of activation: the classical way and the alternative way.

When studying C it is normally advantageous to use immune haemolytic tests. If fresh serum is added to sheep erythrocytes which have previously been allowed to react with specific antibodies, such sensitized erythrocytes (EA) will be lysed. Calcium and magnesium ions are necessary for immune haemolysis to occur:

$$EA + C + Ca^{2+} + Mg^{2+} \quad \text{red cell ghosts} + \text{haemoglobin}.$$

### Nomenclature

The factors which participate in the classical pathway are called C1, C2, C3, C4, C5, C6, C7, C8 and C9. With the exception of C4, which participates in the activation chain between C1 and C2 all C factors are numbered according to the sequence order in which they react in lysis of cells in immune haemolytic systems.

A C component or groups of components with enzyme activity are denoted by a bar over the component. Thus $\overline{C1}$ means that the native C1 factor has been activated and is now enzymatically active, $\overline{C42}$ denotes the enzymatically active form of a complex created between the fragment of the C4 and C2 components respectively.

Fragments of C proteins, which occur upon activation of the native components are denoted by an addition of letters, e.g. C3a and C3b, C5a and C5b. The creation of such fragments is called conversion of the native factor.

In the alternative pathway, also called the properdin system, the factor B, C3, factor D and properdin participate. These factors are also called B, C3 and P respectively.

Fragments of factor B, which occur upon activation, are denoted Ba and Bb respectively.

## The structure of complement factors

All C factors have been purified and in part characterized. In this short review data will be given for only some of the factors, namely C1q, C3, C4 and C5.

C1q is a protein with the molecular weight 410 000. Chemically C1q is similar to collagen, which is unusual for plasma proteins. The molecule consists of six identical subunits. Each subunit consists of three polypeptide chains, i.e. the C1q molecule is in fact composed of 18 chains. Every unit contains three distinct regions: Globular peptides in the N and C terminal regions and, in between, a connecting link within a collagen-like amino acid sequence (*Figure 5.1*). The haemolytic function is rapidly destroyed by collagenase, which shows the importance of the intact collagen region. The globular peptides in the peripheral C terminal region contains structures which can bind to immunoglobulins. Thus every C1q molecule has six Ig-binding sites. C1r

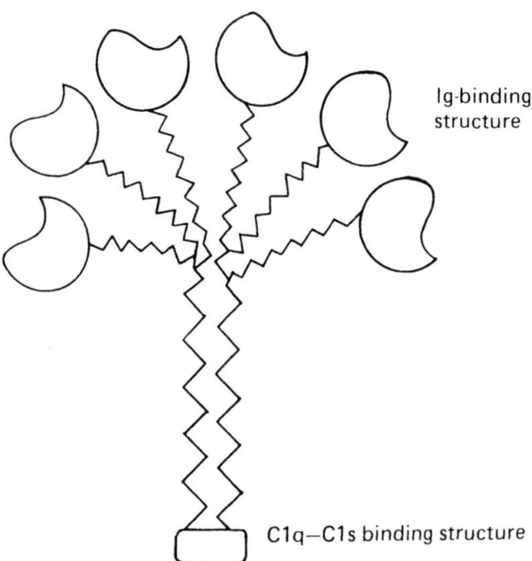


*Figure 5.1* Scheme of the C1q structure

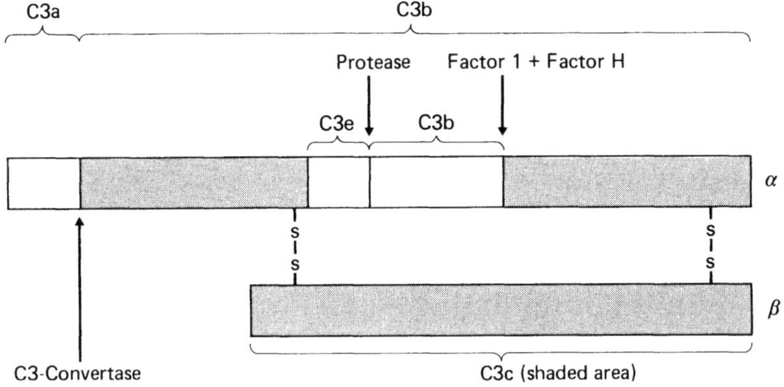



*Figure 5.2* Scheme of the C3 structure

and C1s are bound to the collagen part of C1q and these three proteins together constitute in the presence of calcium, the C1 factor (C1qrs).

C3 and C5 are both composed of two polypeptide chains, $\alpha$ and $\beta$, which are joined by disulphide bridges. When C3 is acted upon by C3 convertases (*see below*), a piece of the $\alpha$ chain is split off and C3a and C3b fragments are created. An enzyme in plasma, factor I (C3b inactivator, C3bINA) can split C3b into two further fragments, C3c and C3d. C3c consists of parts of the $\alpha$ chain and the intact $\beta$ chain. C3d consists of a part of the $\alpha$ chain. It is possible after proteolysis of C3 to isolate the C3e fragment, which is part of the $\alpha$ chain (*Figure 5.2*).

When C5 is activated C5a is split from the $\alpha$ chain, while the rest of the $\alpha$ chain and the intact $\beta$ chain create C5b.

C4 consists of three polypeptide chains, $\alpha$, $\beta$ and $\gamma$, that are joined by disulphide bridges. Activated C1 will split C4 in a minor fragment, C4a, consisting of a part of the $\alpha$ chain and a larger fragment, C4b.

## Activation of complement

### The classical pathway

The term 'classical pathway' refers simply to the fact that this activation chain was the first to be discovered. The reaction steps in the classical pathway (*Figure 5.3*) have been clarified mainly using immune haemolysis as a model system.

The first step is that C1 is bound to the Fc fragment of antibodies bound to the surface of the red blood cells. C1 is only activated by antibodies if they have been able to react with antigen. The C1 factor is a trimolecular $Ca^{2+}$-dependent complex consisting of C1q, C1r and C1s. C1q binds to the antibody in immune complexes, whereupon changes in the macromolecules are induced activating C1. C1r now changes into an enzymatic form and activates C1s to become an esterase (C̄1s). The activated C1, factor C̄1 has as substrate C4 and C2. C̄1 splits C4 into two fragments, a smaller C4a and a larger C4b. C4b has affinity and binds to the cell surface. C2 now binds to C4b and C̄1s in the activated C1 molecule can split C2 in the presence of magnesium. The larger C2 fragment, C2a, together with C4b creates a complex with enzymatic activity called C4b2a, or C̄4̄2̄. When C̄4̄2̄ is produced there is no further requirement for C1 and this molecule does not participate further in the reaction chain.

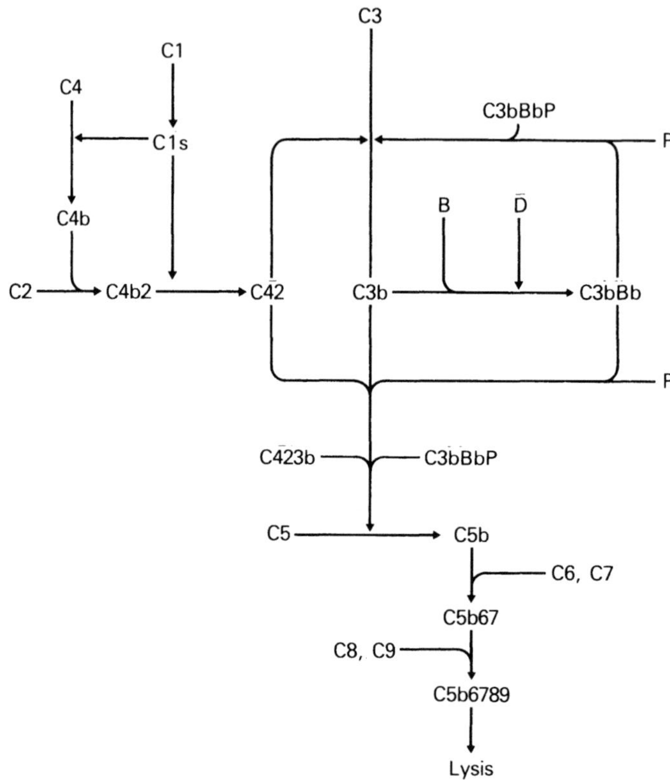


*Figure 5.3* Activation of the complement system via the classical and alternative pathway respectively

C4̄2 cleaves the C3 molecule into a small peptide C3a and a larger C3b. The larger fragment, C3b, binds to the cell membrane. When C3 is split into C3a and C3b an internal thiol-ester is cleaved in the middle of the α chain of the native C3 molecule. As a consequence of this cleavage a reactive thiol group and a carbonyl group is formed. The latter can either be hydrolysed or participate in the complex creation with other plasma proteins.

C4̄2 now together with C3b forms a new enzyme, C5 convertase, or C423b, which has the ability to split C5 into two parts, C5a and C5b. The larger fragment, C5b, binds to the cell surface, where a trimolecular complex of C5b, C6 and C7 is built up, C5̄67. C8 and C9 then react with C5̄67 after which the C5b–C9 is generated. This C5b–C9 complex (membrane attack complex, MAC) forms a channel to the interior of the cell through the phospholipid layers of the cell membranes, which results in leakage and subsequent destruction of the cell.

The classical pathway is activated by immune complexes composed of antibodies of classes IgG1, IgG2 or IgM. Immune complexes comprising IgG4, IgA or IgE antibodies cannot activate the classical pathway.

Activation of the classical pathway can, however, occur in the absence of immune complexes if C1 is bound and activated by certain substances, e.g. DNA, lipid A in the lipopolysaccharides of Gram-negative bacteria and several other polyanions. C-reactive protein in complex with various polysaccharides, e.g. the C polysaccharide in pneumococci can also directly activate the classical pathway.

*The alternative pathway*

The alternative pathway (*Figure 5.3*) is also called the properdin system. It is independent of the early factors in the classical pathway, namely C1, C4 and C2. Instead three distinct plasma proteins in addition to C3, are involved in the early activation steps, namely factor B, factor D and properdin. This activation pathway becomes identical to the classical pathway after the C3 step. The following build-up of the C5b–C9 complex is identical in the two activation pathways.

The alternative pathway is activated without participation of antibodies by substances such as zymosan, inulin, lipopolysaccharides from Gram-negative bacteria, teichoic acid from pneumococci, certain viruses and transformed cells.

A C3b-like molecule is created in a continuous manner via hydrolysis of C3. This molecule can bind to various surface structures or it can exist in a free form in the plasma, but will rapidly be broken down in free solution, inactivated, by the control proteins, namely factor H ($\beta$1H-protein) and factor I (C3b inactivator). If this C3b-like molecule, however, is bound to certain structures on cell surfaces, or other activators, it results in the creation of C3b which is then protected from degradation. Factor B can now be bound to C3b to form a C3bB complex. Factor D, which exists in the serum as an active enzyme will now cleave off a fragment from B, but this will only happen after B has been bound into the C3bB complex. This new C3bBb complex can cleave C3 into C3a and C3b and can thus recruit further C3b molecules. The C3bBb complex is labile due to the fact that Bb rapidly dissociates from C3b, but can be stabilized if properdin (P) is bound to the complex. P also delays the spontaneous destruction of the complex by interfering with the dissociation of Bb, and P protects C3b in C3bBb against degradation into C3c and C3d by the control proteins. C3bBbP functions as a C3 convertase and splits available native C3 into C3a and C3b. This feedback cycle can run until any of the components within it is consumed. By addition of further C3b molecules to the C3bBb complex C3b$_n$Bb and C3b$_n$BbP are formed, which besides C3b converting capacity also have the ability to cleave C5 into C5a and C5b. After this the reaction will proceed as in the classical pathway creating C5b–C9 complexes, which cause damage to the cell membrane and the lysis of the cell.

Proteolytical cleavage of C3 and C5 into C3a, C3b and C5a, C5b respectively can occur in the circulation and in the tissues via plasmin, trypsin or through the granulocyte proteases elastase and collagenase. Such cleavage is relevant during the creation and maintenance of the inflammatory reaction.

**The biological functions of the complement system**

The C system plays an essential role in the elimination of bacteria, certain viruses and immune complexes. This occurs in part through the release of acute inflammation, which limits the spread of bacteria, viruses and other damaging substances and also in part through the increased destruction of such foreign material via phagocytosis.

The deposition of the C5b–C9 complex on the surface of cells and bacteria through the activation of the classical or alternative pathway may lead to cytolysis.

Immune adherence means that particles or immune complexes which carry C3b on their surface may bind to certain cells in the body, which have receptors for C3b. Among such cells are the human red blood cells, neutrophil granulocytes, monocytes and macrophages, thrombocytes, B lymphocytes and cells in the glomeruli of the kidney. Immune adherence to phagocytes is called opsonization, which means that phagocytosis of C3b-coated cells and immune complexes will become more efficient than in situations where complement activation has not occurred.

Virus neutralization can be achieved both through the classical and alternative pathways. Certain viruses also have the ability to activate the classical pathway in the absence of antibodies.

The early factors of the classical pathway play an essential role in inhibiting the aggregation of just formed immune complexes, which could especially be referred to an intact C1 function.

The ability of fresh serum to solubilize immune complexes is a feature predominantly related to the activation of the alternative pathway. These observations, however, have only been made in *in vitro* systems and the biological relevance is still unclear.

The small peptides C3a and C3b which are cleavage products from C3 and C5 during complement activation have both the capacity to release vasoactive amines and histamine, from mast cells and basophil leucocytes. These peptides are anaphylatoxins.

C5a also expresses a chemotactic activity particularly for neutrophil granulocytes. The $C\overline{567}$ complex in free solution has a chemotactic effect on granulocytes and plays an important part in the Arthus' reaction. This is a reaction that can be seen in some immunological diseases, e.g. certain immune complex diseases in the lungs and vaccine reactions. If, for example, an individual has already produced circulating antibodies against an antigen present in a vaccine, renewed administration of that vaccine may cause vasculitis and tissue damage locally at the site of injection. The antigen creates soluble complexes with the antibodies. Immune complexes are localized within and surrounding the small blood vessels, the complement is activated and active $C\overline{567}$ attracts granulocytes to the site. Upon phagocytosis of the immune complexes the granulocyte releases lysosomal enzymes and this leads to the development of an inflammatory reaction. Furthermore, C5a can aggregate neutrophil granulocytes, which leads to release of superoxides from these cells.

C3e is a fragment which can be split from C3 upon activation (*Figure 5.2*) and has been reported as being capable of mobilizing granulocytes from the bone marrow, thus increasing the number of circulating granulocytes. The physiological importance of C3e has, however, not yet been finally determined.


**Regulatory substances during complement activation**

Both $C\overline{42}$ and $C\overline{3bBb}$ have a short half-life in circulation due to dissociation of these complexes. The membrane binding structures in these complexes are also short-lived in solution, which limits the effect of complement activation. The short life-span also hinders the destruction of bystander cells upon local complement activation. Activation of complement is also regulated by certain normally occurring specific control proteins, which function at definite steps in the activation sequence.

The $C\overline{1}$ inactivator, $C\overline{1}IA$, which is also called C1 esterase inhibitor, binds in an irreversible manner to C1s and thereby blocks the activation of C4 and C2. $C\overline{1}INA$ also inhibits $C\overline{1}r$ and other proteases outside the complement system such as plasma kallikrein, plasmin and activated Hageman factor.

When C3 is split by C3 convertases this leads to C3a and C3b, which are both biologically highly active molecules (*see above*). C3b plays a threefold role. It is a necessary factor in the feedback system during the activation of the alternative pathway; it is necessary for the activation of C5–C9 by participating in the C5 convertases (C$\overline{423b}$ and C$\overline{3bBbP}$); and it has an opsonizing capacity. C3a like C5a is an anaphylatoxin and C5a has in addition a chemotactic capacity.

In plasma there are normally proteins which can regulate or modify the activity of the factors, described above.

Factor I (C3b inactivator, C3bINA), is an enzyme which splits C3b into two fragments, C3c and C3d. This cleavage is enhanced by a co-factor, factor H (B1H protein) which binds to C3b whereupon the complex binding between C3b and factor B is blocked. Factor I is of particular importance in keeping the C3b-dependent feedback system in the alternative complement pathway under control. Factor I can also, in collaboration with another normally occurring protein the C4-binding protein (C4BP), split C4b into the functionally inactive fragments, C4c and C4d.

The anaphylatoxin inactivator is a carboxypeptidase which splits arginine from C3a as well as from C5a, whereupon these peptides lose their capacity to release histamine and they also lose the chemotactic ability. C5a is also inactivated by being taken up by the cells to which it has been bound, e.g. by the granulocytes.

The anchoring of the C5b and C5b–C9 complexes onto cell surfaces is inhibited by the S protein.

## The relation between complement and the coagulation, fibrinolysis and kinin systems

Although the interplay between the complement and the coagulation systems is not known fully, a few features demonstrating such an interplay will be described. Upon intensive activation of the complement chain up to C6 the coagulation process may be activated, which will then affect the thrombocytes. It seems to be one of the mechanisms underlying disseminated intravasal coagulation. The activated Hageman factor in the coagulation system can interact with proenzymes in plasma and initiate fibrinolysis by converting plasminogen to plasmin. Activated Hageman factor can also change pre-kallikrein into kallikrein, an enzyme which splits bradykinin from certain serum proteins.

Plasmin can activate C1 to C1 esterase. Plasmin can further split C3a and C3b from C3 and C5 respectively. The C1 esterase inhibitor, which is the only natural inhibitor of C1 esterase, is also able to inhibit the activated Hageman factor and kallikrein. It is the most important inhibitor in plasma of these two enzymes. It can also inhibit plasmin but more efficient inhibitors are normally the main regulators of that enzyme.

The complicated interplay which results in biologically extremely active products (anaphylatoxin, bradykinin, C3b, chemotactic factors), is not yet known in detail but it is clear that the body contains control mechanisms which eliminate a too intense inflammatory response. If these control proteins are lacking or are being swamped this may lead to different manifestations of inflammatory disturbances.

## The synthesis of the complement factors

C1q, C1r and C1s are synthesized by the epithelial cells of the small intestine. They can also be produced by macrophages and fibroblasts. C4, C2, C3, C5 and factor B are produced by macrophages. The synthesis of C3 predominantly occurs in the liver in the hepatocytes, where the C$\overline{1}$ inactivator is also produced.

An important discovery was the finding that the synthesis of C4, C2 and factor B is regulated by genes within the HLA region. The actual meaning of this linkage between the immunologically highly important HLA region and proteins of the complement system is not yet known.

Several of the C factors, in particular C1s, C3, C4 and factor B belong to the acute phase proteins, which means an increased synthesis in a state of inflammation.

## Membrane receptors for complement

Receptors for complement factors and their fragments on cell membranes have been studied intensively during the last few years. So far seven distinct receptors have been identified as indicated in *Table 5.1*.

C receptor type 1, CR1, is the structure which causes immune adherence of complement coated immune complexes. CR1 reacts with C3c and C3b, in the latter case with the part of the molecule which contains C3c, and it is also able to bind C4b and C5b. CR1 is present on all B lymphocytes and possibly also on non-identified subpopulations of lymphocytes. If C3b bound to immune complexes is exposed to purified CR1, C3b is rapidly degraded by factor I (C3bIA), which probably means that CR1 does function as a co-factor for factor I, resembling factor H. It is likely that CR1 plays an important role in the elimination of soluble immune complexes. Interesting new discoveries suggest that patients with systemic lupus erythematosus may have a reduced number of CR1 structures on their erythrocytes, which may add to the development of this classical immune complex disease (chapter 10). CR1 is also responsible for the immune adherence of opsonized immune complexes to neutrophil granulocytes and upon binding of C3b the cells release neutrophil lysosomal enzymes and superoxides.

C receptor type 2, CR2, binds specifically to a structure in C3d and in the C3b molecule after cleavage of the internal thiol-ester. CR2 has so far only been discovered on B lymphocytes and it seems to act as a suppressor of certain lymphocyte reactions, e.g. in the MLC reaction. The underlying mechanism is unknown.

C receptor type 3 has been described recently. It is claimed to bind to certain parts of the C3 region and to be of importance during phagocytosis.

The C1q receptor reacts with the collagen part in the free C1q molecule but not with native C1, where the reactive structure is covered by C1r and C1s. Cells carrying C1q receptors can thus bind C1q-carrying immune complex to the surfaces. Reaction between C1q and the C1q receptor on granulocytes and monocytes leads to a stimulation of the oxidative metabolism of the cells. It is likely that this is of importance in the defence against infections and at the level of the inflammatory reaction.

Factor H receptors (H–R) exist on B lymphocytes and monocytes. Factor H in complex with C3b causes a secretion of stored factor I from these cells.

C3a receptors, C3a–R will bind C3a and also C4a, but with lower affinity. If the arginine in C3a is split by the anaphylatoxin inactivator the binding capacity to C3a–R

**TABLE 5.1. Membrane receptors for complement**

| Receptor | Specificity | Cell distribution |
| --- | --- | --- |
| CR1 | C4b, C3b, C3c, C5b | Erythrocytes, macrophages, neutrophil granulocytes, lymphocytes |
| CR2 | C3d | B lymphocytes |
| CR3 | C3d | Erythrocytes, macrophages, neutrophil granulocytes, lymphocytes |
| C1q–R | C1q (collagen region) | Neutrophil granulocytes, lymphocytes, monocytes |
| H–R | Factor H | Neutrophil granulocytes, lymphocytes, monocytes |
| C3a–R | C3a, C4a | Mast cells, monocytes |
| C5a–R | C5a, C5a$_{desArg}$ | Mast cells, monocytes, neutrophil granulocytes |

is destroyed. The binding between C3a and C3a–R on mast cells will cause a release of histamine.

C5a receptors, C5a–R, are present on neutrophil granulocytes, mast cells and macrophages. Upon binding of C5a to granulocytes they are stimulated to chemotaxis, whereas the reaction between C5a–R and C5a on mast cells will cause histamine release. When C5a is bound to C5a–R on macrophages they are stimulated to the secretion of interleukin 1, which then causes an increase in the production of the acute phase proteins. Interleukin 1 also has an important capacity during the activation of T lymphocytes. Binding of C5a to neutrophil granulocytes leads to the release of lysosomal enzymes as well as increased superoxide synthesis.

**The complement binding reaction**

The ability of the complement to bind to antigen–antibody complexes makes it possible to use this reaction to detect and measure antigen or antibodies in complex mixtures. The most famous complement binding test used in medicine is the Wasserman reaction, which is still used to diagnose syphilis. In virology the complement binding reaction has found widespread application partly in identifying certain viruses using known antisera and partly in detecting specific virus antibodies in sera.

Immune complexes formed when antigen reacts with specific antibody, will bind complement. The complement consumption can be revealed by the addition of sensitized red blood cells to the mixture as indicated below:

*Reaction 1.* Antigen + antibody + complement + $Ca^{++}$ and $Mg^{++}$ will lead to complement binding.
*Reaction 2.* Reaction mixture 1 + antibody-coated sheep red blood cells are mixed. In the present case this will not lead to haemolysis.

In reaction 1 complement is consumed by the antigen–antibody complexes. No complement will be left to cause haemolysis of the antibody-coated sheep erythrocytes. This means a positive complement binding reaction. If antigen or antibody were lacking in the first reaction mixture, complement would not be consumed and haemolysis would appear in reaction step 2. In the latter case the complement binding reaction is negative.

# Bibliography


FEY, G. and COLTEN, H. R. (1981). Biosynthesis of complement components. *Federation Proc.*, **40**, 2099.
HUGLI, T. E. and MÜLLER-EBERHARD, H. J. (1978). The anaphylatoxins: C3a and C5a. *Adv. Immunol.*, **26**, 1.
KAZATCHKINE, M. D. and NYDEGGER, U. E. (1982). The human alternative complement pathway. Biology and immunopathology of activation and regulation. *Progr. Allergy*, **30**, 199.
LOOS, M. (1982). The classical component pathway: Mechanism of activation of the first component by antigen–antibody complexes. *Progr. Allergy*, **30**, 135.
MÜLLER-EBERHARD, H. J. and SCHREIBER, R. D. (1980). Molecular biology and chemistry of the alternative pathway of complement. *Adv. Immunol.*, **29**, 2.
PANGBURN, M. K. and MULLER-EBERHARD, H. J. (1984). The alternative pathway of complement. *Springer Semin. Immunolpathol.* **7**, 163.
REID, K. B. M. and PORTER, R. R. (1981). The proteolytic activation systems of complement. *Ann. Rev. Biochem.*, **50**, 433.
ROSS, G. D. (1982). Structure and function of membrane complement receptors. *Federation Proc.*, **41**, 3089.
SCHIFFERLI, J. A. and PETERS, D. K. (1983). Complement, the immune-complex lattice and the pathophysiology of complement-deficiency syndromes. *Lancet*, **II**, 957.

# Chapter 6

# Production of antibodies

Hans Wigzell

Circulating antigen-specific antibodies are immunoglobulins with regard to their biochemistry. These molecules result from a complicated chain of events which begins with a reaction between specific immunocompetent lymphocytes that recognize an immunogen. B lymphocytes as well as T lymphocytes frequently participate during the induction of antibody production together with macrophages. But only B lymphocytes and their differentiated descendants (B lymphoblasts and plasma cells) have the capacity to synthesize humoral immunoglobulin molecules. An individual who lacks the capacity to produce circulating antibodies has a severe handicap and will accordingly display an increased susceptibility to infection caused by several different micro-organisms (*see* chapter 13).

The number of lymphocytes in an adult human is in the order of $10^{12}$ cells with an approximately equal distribution between T and B lymphocytes. The frequency of cells with specific capacity to react against an antigenic determinant previously not encountered varies according to the situation, but can be less than one cell out of 50 000 lymphocytes. Against certain antigens a much higher frequency of reactive cells can be shown, but this may mean that previous immunization against these or cross-reactive antigens has taken place. One consequence of immunization is that the number as well as the frequency of immunologically reactive lymphocytes against the relevant antigen may increase.

The capacity of B and T lymphocytes to react against specific immunogens is caused by the fact that these cell types have, on their outer cell surface, receptors with a selective capacity to bind to antigenic determinants of various kinds. The receptors for antigen on the B lymphocytes are made up of immunoglobulins while the chemistry of the corresponding receptors on the T lymphocytes still remains largely unknown (*see* chapter 7). These receptors constitute a recognition mechanism through which the individual can differentiate between his own and foreign structures, i.e. between self and non-self. This discriminatory power is however not without faults, which may sometimes cause autoimmune (self-immune) reactions (*see* chapter 8).

After tight binding between antigenic determinants of the foreign structure and receptors of the lymphocyte, various activities may be induced in the immuno-competent cell. Exactly what activity, if any, will result is dependent upon the mode of presentation, concentration of the antigen, the cell types surrounding the lymphocytes, etc., in a complicated interplay. In principle, two major possible chains of activation can be initiated, which lead to opposite consequences as indicated in *Figure 6.1*. One pathway leads to an active immune response where antibody production plays an important part. The result is immunity. Immunity can be defined as a selectively

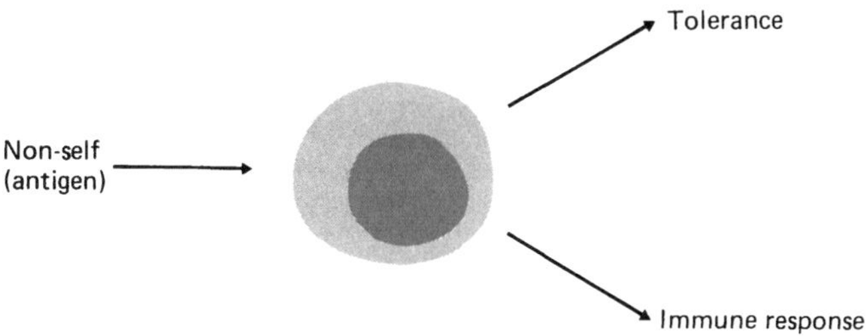


*Figure 6.1* An immunocompetent lymphocyte can after contact with antigen develop according to two different pathways, one leading to immunity and the other leading to specific tolerance

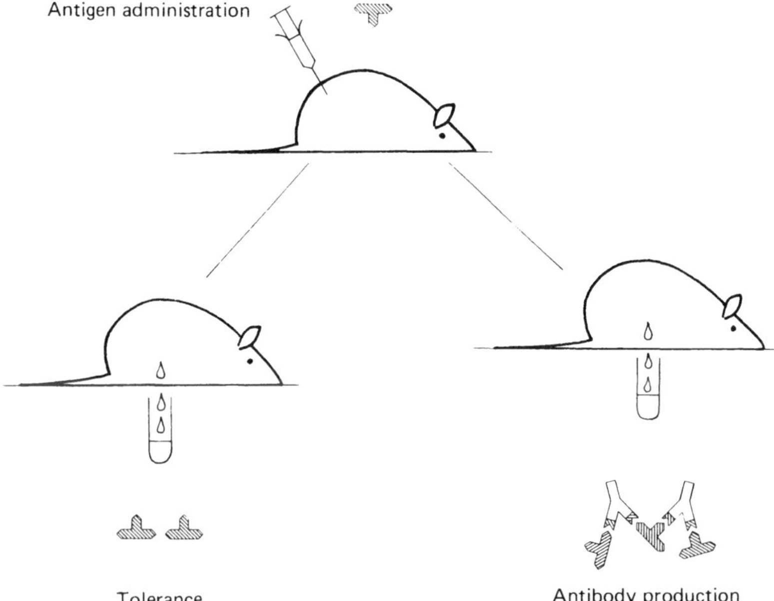


*Figure 6.2* Administration of antigen in an individual can lead to antibody formation or the selective lack of antibody formation, i.e. tolerance

increased immune capacity against a defined antigen, while the ability of the individual to react immunologically against other antigens remains unaltered.

The other pathway leads to a lack of an active immune response against the antigen. It is called immunological tolerance and is defined as a selective inability of the individual to react in an immunological manner against a relevant immunogen while normal capacity remains against other antigens.

Some conditions which determine whether lymphocytes are induced into an immune or tolerance mode of response are described in this chapter, as well as in chapters 7 and 8. It should be stressed, however, that upon administration of an antigen to an individual there may be a parallel induction of tolerance in some cells and immunity in other lymphocytes. Normally it is only possible to detect the active part (immunity), i.e. the normal consequence of stimulation by antigen in an immunocompetent individual (*see Figure 6.2*). This results in immunity with antibody production as one part of this response pattern.

## The cellular background of antibody production

Antibody production primarily occurs in the peripheral lymphoid organs of the body, lymph nodes and spleen. In the human there may also be a very sizable antibody production in the bone marrow. The common denominator for these organs and tissues is that they have a specialized anatomy and histology where different cell types can travel or remain strategically placed, and are capable of capturing, in an efficient manner, foreign structures and presenting immunogens to the competent lymphocytes. (For details in the construction of such a tissue, *see* chapter 1.)

As previously mentioned it is possible to schematically subdivide immunogens into two major groups depending on their requirement for T lymphocyte involvement. Many immunogens require a simultaneous presence of helper T cells reacting against the antigen in order to be able to activate antigen specific B lymphocytes to produce high levels of antibody. Such immunogens are called thymus dependent (TD) antigens. Other antigens do not require such T cell involvement but have the unique capacity to directly activate specific B lymphocytes into antibody synthesis. The latter type of immunogens are called thymus independent or TI antigens.

When thymus dependent (TD) antigens are used for immunization an important initial phase consists of an uptake of antigen into macrophages present in the various peripheral lymphoid tissues. This uptake may occur in the form of fragments of the initial immunogenic molecule. In order for such fragments to become immunogenic for T lymphocytes they should have the ability to associate more or less avidly with certain cell-surface glycoproteins. These glycoproteins may vary in their chemical composition between individuals. They were first recognized for their ability to invoke strong transplantation immune reactions when tissue was grafted between individuals carrying different variants of these surface proteins. The name of the genetic system coding for these glycoproteins in man is the HLA system (Human Leucocyte Antigen, group A). These molecules and their relevance are described in more detail in chapters 7 and 9. Complexes between fragmented immunogens and HLA molecules on macrophages would seem to constitute the predominant type of specific stimulating immunogen for antigen-specific human helper T cells. T lymphocytes activated by this kind of immunogen may, among other things have the ability to help B lymphocytes to start producing antibodies at high rate against the antigen. Such T lymphocytes were therefore originally called helper T cells. Exact details of the help they provide is still largely unclear. It has been possible to prove, in *in vitro* experiments, that helper T cells can produce molecules with the ability to bind to B lymphocytes which themselves have bound immunogen. These T cell-derived molecules seem to be particularly good at reacting with the antigen if it is present on the surface of the B cell in a complex together with the same type of HLA molecules that are present on the initial antigen-presenting macrophage.

When helper T cells and B cells, which react against the same immunogen, are analysed for their specificity, it is frequently found that they react with different determinants on the same immunogenic macromolecule. Helper T cells with a certain specificity can thus help B cells with entirely different antigen-binding reactivity. This capacity for collaboration between T and B lymphocytes with different antigen-binding specificity, is not only positive but can also serve as a basis for the induction of autoimmunity (*see* chapter 8). Besides producing antigen-specific molecules the helper T cell is also able, upon activation, to release several different kinds of lymphokines (pharmacologically active proteins). Some of these have been reported to have an antigen non-specific capacity to stimulate B lymphocytes into increased activity. This

**TABLE 6.1. T cells helping B lymphocytes to produce antibody**

| | |
|---|---|
| *Phase I* | Antigen specific helper T cells react with an antigen sitting on the surface of macrophages. The helper T cells are then activated and may go into division. |
| *Phase II* | Activated helper T cells now release several different lymphokines, some of which may help B cell proliferation. The antigen-specific helper T cell or a soluble molecule from that cell may react with B lymphocytes if these cells have bound antigen and at the same time have the same type of class II MHC molecules as the antigen-presenting macrophage. |
| *Phase III* | The B cell is now activated via the contact with an antigen-specific T cell or T cell derived molecule. If the B cell is at the same time presented with antigen-non-specific lymphokines this further increase the activation. Non-specific molecules can also allow other previously activated B lymphocytes to continue to be active. |
| *Phase IV* | The B cell is now a large cell, a blast, and is dividing rapidly and producing immunoglobulin molecules for export at a high rate. |

capacity to stimulate B cells would seem to function especially well if the B cells have already been activated via binding to antigen and contact with the antigen specific molecules derived from the helper T cells. One of these lymphokines has been reported in certain systems to be able to fully replace the helper T cells and has thus been called TRF (*T* cell *R*eplacing *F*actor). It is likely that several T lymphocyte-derived lymphokines exist with a more or less selective ability to regulate B cell function. *Table 6.1* summarizes the present state of knowledge with regard to the various phases in helper T cell activation of B lymphocytes and the initiation of high levels of antibody production.

Thymus independent or TI antigens have the ability, as previously mentioned, to directly activate B lymphocytes to antibody synthesis without the requirement for helper T cells. It is, however, likely from several sets of experiments that macrophages may enhance the ability of TI antigens to activate B cells. On immunization with a thymus independent antigen it can be seen that proliferation will only occur in the B cell areas of the peripheral lymphoid tissues. The mechanism underlying the unique capacity of the TI antigens to activate B cells is now partially understood. Besides having conventional antigenic groups such TI antigens also carry the innate capacity to provoke cellular proliferation in B lymphocytes. This mitogenic (mitosis = cellular division) capacity of the TI antigens means that any B lymphocyte with antigen-binding receptors for any of the antigenic groups on the antigen will now bind to its surface a B cell mitogen. Low concentrations of TI antigen lead to a selective activation of B cells with genetically predetermined antigen-binding specific receptors for the antigen in question. If the concentration of a TI antigen becomes very high, this may allow the antigen to bind directly via weakly binding, hypothetical mitogen receptors to all B cells. This is regardless of whether the antibodies on the lymphocytes do or do not display any significant binding force to the immunogen. This now results in a polyclonal immune response (many B lymphocytes with various antibody specificities are now activated in a non-specific manner = poly; they give rise to descendants via cellular proliferation and thus create many clones). It is possible that such a polyclonal activation of a large number of B lymphocytes may occur in certain clinical situations, e.g. in massive infections with Gram-negative bacteria. TI antigens are bacterial polysaccharides such as endotoxin, dextran, etc. TD antigens on the other hand, are frequently protein in nature. Other characteristic features of TD and TI antigens are summarized in *Table 6.2*. Upon immunization with TD antigens in particular, but also to a lesser degree with TI immunogens, a gradual differentiation of the participating immunocompetent lymphocytes occurs. This is most clearly shown at the level of the B

**TABLE 6.2. TI and TD antigens. Features and consequences upon immunization**

*A. Thymus dependent antigens*
Biochemistry: Frequently proteins, but can be complex molecules, e.g. polysaccharide–protein complexes. Provokes initial IgM synthesis but then normally switches to IgG, IgA or IgE if specific helper T cells are present. Secondary immune response is dominated by IgG, IgA or IgE, while IgM is relatively diminished. The binding capacity of the produced antibodies increases with the time after immunization, i.e. avidity and affinity will increase. Provokes long-lasting and strong immunological memory demonstrable both at the T and B cell level.

*B. Thymus independent antigens*
Biochemistry: Frequently polysaccharides. Provokes initial IgM synthesis and this may not switch to other Ig classes with time. A second contact with the antigen normally results in an antibody response still dominated by IgM antibodies. Antibodies produced early during the immunization have a similar binding capacity as those produced later, i.e. no rise in avidity or affinity with time occurs. Provokes poor and short-lived immunological memory at the level of B lymphocytes. Thymus independent antigens are by definition poor inducers of helper T cells but may induce significant T suppressor activity.

lymphocytes where more and more specialized forms occur in regard to their capacity to produce antibodies at a high rate. Originating from small resting lymphocytes the first antibody-exporting B cells appear in the form of large cells of lymphoblastoid type. Such cells normally primarily produce IgM antibodies but may then switch to another class, such as IgG, IgE or IgA. This switch seems to occur predominantly after immunization with TD antigens. In parallel to the class switch there may also be a gradual change of the cells to a cellular form which is extremely suitable for protein synthesis, i.e. the plasma cells. These cells have a very well-developed endoplasmic reticulum full of ribosomes and also a well-developed Golgi complex.

Upon immunization with TD as well as TI antigens the first antibodies produced normally belong to the IgM class. If the immunogen was a thymus dependent antigen there is subsequently normally an efficient switch of antibody classes particularly to IgG and IgA. We now know that the first immunoglobulin which appears on the surface of the differentiating B lymphocyte is of IgM class in the form of two heavy and two light chains in one molecule. The cell-bound IgM immunoglobulin is substantially smaller than the IgM found in the serum. B lymphocytes with IgM antibodies on the cell surface, can react with immunogens but are relatively immature at this stage. Later in the differentiation, which occurs in the absence of antigen IgD also appears on the cell surface together with IgM. All IgM and IgD molecules present on a single B lymphocyte express the same antigen-binding specificity. Upon immunization B lymphocytes triggered into activation by immunogen enlarge and start to produce antibodies for export at a high rate, several thousandfold higher than that of synthesis in the resting newly formed B cell. In parallel many of these lymphocytes also start to divide rapidly. If the immunization is carried out using a TD antigen with time many of the IgM-producing dividing cells may change their immunoglobulin class to IgG, IgE or IgA. This normally occurs with the maintenance of the same antigen-binding specificity of the antibody molecules produced. The change in immunoglobulin classes from IgM to other classes will thus occur within the lymphocyte clones, originally initiated from the start of the immunization. If the immunization is carried out with a TI antigen this switch from IgM to other classes is significantly reduced. *Figure 6.4* shows in a schematic manner how a B lymphocyte differentiates within the body.

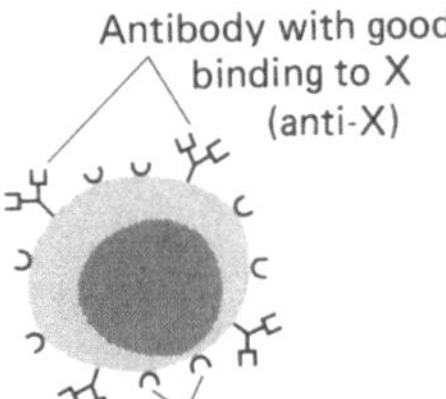


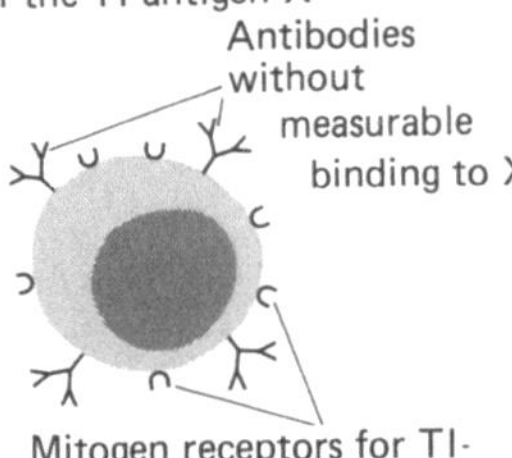


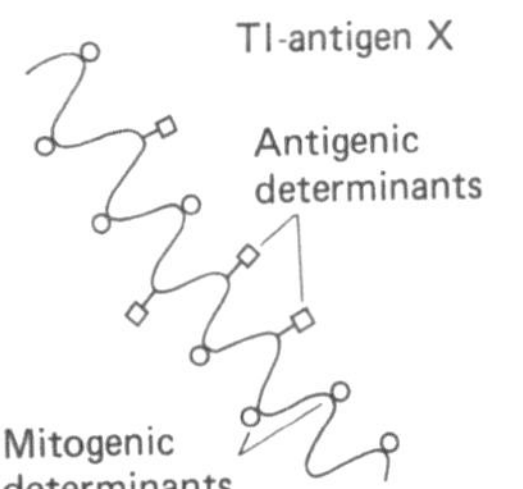


*Figure 6.3* Specific antibody induction of thymus independent antigens at a low concentration of antigen and non-specific induction at a high concentration of the same antigen. TI antigens have besides antigenic determinants, mitogenic structures for B cells in general

## Kinetics of antibody formation

The initial contact between an immunogen and a corresponding immunocompetent lymphocyte leads to a detectable antibody response. If the antigen is of the TD type, this also leads to the development of immunological memory by the immune system. If such a memory is allowed to develop this will be reflected in the immune response upon renewed contact with the same antigen in the form of a socalled secondary or anamnestic antibody response. A prominent part in this memory seems to be the number of immunocompetent B lymphocytes capable of reaction with the relevant TD antigens which have increased in number upon the first contact. Likewise, it is possible to show that T memory cells are induced and necessary for any prolonged immunological memory. The memory cells frequently display features with distinctly different qualities compared with the immunologically virgin lymphocytes present during the first immunization period. It is informative to study the kinetics of antibody

Antigen independent

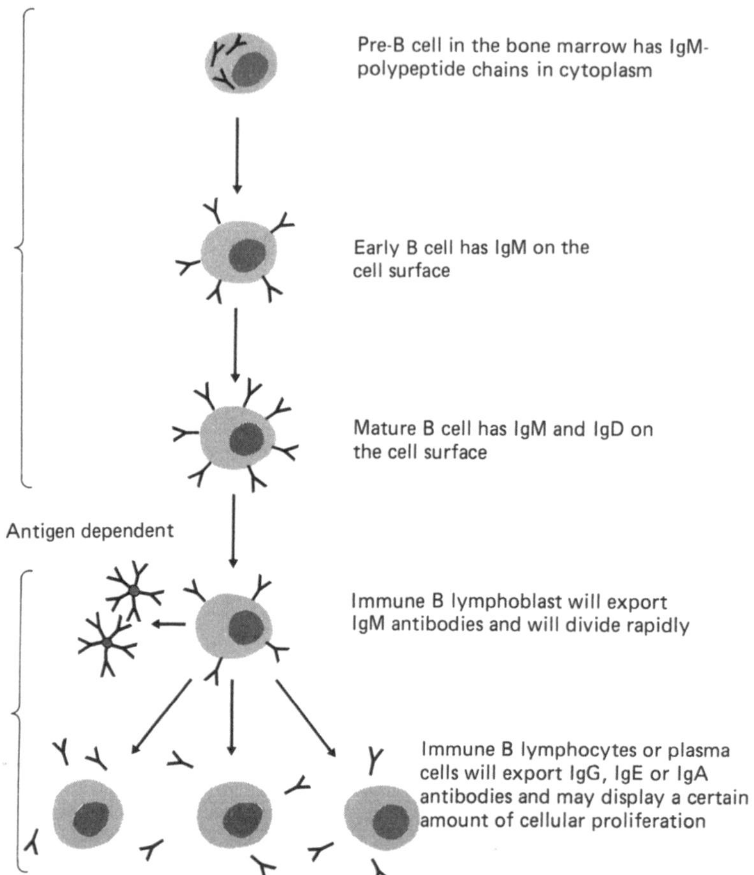


*Figure 6.4* B cell differentiation in the presence and absence of antigen

synthesis during primary and secondary immune reactions against thymus dependent and thymus independent antigens.

## Primary antibody response

In the primary antibody response against a thymus dependent antigen it is possible to distinguish two major kinds of components, i.e. an antibody response of IgM type and a corresponding one of IgG antibodies (*Figure 6.5*). What is true for IgG is also true for IgA and IgE antibody responses. The IgM response is the oldest one from the point of the phylogeny (*see* chapter 1) and can frequently be induced using lower antigen doses than those required to initiate an IgG response. Aggregated and particulate antigens frequently provoke a more rapid and stronger IgM response than soluble antigens in a non-aggregated form. The IgM response has a short induction period, in certain cases less than 24 hours. This is followed by a logarithmic phase where the antibody concentration in the serum may rise very rapidly. After maximum titres have been

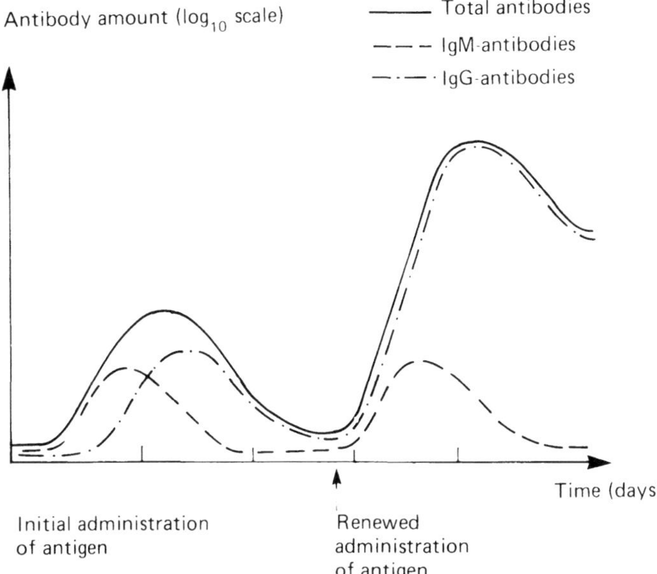


*Figure 6.5* Primary and secondary serum antibody response against a
thymus dependent antigen

reached the concentration may start to decline, initially quite slowly, then at a more
rapid but constant rate. This is probably caused by the fact that there is a very small
production of IgM antibodies after a certain period because the antigen is no longer in
an immunogenic form.

The IgG response has a longer induction phase than the IgM response. IgG
antibodies can frequently be demonstrated in serum only after the IgM response has
reached its maximum or is in decline. Under the logarithmic part of the IgG response
the antibody titres can double as often as every eight to ten hours. This logarithmic
phase in many cases coincides with the declining phase of the IgM response. The
maximal IgG concentration is normally reached one to a few days after the end of the
logarithmic phase. Subsequently, the antibody concentration starts to decline but in
contrast to the IgM response the production of IgG antibodies is reduced at a slower
pace and frequently continues at a low rate for years.

When the antigen is a thymus independent immunogen the IgM synthesis frequently
dominates during the whole immune response period (*Figure 6.6*). Although immunoglobulin classes other than IgM are induced by thymus independent antigens they
normally fail to show the same clear shift in dominance with time as occurs when the
immunogen is a TD antigen.

## Secondary antibody response

Two to four weeks after immunization with a thymus dependent antigen it is normally
possible to induce a secondary type of antibody response if a renewed stimulation with
the same antigen is carried out. The first contact with the antigen has caused the
induction of an immunological memory. In the human immunological memory IgG
antibody production against certain thymus dependent antigens may remain many

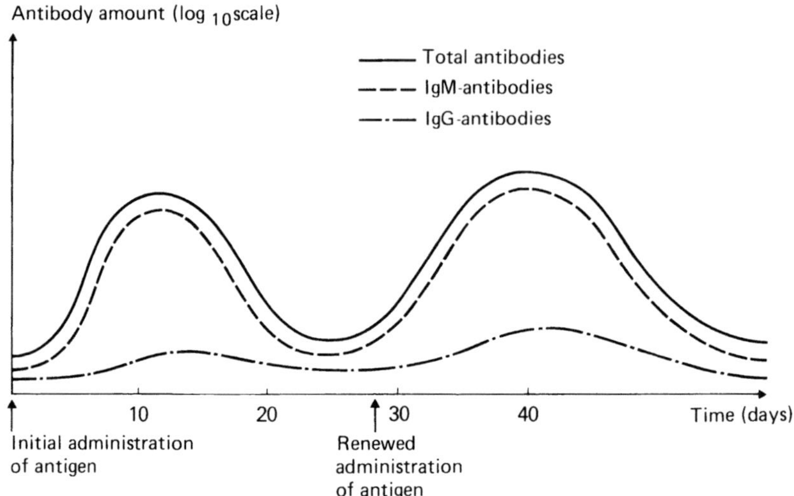


*Figure 6.6* Primary and secondary antibody response against a thymus independent antigen

decades after the primary stimulation. It is also possible to demonstrate an immunological memory for the IgM antibody response.

The secondary antibody response is, however, normally considerably lower for the IgM antibodies compared to the IgG response. The secondary antibody response differs from the primary one in several ways if the immunogen is a thymus dependent antigen (*Figure 6.5*). The induction phase is shorter and a higher concentration of antibodies appears more rapidly in the circulation. While the IgM antibodies dominated in the primary immune response there is now an immediate production of IgG antibodies in high concentrations. Under the logarithmic phase the antibody titres may now in optimal situations double every seventh hour and maximal antibody titres are normally reached within less than two weeks. The titre then starts to decrease and after a month or two it frequently stabilizes at a quite low plateau level. If one compares the quality of the antibodies within the same immunoglobulin class there is another difference between the primary and secondary antibody responses. On primary immunization with a TD antigen there occurs with time the production of antibodies with increasing binding strength, i.e. higher avidity for the antibody in question. This maturation in binding capacity is to a large degree dependent on clonal selection under conditions of decreasing antigen concentrations *in vivo* of genetically predetermined lymphocytes carrying receptors with high antigen binding capacity (*see later*). However, with a secondary antibody response even the early produced antibodies now express high avidity, i.e. they are most likely derived from memory B cells with a corresponding binding capacity on their cell-bound antibodies.

In contrast thymus independent, TI antigens do not normally lead to the induction of an efficient immunological memory and also fail upon renewed contact to result in an antibody response of a secondary type as exemplified in *Figure 6.6*. Here the secondary response is frequently very similar to that of the primary one with IgM as the dominating immunoglobulin class. Also there is normally no significant maturation in affinity with time of the antibodies produced when the antigen is a TI immunogen. This is probably because thymus independent antigens are poor inducers of memory cells.

## Endogenous regulation of the antibody response

The antibody response, which is initiated upon immunization is regulated in many ways *in vivo*. The immunogen which has been administered or introduced into the body via infections is normally degraded with time. This means that the specific exogenous stimulus, which initiated the immune response has now disappeared. Antibodies which are produced play an important role in the regulation of the immune response. The early produced IgM antibodies have a unique capacity to help enhance the production of further antibodies via an improved recruitment of helper T cells. The exact underlying mechanism of this phenomenon is unknown. IgG antibodies on the other hand normally have a capacity to abrogate the immune response. They tend to suppress in a specific manner an ongoing response, possibly by blocking of antigenic determinants coupled with increased metabolism and breakdown of the immunogen. It has also been reported that suppressor T cells may tend to be induced in situations where immune complexes between antigen and IgG antibodies are being formed. The actual validity of this latter claim, however, remains to be further verified.

One of the above indicated regulatory parameters, the ability of IgG antibodies to inhibit immunization, is used with great success as a clinical procedure to stop immunization of mothers who lack a blood group antigen, Rh, from making antibodies against this antigen when the fetus is Rh positive, i.e. has the antigen in question. Such IgG anti-Rh antibodies are given to these mothers after delivery. During delivery erythrocytes from the child are often passed into the blood circulation of the mother, which may lead to immunization. The administered IgG anti-Rh antibodies bind to the erythrocytes of the child which are present in the circulation of the mother and this causes a rapid breakdown of these red cells before they are able to immunize the woman. Through such a specific antibody regulation it is now possible for most Rh-negative women to deliver several Rh-positive children (*see* chapter 9).

## Creation of antibody specificity

An adult human being is probably able at any given moment to produce more than $10^9$ different antibody types as far as antigen-binding specificity is concerned. At the same time it is known that in human DNA there is probably not enough space for more than one million conventionally defined genes. Antibodies are proteins, whose amino acid sequences are determined in a conventional manner via the transcription and translation of DNA and RNA. How is it possible to create such a very high number of protein variations within a single individual?

Earlier in this chapter we discussed the kinetics of antibody production. A very important part in explaining the dynamics is the fact that in our body there are, at the time of administration of antigen, lymphocytes with predetermined specificity for the immunogen in question. The binding capacity of these cells to the immunogen varies with most of them expressing weak but detectable binding whilst only a few react strongly with the immunogen. The immunization normally leads to an increase and selection for those lymphocytes which have the strongest binding to the relevant antigen. The induction of immunity at the lymphocyte level is mainly a matter of selection and clonal expansion of predetermined specific lymphocytes and their descendants.

Three chromosome pairs directly participate at the structural level in the creation of genes encoding the protein parts of the immunoglobulins in a single B lymphocyte (two chromosomes for the heavy, two chromosomes for the $\kappa$ and for the $\lambda$ chains respectively). In the single lymphocyte only two of the six chromosomes are used, namely one of the two which are potentially able to produce heavy chains and one of the four which can determine the synthesis of light immunoglobulin chains. This means that four chromosomes in this regard are 'silent' and they will normally remain so during the life-span of this B lymphocyte and its descendants. It is possible to describe the B lymphocyte during the various differentiation phases as exemplified in *Figure 6.4*, not only at the protein (immunoglobulin) level but also at the DNA level.

The principal design of the structural genes for immunoglobulins is exemplified by the heavy immunoglobulin chains in *Figure 6.7*. Stretched out like a string of pearls are the various specific parts of DNA on the single chromosome in which each region determines a certain part in the protein sequence. As previously mentioned (chapter 2) the heavy immunoglobulin chain consists of a variable and a constant region. The genes responsible for the variable region are distributed in three different groups; V, D and J groups. The exact number of V, D and J genes varies for different species. In the human, a reasonable estimate is that there are about 100 V, maybe 50 D and 4 J genes. As far as the structural genes for the constant regions are concerned, i.e. those which determine class, there is only one gene for each class or subclass.

When a B lymphocyte is produced from stem cells in the bone marrow it is first seen at the protein level by the fact that the cell starts to produce free heavy IgM chains in the cytoplasm. At the DNA level in the single cell the following events have already occurred (*see Figure 6.7*). Out of the V, D and J groups one single representative of each has been cut out and joined together to form a unit by inherent cell hybrid–DNA technology, i.e. the cell is using restriction enzymes to cut and link together one V with one D and one J gene. This VDJ combination can now, together with the region coding for the constant part of the IgM chain, produce an IgM polypeptide chain which is unique and representative for this B cell. This occurs through the production of an RNA molecule, which is initially large, but after trimming this results in a messenger RNA which now only contains RNA stretches relevant for the protein structure in question. This hybrid DNA activity coupled with a compartmentalization of the structural genes of the variable region to three gene groups in itself gives rise to a large number of variable combinations, here exemplified as $100 \times 50 \times 4 = 20\,000$ combinations at structural gene level. Furthermore, during the process of linking together V, D and J genes additional variations can arise. Calculations have been made suggesting that through such chemical misfits at least 30 new variants may arise. This means that around $600\,000$ variants of polypeptide chains within the heavy chain class can be made using only genes of one of the two relevant chromosomes. Since the structural genes for the V and D segments may vary between the two chromosomes this means that the potential number of IgM chain variants is even higher at the level of the individual. The structural genes for the light chains, i.e. $\kappa$ and $\lambda$ chains, generate variants in a similar manner among these polypeptides. A 'heavy' variable region of the antibody is combined with a 'light' variable region to create the antigen binding domain (*see* chapter 2). Thus, the number of variants within the $\kappa$ and $\lambda$ chains should be multiplied with those of the heavy Ig chains, in order to give the final potential variation at the level of the intact antibody molecules within an individual. It should, however, be realized that it is unknown whether any heavy chain is able to associate with any light chain to produce a functional antibody molecule.

Later during antibody formation when, for example, a B lymphoblast making IgM with $\kappa$ light chains switches to, let us say, the formation of the IgG subclasses (while retaining the $\kappa$ chains) further rearrangement at the DNA level occurs in the heavy

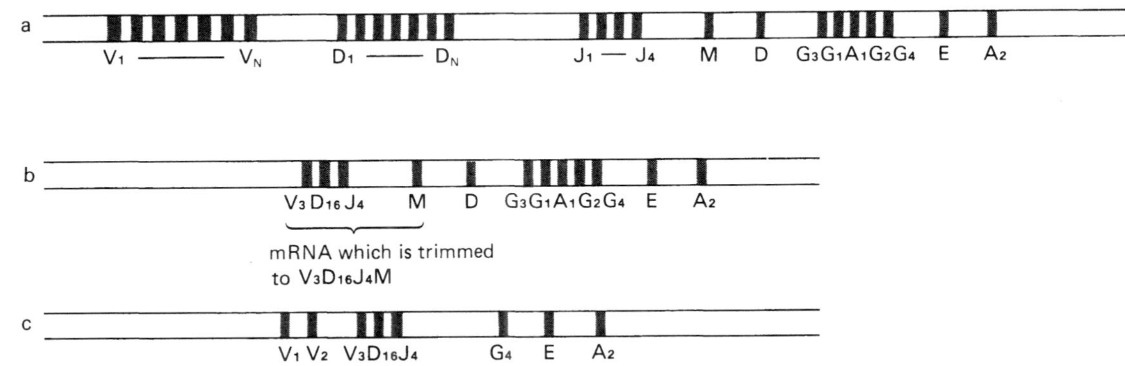



*Figure 6.7* Distribution of structural genes coding for heavy chain Ig genes. (a) DNA is present in all normal cells as far as heavy chain Ig genes are concerned. (b) DNA on the 'Ig active chromosome' in a single B cell produces an IgM chain using $V^3D^{16}J^4$ genes to produce its variable part. (c) DNA on the Ig active chromosome in a single B cell of type b, which now gives rise to cells producing IgG4 antibodies

chain Ig genes as depicted in *Figure 6.7(c)*. The same VDJ group which previously had been put together with a constant region of IgM now moves close to the IgG subclass gene and this is expressed at the protein level. At the same time the constant genes, which previously resided between the VDJ and the relevant Ig gene on the active chromosomes are deleted. This means that the normal change in immunoglobulin class, which can be seen upon immunization, occurs in a certain predetermined direction. The actual direction cannot be changed but 'jumps' may occur which quicken the arrival at the 'final goal' (here the $IgA_2$ gene). When Ig class switches are initiated evidence exists indicating that additional point mutations can be introduced in the VDJ segments, thus creating further possibilities for antibody variability.

Thus, the normal Ig differentiation pathway of the human B cell at the DNA level seems to be the following: initially IgM chains are expressed in the cytoplasm after the successful rearrangement of DNA in the heavy chain Ig genes on one of the two relevant chromosomes. Subsequently the B cell tries to obtain a functional rearrangement of its $\kappa$ chain genes. If this fails it still has the possibility of trying a rearrangement in the $\lambda$ genes. If this also fails (the DNA redistribution can fail although the frequence of this failure is unknown) such pre-B cells probably never mature into immunocompetent lymphocytes. As the bone marrow of a healthy individual produces several million new lymphocytes per minute there is, however, room for failure.

In summary, the variation of antigen-binding specificity of antibody molecules is reached in two steps:

(1)   via a compartmentalization of several groups of variable genes which can be linked together and thus create a large number of possibilities;
(2)   the combination of two variable polypeptide chains which results in a multiplication of the number of variations within two different chromosomal systems (heavy and light Ig chain genes).


## Monoclonal eternal antibodies

B lymphocytes which produce antibodies cannot be grown in tissue culture for any length of time. In 1975 an ingenious method was developed by the scientists Köhler and Milstein to eternalize single antibody-forming B cells using a hybridoma technique. The principle takes advantage of a tumour cell, which because of its malignancy, is eternal in tissue culture and allows it to fuse with antibody-producing B cells. Before fusion the tumour cells are selected to lack certain enzymes necessary for growth, thus ensuring that the tumour cells only grow in certain special media. The tumour partner is chosen so that it predominantly fuses with B cells and allows Ig synthesis. If now, for example, spleen cells from an immunized mouse are mixed with the tumour cells under fusing conditions, by chance certain cells consisting of hybrids between a normal and a malignant cell will be generated. If this cell mixture is put in a selective tissue culture medium, normal tumour cells cannot grow because of their enzymatic defects. Normal B cells cannot grow either. The only cells which can grow are the hybrids as they have normal enzymes (derived from the B cell) and they have the eternal principle (derived from the tumour cell). Various specificity tests to select the special antibody-forming hybrid required can then be performed. With this method it is now possible to obtain tailor-made antibodies against virtually anything. The reagents can subsequently be used in a standardized manner around the world. Human monoclonal antibodies using the same principle have also been produced and some are already used in clinical practice. The results of this methodology have already led to progress in most areas where conventional antisera are now used.

## Bibliography

GOLUB, E. S. (1977). *The cellular basis of the immune response*. Sinauer Ass. Inc., New York.
FOUGERAU, M. and DAUSSET, J. (1980). *Immunology 80*. Academic Press; New York, London.

# Chapter 7

# Cell-mediated immune reactions

**Hans Wigzell**

Situations where cells actively participate locally in an aggressive manner in the immune response, are called cell-mediated immune reactions. In these reactions, by definition, humoral factors, such as complement and antibodies, are of secondary importance. However, no absolute borders exist between humoral and cellular immunity and antibodies can in certain cases recruit cells to function in a cytotoxic manner against antibody-coated organisms. The consequences of cell-mediated immune reactions will frequently involve tissue damage.

Many different cell types ranging from the phylogenetically old macrophages to granulocytes and specialized lymphocytes are able to participate in cell-mediated immunity. In many cases T lymphocytes play a primary role in these reactions either directly or via the recruitment of other cell types in the local immune response. Mature T cells which leave the thymus after differentiation in this organ, can be subdivided into three major groups; helper, killer and suppressor T cells. Additional subgroups exist to the three major entities. The three major groups of T cells constitute distinct cell groups which seemingly cannot change from one type to another. They have on their surface unique differentiation related markers which can be used as antigen and thus allow a rapid quantitative estimate of the respective T cell types in blood and tissues.

## Role of the thymus during T lymphocyte differentiation

The thymus, which is situated behind the breast bone, consists of two parts. One, the epithelial part, is created from anlagen at the gill pouches. These cells constitute the basic structure of the thymus. They participate, for example, in the creation of the Hassal's corpuscles whose functions are still largely unknown. The epithelial cells are able to produce certain types of thymus hormones, some of whose entire structure are known (e.g. thymopoietin). These thymus hormones have the ability to assist in the maturation of thymocytes during their differentiation within the organ. Administration of such hormones to individuals who lack the epithelial thymus anlage will, however, normally only partially correct the T cell deficiency in such individuals.

The second group of cells in the thymus are derived from the bone marrow and consist of two cell types. The first, the thymocytes, leave the bone marrow in the form of prothymocytes and enter the thymus and mature within this organ to immuno-competent T lymphocytes. These cells constitute a numerically dominant cell type within the functional thymus. The second cell type is similar to a dendritic macrophage. These latter cells seem to have a turnover in the thymus which is significantly slower than that of the thymocytes. Upon ionizing radiation or treatment with cytotoxic drugs the bone marrow derived cells in the thymus are selectively wiped out while the epithelial cells survive. The latter may then help if new cells from the bone marrow come to repopulate the thymus. Upon differentiation of the immature prothymocytes to immunocompetent T cells within the thymus there is a special kind of 'teaching' of the T cells in order for them to function in an optimal manner in the tissues of the periphery. Within the thymus the various T cell groups are selected to be close to auto-immune where the specificity in part is directed against the individual's own major histocompatibility complex (MHC) molecules.

The HLA system does comprise the MHC of man. A human being thus has helper and cytolytic T lymphocytes that have a part of their specificity directed against their own HLA molecules. The helper T cells will predominantly be selected for reactivity against class II MHC molecules (*see* chapter 9). Killer T cells for their part are selected predominantly against class I MHC molecules. The specificity and reactivity of suppressor T cells are also partially regulated by differentiation within the thymus but much still remains unclear.

Several experimental results indicate that dendritic macrophages within the thymus may help in teaching the thymocytes to display some specificity for self-MHC. These dendritic cells also have a high concentration of class I and class II MHC antigens on their surface. *Figure 7.1* exemplifies the probable role of the various thymus components during the differentiation and selection of immunocompetent antigen specific T cells within the thymus resulting in T cells with optimal capacity to see antigens together with self-MHC molecules.

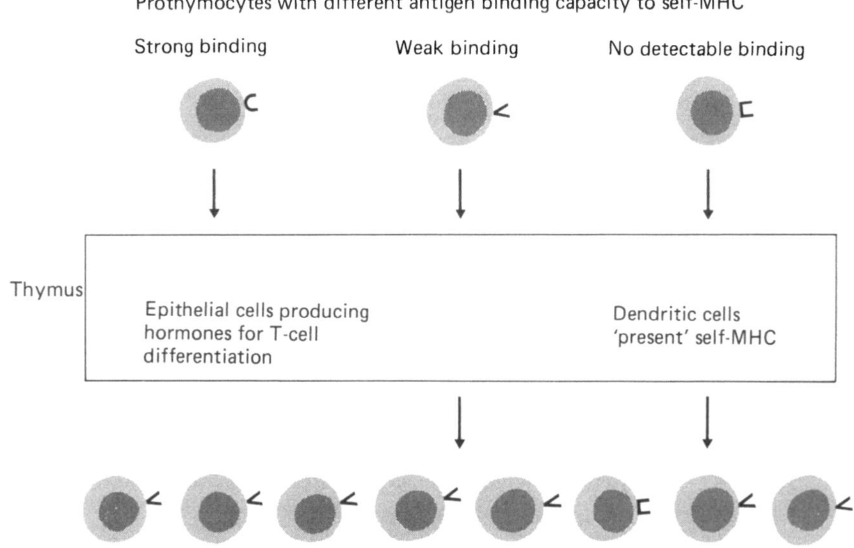


*Figure 7.1* Selection for weak reactivity against self-MHC in the thymus

This specificity does not have the strength to lead to overt autoimmunity, but has as a positive consequence that minor changes in the normal MHC molecules caused by the association of these molecules to small antigenic fragments may lead to increased binding strength of the specific T cells and a subsequent activation of relevant lymphocytes. Experimental studies using thymic grafts have shown the education of T cells to recognize self-MHC in such a manner is governed by the dendritic cells within the thymus. If an animal, lacking thymus, receives a thymic graft from a donor with a different MHC composition, this will lead to the education of the first prothymocytes coming from the marrow into the thymic graft to recognize the MHC structures of the thymus as self-MHC. This means that the first T cells which subsequently leave the thymus will 'see' in the peripheral tissues the 'wrong' MHC molecules which may lead to a suboptimal sensitivity with regard to recognition of foreign material. However, after a few months the dendritic macrophages in the thymic graft are replaced by new cells from the marrow, carrying the MHC structures of the host, which now results in a 'teaching' of T cells in a 'correct' manner. It is likely that this phenomenon partially explains why after thymus grafts to T cell-deficient children it may frequently take up to a year before full T cell competence is achieved.

## Specificity of T lymphocytes

T lymphocytes like B cells have their own antigen-binding capacity where the richness of variability would seem to be in the same order of magnitude as that of the B lymphocytes. Despite this we know less about the structure of the T cell receptors. They are present on the surface of T lymphocytes as a two-chain molecule, held together by covalent bonds. Both chains seem to be constructed in the same manner as heavy chains of B cell immunoglobulin, that is they contain V, D, J and C regions. Evidence of a third variable chain is also available, but so far only at the level of mRNA. Closely attached to the antigen-binding two-chain molecule in the cell membrane are three smaller, non-variant proteins, the function of which is to trigger the lymphocyte into activation upon contact with proper immunogen. Antigen-specific molecules released from T cells have also been described with reported capacity to influence other lymphocytes in a positive or negative manner. The latter molecules require, however, further characterization before firm conclusions as to their functional roles and relationship to the cell-bound antigen-specific T cell receptors can be drawn.

The specificity of human T lymphocytes is different from that normally found to be typical of B cells. Both helper and killer T cells seem to predominantly 'see' foreign structures together with one or another of their class I or class II MHC molecules. As stated before, in the human, class II MHC structures (HLA DR) seem to be the dominating antigen presenting structures of relevance for the helper T cells and their specificity. In contrast killer T cells to a major degree seem to see foreign structures, in the context of the class I MHC molecules (HLA, B or C). This restriction with regard to class I or class II MHC molecules is however not absolute. Suppressor T cells have in some experiments been reported to be more like conventional B cell antibodies in their antigen-binding specificity but there is substantial evidence indicating that suppressor T cells exist with specificities restricted by MHC molecules. Besides having antigen-binding specificity directed against MHC molecules (altered self-MHC) there also exist T lymphocytes from all three major groups with a specificity which is anti-idiotypic, i.e. directed against the antigen-binding areas on T cell receptors or antibody molecules (*see* chapter 2). Such T lymphocytes can play an important part during specific immune regulation and are further discussed in chapter 8.

The fact that the dominating T cell specificity is focused on MHC class I and II molecules may also explain why such molecules are the strongest histocompatibility antigens within the species. The T lymphocytes have receptors selected for a weak affinity for self-MHC structures. This will not in itself lead to specific triggering of the T cells. However, if such MHC structures are modified by the binding of, for example, a peptide fragment from a virus, this complex fragment-MHC molecule can now in certain situations achieve enough binding strength to the antigen binding areas of the T cell receptor to trigger that T cell into action. It is also clear that those T cells which can react in the human body against self-MHC structures complexed to a proper antigenic fragment, may also react against certain foreign MHC molecules in the absence of additional antigen. This would explain why foreign MHC structures, in the human the HLA antigens, constitute such powerful transplantation antigens; they are recognized within the human body in the same manner as self-MHC structures modified by antigenic fragments.

The discovery that T lymphocyte activation normally requires antigen to be presented in the context of self-MHC molecules on the surface of a cell is of both theoretical and practical interest. The capacity of these molecules to combine with various antigenic molecules which may appear on the surface of a cell, is a likely explanation of the great polymorphism in the MHC systems which have been observed, e.g. in the H-2 system in the mouse and the HLA system in the human (*see* chapter 9). It can be argued that through this variation within the species there may always be some individuals whose MHC structures carry the capacity to combine efficiently with, for example, new virus antigen and thereby permit an effective cell-mediated immune reaction. The finding that the T cell specificity is partially anti-MHC and partially antigen specific in a complex, also explains why the same antigenic fragment when placed on different MHC backgrounds yields cell mediated immune reactivity with entirely different specificity requirements. The same virus induced antigen in two individuals with different MHC genes will thus induce specific immune T cells with largely non-overlapping specificities.


**Helper T cells**

Helper, or, sometimes termed inducer T cells, were originally detected by the discovery that T lymphocytes could help, catalyse, the capacity of B cells to produce antibodies. The principal ways through which this occurs have already been described in chapter 6 (*Table 6.1*). We now know that within this group of helper T cells there probably exist several subgroups of functionally distinct cells. Besides being able to help B cells produce antibodies against the thymus dependent antigens, helper T cells also have a corresponding capacity to enhance the activation of killer T cells. Other helper T cells react against foreign substances by inducing a delayed-type hypersensitivity reaction (discussed later in chapter 16) and may release substances which activate osteoclasts thereby starting bone resorption. They also have the capacity to produce specific growth factors for the cell-dependent form of mast cells. Finally there are special helper T cells which have the capacity to induce suppressor T cells, which in turn may have the capacity to inhibit other helper T cell types. If helper T cells are lacking, a major part of the specific immune response will be lacking.

A central role in the activation of helper T cells is played by the antigen-presenting form of macrophages. These cells have a particularly good capacity to present antigenic fragments on the cell surface in a manner easily accessible to helper T cells and where class II MHC molecules may play a crucial role (*see* chapter 9). During the reaction

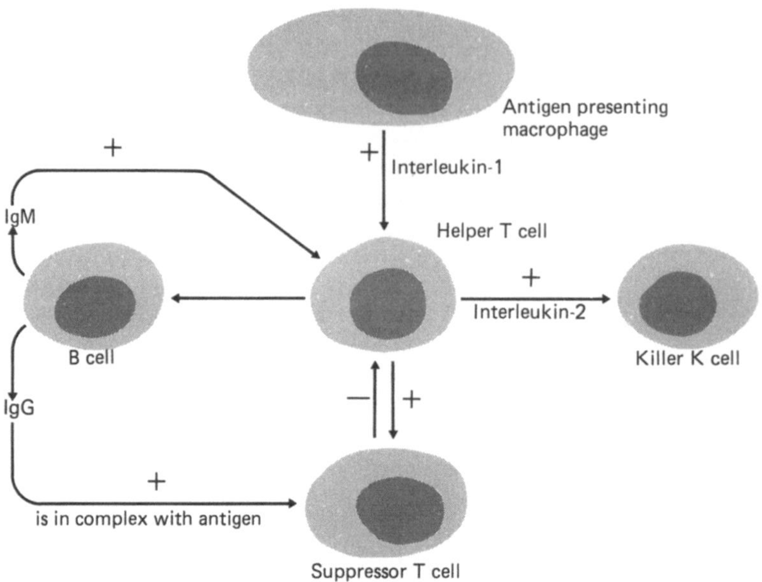


*Figure 7.2* Scheme depicting the three major T cells groups and their main reactions within the lymphocyte population. + = stimulation; − = inhibition

between the antigen-specific receptors on the T cells with the antigenic complex on the surface of the macrophage the latter will produce a pharmacologically highly potent polypeptide, the interleukin-1 of LAF (lymphocyte activating factor). Interleukin-1 has a good capacity to activate helper T cells upon binding to antigen thereby inducing proliferation and production of pharmacologically active substances. Interleukin-1 has also been called the body's own endotoxin because it has the capacity to provoke reactions, normally linked to the presence of endotoxins from Gram-negative bacteria within our body.

Via interleukin-1 and antigen, T helper cells are thus activated to produce their pharmacologically active substances and this starts a number of reactions with other cells (*see Figure 7.2*). Of special interest is the polypeptide interleukin-2, which is produced predominantly by helper T cells and which can function as a specific growth hormone for all T cells, in particular killer and suppressor T cells. With the help of interleukin-2 added to tissue culture it is now possible to grow T lymphocytes in large amounts *in vitro*.

## Suppressor T cells

It is possible to regulate the immune response in many ways, e.g. via limitation of an accessible antigen, via antibody induced redistribution of antigen (chapter 6) and via the production of specific immunological tolerance (chapter 8). It is also possible to regulate immune reactions via specific suppressor T cells, which may act in a selective manner to inhibit the function of other cells. The best known function of suppressor T cells is inhibition of helper T cells. The exact mechanism underlying this inhibitory capacity is unknown, but it has been possible to prove in experimental systems that suppressor T cells can produce specific molecules with ability to bind to the relevant helper T cells. Furthermore there are suppressor T cells which can inhibit killer T cells or the immunoglobulin-producing capacity of B cells in a similar direct manner. The specificity of such suppressor T cells has been shown to be directed against a defined antigen, frequently in the context of MHC of the target cell. Alternatively, the specificity of the suppressor T cells may be directed against the antigen-binding areas of the target lymphocyte, i.e. having an anti-idiotypic specificity.

Suppressor T cells can be induced in many different ways. Efficient induction of these lymphocytes can be obtained by administration of immunogen at a high concentration leaving a certain amount soluble in the body fluids. Immune complexes, especially between IgG antibodies and antigens have also been reported as efficient molecules in recruiting the suppressor T cells. It is believed that certain rare immune deficiencies in man result from excessive suppressor T cell function making normal B and T cell function in such patients impossible. A lack of suppressor T cells has shown in experimental systems to result in an increased incidence of autoimmune antibodies coupled with an increased tendency to develop glomerulonephritis.


## Killer T cells

A very important group of cells within the cell-mediated immune system are T cells with cytolytic capacity, termed killer T cells. These cells act via lysis of the target cells by a direct cellular contact between the killer cell and its target. Such T cells have exquisite specificity and will, in a mixed cellular population, only kill those cells which carry on their surface antigens which fit the antigen-binding receptors on the killer T cell. Thus the lytic mechanism is indeed limited to intimate contact and does not contain humoral cytotoxic mechanisms of long duration.

Specificity of killer T cells is mostly directed, as previously mentioned, against antigen seen in the context of self-MHC molecules of class I (in the human HLA-A, B or C, *see also* chapter 9). It is, however, possible for some cytotoxic T cells to also 'see' antigens in relation to class II MHC molecules. If a human being is infected by a virus there will frequently develop within the body cytotoxic T cells with a specificity for various peptides in conjunction with one or more HLA antigen, as described above (*see Figure 7.3*). The reason why killer T cells in all animal species so far studied display this unique preference to 'see' antigen in contact with class I MHC molecules while the helper T cells predominantly 'see' antigen together with class II MHC molecules is still unclear. As mentioned above the great polymorphism of class I and II MHC genes within the species can be explained by this tendency of T cells to see antigen only in the context of MHC molecules. The capacity of the immune system at the level of T cells to respond to a particular antigen, is thus dependent on the possibility of the cells reacting against fragments of that antigen associating with MHC structures within the individual in question.

Killer T cells are considered to be relevant, particularly during the elimination of viruses via the killing of cells containing such infectious agents. Such an elimination results in the death of the infected cells and this may be the reason for the dominating symptoms during certain types of infection. In fact there are examples in experimental systems where the death of an infected animal is not due to the virus itself but to elimination of the cells infected by the virus by killer T cells. The capacity of T cells to kill is not always of benefit to the multicellular organism. Killer T cells like helper T cells also play an important part in the rejection of foreign transplanted tissue and are able to kill tumour cells carrying unique antigens in experimental systems.

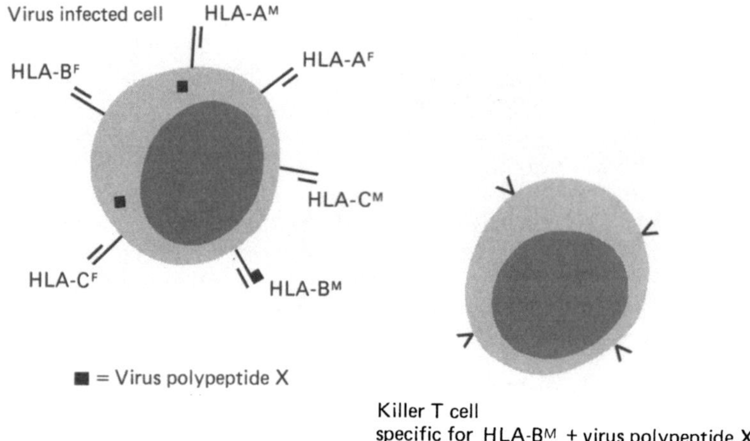



*Figure 7.3* The specificity of killer T cells. A nucleated cell in a human being normally has six different class I MHC molecules (HLA, B and C molecules). A certain virus polypeptide may for example only be 'seen' by one particular killer T cell together with a special HLA-B molecule, the gene for which was inherited from the mother. F, from the father, M, from the mother

## Other cell-mediated cytotoxic reactions

Other cells with cytolytic capacity exist besides killer T cells. One important principal mechanism in the generation of many types of effector cells is based on the fact that several different cell types have Fc receptors on their surface, i.e. structures which can bind to constant regions on immunoglobulin molecules. These receptors can have different specificity, e.g. for IgM, IgA, IgE or IgG, even for subclasses of IgG. Cells carrying such receptors may become passively 'armed' by specific antibodies binding to these receptors. Some of these cells can subsequently function as killer cells with a specificity given to them by the cellbound antibodies. Alternatively, a cell can be coated by antibodies on its surface with specificity against the antigens. Such Ig-coated cells function as attractive targets for cells with killer capacity and suitable Fc receptors. A common name for cells which can function via this antibody-dependent cell-mediated cytotoxicity (ADCC) is K cells (killer cells). Many different types of cells are, however, encompassed in that definition. It is possible to show that IgG or IgA coated parasites can be lysed by eosinophil granulocytes. T cells and natural killer cells may constitute a large part of the K cells against IgG coated nucleated target cells. Monocytes and macrophages can also function effectively against IgG coated erythrocytes through a mixture of contact mediated cytolysis and antibody-induced phagocytosis. IgE has also been reported to be able to induce aggressive macrophages against certain types of parasites.

Besides antibody-induced cell-mediated cytotoxicity and killer T cells a third group of cells called natural killer (NK) cells, have been demonstrated in many different species, including man. These natural killer cells look like large lymphocytes but the majority do not seem to belong to any of the 'classical' cell types. In their cytoplasm they have weakly eosinophilic granules and constitute about 5% of the lymphocytic cells in human peripheral blood. NK cells have their own unique organ distribution pattern and are present in normal numbers in thymus-deficient individuals. These cells can function in a similar manner to killer T cells, i.e. by direct contact, without addition of antibodies. The majority of natural killer cells are however not thymus dependent (*see* chapter 1). Average NK cells in the same animal species all seem to have a similar selective binding capacity. This specificity is a feature which can also be expressed by several 'classical' cell types as well. Killer T cells during certain stages of activation may, for instance, be able to add NK specificity to the unique specificity of the individual killer T cells.

NK cells have attracted attention due to their capacity to kill several different types of tumour cells *in vitro*. In animal experiments they have been found to play a role in the natural resistance *in vivo* against certain tumour cells if transplanted. NK cells also have the capacity to react against stem cells within the bone marrow of the same individual and against immature thymocytes. One may hypothesize from the distribution pattern of NK cells within the body (high in blood and spleen, low in bone marrow and thymus), that one function of these cells could be to inhibit immature cells from leaving their normal places in the tissues for other parts of the body. NK cells also have been found to be of relevance with regard to the defence against certain infections of both viral and parasitic origin. It is likely that NK cells represent a phylogenetically older defence system than the antigen-specific T and B lymphocytes.

## Two examples of T cell dependent cell-mediated immunity

### Delayed-type hypersensitivity reactions

Classical delayed-type hypersensitivity reactions are provoked in already immune individuals after contact with certain antigens, and will only be visible after a period ranging from 24 to 48 hours. A classical example of delayed hypersensitivity reaction in man is the tuberculin reaction. In people immune to antigens from the tuberculosis bacteria an intracutaneous injection of antigen (tuberculin) will, after one to two days, lead to a temporary redness and induration at the site of injection. Microscopically it is possible to demonstrate an invasion of lymphoid cells followed by an accumulation of (predominantly) macrophages and monocytes at the site of injection. What happens is that helper T cells, immune to tuberculin first migrate into the inoculated tissue. Here they react with antigen which has been bound to specialized macrophage-like cells in the skin (Langerhans cells). These reactions induce the lymphocytes to release, among other things, lymphokines (pharamacologically active molecules). One of these molecules (MIF, macrophage migration inhibition factor) has the ability to locally enrich macrophages in the tissue. Another molecule (MAF, macrophage activation factor) activates the enzymatic machinery of the macrophages, making them more aggressive. These reactions mean that at the local 'hypersensitive' area there is an enrichment of immune T cells as well as non-specific but aggressive macrophages which together function as an efficient defence mechanism against infections.

Delayed-type hypersensitivity may appear following many different types of infections. The above described test using relevant antigen can then be used to test whether T cell immunity against the micro-organism has developed. The existence of such cells does not necessarily mean that protective immunity against the organism has developed. Delayed-type hypersensitivity can also be induced against certain chemical substances capable of reacting with the tissues of the body, in particular cells of the skin. Such skin reactions are then called contact allergies or allergic contact eczemas. They have the same cellular background as the delayed-type hypersensitivity reactions against inoculated antigens as stated above.

**Rejection reactions against foreign tissues (the allograft reaction)**

Our knowledge about specific cell mediated immunity has to a large degree come from studies of immune reactions induced by transplantation of tissue from one individual to another. All individuals have on the surface of their cells genetically determined transplantation antigens. If they are foreign for the recipient of a transplanted tissue an immune reaction will be induced against these antigens. This will normally lead to the rejection of the transplant. Such a rejection in the case of a first set transplant only occurs after a week or more, thus permitting the foreign transplant to first heal, followed by a subsequent rejection. If, however, one then attempts to transfer a second transplant from the same donor this is now rejected much faster (second set rejection), without initial healing. This is due to the fact that the first transplant has induced immunological memory against the foreign transplantation antigens.

Despite the fact that T as well as B lymphocytes and their products participate during the rejection it is normally T cells which play the dominating roles in tissue rejection (for a detailed discussion of transplantation immunology, *see* chapters 9 and 14). In animals it is possible, by thymectomy (removal of the thymus) early during development, to create an individual without T lymphocytes. In a similar manner defects during the development of the fetus may lead to a child who is born without T lymphocytes. Such individuals lack the capacity to reject foreign tissue and it is possible even to transfer tissue from one species to another, which may then permanently heal. In mice with a complete thymic deficiency it is possible to transplant skin from a fowl to a mouse leading to the subsequent growth of feathers, etc. This is because transplantation antigens like most other macromolecules within our bodies belong to the TD antigens (*see* chapter 6).

T cells are essential for the induction of allograft reaction (reaction against different transplantation antigens within the species) and also play a very important role during second set reactions. It should however be realized that antibodies (produced via helper T cells activating B cells) and complement in later stages of allograft reaction may contribute significantly in the rejection of the graft. The concentration of relevant transplantation antigens on the surface of the target cell plays an important role in deciding the consequences of such antibodies. If IgG antibodies react with a cell they can only fix complement and cause cellular lysis if two IgG molecules come into close enough contact with each other on the surface of the target cell. This means that below certain concentrations of surface antigens it may be very difficult or close to impossible to kill such cells using IgG antibodies and complement. Killer T cells have seemingly a much higher sensitivity and can kill target cells with very low antigen concentrations on their cell surface. Antibodies of IgG type may in fact under these conditions sometimes prevent killer T cells from being able to lyse the target cells.

The allograft reaction thus consists in its effector phase of a complicated immune response with several different possible pathways leading to damage of the transplanted cells. This reaction is also called a host-versus-graft reaction, to distinguish it from graft-versus-host reactions, which may be produced if immunocompetent T cells are inoculated into a foreign recipient that lacks T lymphocytes. In the latter case the inoculated cells do consider the transplantation antigens of the recipient as foreign and will try to 'reject' these cells, i.e. eliminate the host. Such graft-versus-host reactions are especially problematic in the clinical situation when attempts are made to treat various immunodeficient diseases using bone marrow cells (*see* chapter 14). The reaction will produce diarrhoea, skin lesions, loss of hair, fever and possible death.

# Test of T cell functions

It is of interest in several clinical situations to be able to measure and ascertain if a patient has normally functioning T lymphocytes. Besides performing a direct measurement of the number of T lymphocytes in the body using various markers as specific antibodies, there are also a number of *in vitro* or *in vivo* tests.

### *In vitro* activation

Certain substances have the capacity to selectively provoke mitosis among the majority of T lymphocytes. Two well characterized substances in this context are PHA (phytohaemagglutinin) and concanavalin A, both of which are proteins extracted from different species of beans. The mitogenic effect is measured most easily by the incorporation of radiolabelled thymidine into the DNA of the dividing T lymphocytes. Alternatively, instead of mitogens one may carry out lymphocyte stimulation tests, where the tested cell population is analysed for its ability to respond *in vitro* against foreign strong histocompatibility antigens (*see* chapter 9).

While the above tests are relatively easy to standardize, the socalled migration inhibition test of macrophages is technically more difficult to carry out in a quantitative manner. If macrophages are put in a capillary tube they will migrate from this tube in a typical manner. If immune T lymphocytes plus soluble antigen are added *in vitro* the lymphocytes may produce MIF, which will inhibit the migration of the macrophages and thus limit the area coated by macrophages.

### *In vivo* activation

Depending on the vaccination policy of the country, it is frequently possible to predict that the major part of the adult population may be immune, at the T cell level, to certain types of antigens. Such antigens can be used as rapid *in vivo* tests for the presence of immune, functioning T cells in most people. One can also try to induce delayed hypersensitivity reactions in normal individuals. One efficient chemical in this context, which is normally not found in the surroundings, is dinitrochlorobenzene. If this substance is painted on the skin, it will lead to immunity and subsequent reactions of delayed type in around 95% of the individuals with functioning T lymphocytes. This constitutes a safe, although more time-consuming method of analysing whether an individual has functioning T lymphocytes.

## Bibliography

FOUGERAU, M. and DAUSSET, J. (1980). *Immunology 80*. Academic Press, New York
KATZ, D. H. (1977). *Lymphocyte, Differentiation, Recognition and Regulation*. Academic Press, New York
STUTMAN, O. (ed.) (1977). T lymphocytes, *I Contemporary Topics in Immunobiology*, Plenum Publ. Corp., New York

# Chapter 8

# Immune tolerance and autoimmunity

**Hans Wigzell**

*Immune tolerance* is defined as a specific lack of immune reactivity against one particular antigen, while retaining normal reactivity against all other immunogens. This specific tolerance resides at the level of the lymphocytes and may comprise various lymphocyte groups but not necessarily all types of lymphocytes. Partial tolerance can thus exist.

*Autoimmunity* means immune reactions against 'self' components. Such processes may lead to damage of tissue and will then be called autoimmune disease. It is, however, important to realize that autoimmune reactions do not need to create damage. Certain autoimmune reactions may exist normally during immunization and may even have positive value.

## Immune tolerance

### Tolerance induction during fetal life

It has long been known that specific immune tolerance is particularly easy to induce during fetal life. The original discovery was that bizygotic twins in cattle frequently are tolerant of each other's histocompatibility antigens. Skin transplant exchanged between such twins will thus frequently be accepted in a permanent manner while skin from a third unrelated cow will be rejected with normal speed. It was possible to prove that the underlying basis for this tolerance in cattle with regard to bizygotic twins was caused by a common blood circulation via the placenta between the two fetuses. This meant that such calves, when born, would have a bone marrow consisting of a mixture of their own cells and those of the twin and thus a corresponding mixture at the level of peripheral blood. In man similar consequences may occur in bizygotic twins but this is very rare as they would normally not have a common blood circulation via the placenta.

It is considered that one reason why it is especially easy to provoke tolerance during fetal life is because lymphocytes during their differentiation may be exceptionally sensitive to antigen contact when they have just acquired their antigen-binding receptors on the cell surface. It is possible to demonstrate that contact with antigen during these critical periods may easily lead to a subsequent lack of immune reactivity in the reactive lymphocyte. In B cells such an early contact has been shown to create a halt in the synthesis of immunoglobulin molecules and thus a lack of antigen-binding receptors. Somewhat later during differentiation the B lymphocytes will significantly increase their resistance towards tolerance induction and in experimental systems a

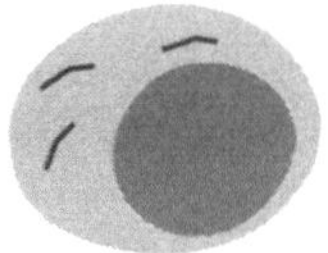

No antigen receptors
Resistant

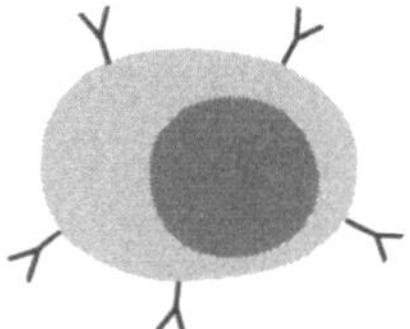

Early B cell: IgM receptors
Highly susceptible for tolerance
induction

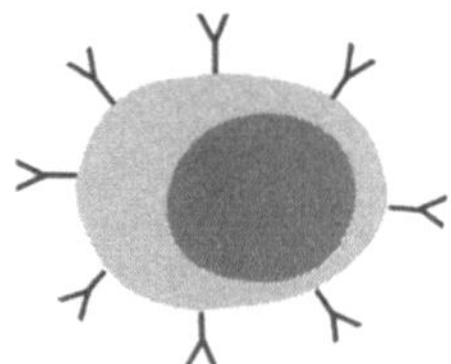

Mature B cell: IgM and
IgD receptors. Relatively
resistant

*Figure 8.1* Different susceptibility for tolerance induction in lymphocytes during differentiation. Example: B lymphocyte

more than 10 000 times higher antigen concentration will now be needed to provoke tolerance instead of immunity compared to the situation with a more immature B cell. *Figure 8.1* summarizes schematically how such a development will occur. It is likely, but not proved, that the same kind of development may exist within the T lymphocyte population during differentiation. This would mean that lymphocytes that mature in the presence of potential antigen, which would then normally automatically be substances within the body, now would have a greater chance to become tolerant.

It is important to understand that all genetic possibilities exist at the DNA level to provide B as well as T cells having antigen-binding receptors with an efficient capacity to react with 'self' molecules.

**Varying degrees of tolerance against 'self' antigens**

The proposed automatic process to produce tolerance against 'self' components as indicated above is not without flaws. One such reason is quantitative. In order for a significant degree of tolerance to be achieved there is normally a requirement for a critical concentration of the molecule in question, besides fulfilling the normal requirements for antigen as depicted in chapter 3. *Figure 8.2* describes how it is possible, in principle, to subdivide our 'self' antigens into three groups depending upon the tolerance-producing capacity in relation to the concentration of the molecules in question. The figure also stresses another fact, namely that it is normally much easier to

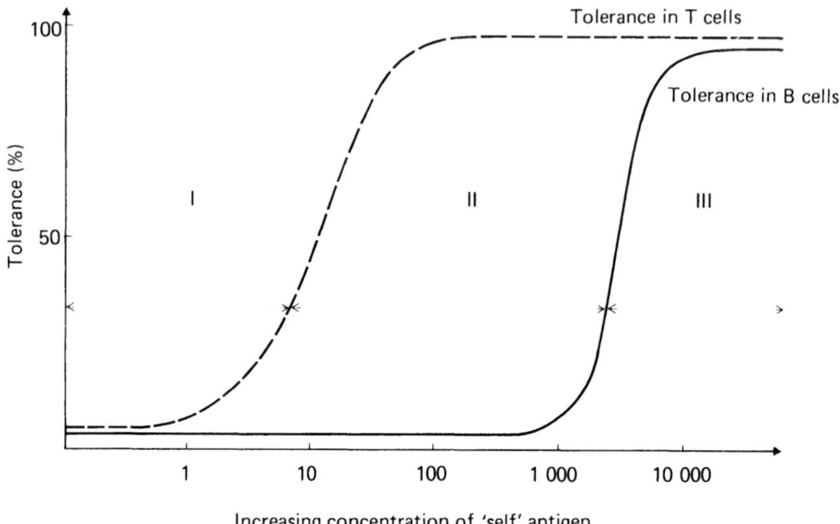



*Figure 8.2* Dose-dependent induction of tolerance against 'self' antigens of thymus dependent nature

provoke functional tolerance in T lymphocytes than in B cells. As virtually all of the potential immunogens within our body belong to the groups of T dependent antigens, the immune response normally requires both helper T cells as well as B cells in order for autoantibodies to be produced upon contact with the molecule in question. The autoantigens of the body are thus subdivided into three major groups. There will be one group of antigens (group I) which will normally exist in such a low concentration where lymphocytes are found that neither T nor B cells will be functionally tolerant. Such group I substances may leak out into the circulation and thus lead to a direct immune reaction of a complete type. Such molecules are normally concealed from the immune system, e.g. are present intracellularly but can be released upon tissue damage such as burns, myocardial infarctions, etc. In many cases autoimmune reaction will then lead to production of antibodies within a week or so after the damage, but such antibodies may have no negative consequences. It is in fact even possible that the reactions of the antibodies may lead to a more rapid cleaning up of the dead tissue. These antibodies cannot react with normal tissue because the antigens are localized inside the cells. In other situations tissue damage in certain organs, e.g. the eye, may lead to a release of tissue antigens which can directly lead to autoantibody production. If some of these antigens, even in normal tissue, are accessible to antibodies the autoantibodies may now be able to damage previously undamaged tissue, e.g. by destroying the clarity of parts of the optical systems of the eyes.

Group II autoantigens (*Figure 8.2*) are made up of 'self' antigens present in such a concentration that helper T cells are lacking due to tolerance, while normal numbers of functional B cells against the same antigens are available. This would, however, normally not lead to autoimmunity due to the thymus-dependent nature of the antigens. The situation is, however, decidedly dangerous and autoimmunity may occur if the B cells receive help in other ways (*see below*).

Group III would finally, according to this scheme, consist of molecules which are present in such a high concentration that it is difficult to prove functional T and B lymphocytes with reactivity against them. It must, however, be stressed that even here antigen-specific B cells may be present in the body, but the high concentration of antigen which normally exists will block the accessibility of the antigen-binding molecules on these cells in a competitive manner and would thus largely exclude a dangerous activation of the type which may dominate for group II antigens (*see below*). Group III antigens are thus in most cases uninteresting as far as autoimmunity goes.

Tolerance normally requires the permanent existence of antigens in order to be sustained. That explains why many substances present during fetal life at a high concentration, but then nor produced any longer, can subsequently be used as antigens in the adult. If an autoantigen has stopped being produced within the body it is merely a matter of time before the tolerance against this structure is broken. A renewed contact with this antigen later in life will result in an immune response.

## Suppressor T cells as inducers of immune tolerance

In addition to the forms of tolerance which are induced by antigen via direct contact with the antigen-specific receptors of the lymphocytes resulting in clonal elimination or blocking, there exists a form of active immunotolerance. This type was originally described in experimental systems where adult immunocompetent mice were inoculated with a thymus dependent antigen in the form of sheep erythrocytes using high concentrations. This amount of antigen resulted relatively rapidly in a failure of these mice to produce antibodies against sheep erythrocytes. They could however produce antibodies against other antigens and were thus by definition immunotolerant against sheep erythrocytes. Interestingly enough in contrast to the earlier 'passive' forms of tolerance this tolerance was possible to transfer to normal adult mice of the same strain using spleen cells from the tolerant animals. When the tolerance-inducing cells of the spleen were analysed as to subsets it could be shown that they belong to the T cell groups. As they have the capacity to suppress, they were thus called suppressor T cells with a specific capacity to induce tolerance, in this case against sheep erythrocytes. It has since been possible in many systems to prove that the tolerance which is induced after the production of a functioning immune response in an individual, will often have as an underlying basis the presence of specific suppressor T cells. The suppressor T cells and their corresponding helper or inducer cells for suppressor cells have been shown to either have as their specificity a relevant antigen in the context of MHC molecules or alternatively the antigen-binding areas of the receptors on the relevant T or B lymphocytes (anti-idiotypic suppressor T cells).

## Immune tolerance against microbiological antigens

There are no fundamental biochemical differences between most 'self' molecules and those which can be brought in from outside in the form of exogenous immunogens. Likewise immune tolerance can be induced against, for example, viral antigens in the same manner as against 'self' components. If a fetus is infected *in utero*, this may provoke a tolerance in the fetus against the antigens of the infecting organism. A clearcut example is infection with LCM-virus (Lymphocytic Choriomeningitis virus) which, in small rodents, can produce a severe meningitis in adult animals. The virus may also affect human beings. Infection of pregnant mice will lead to a virus infection of the fetus. This will not kill the fetuses but frequently they will be born as carriers of live LCM virus but without any signs of meningitis or other symptoms of disease.

If these experiments are carried out on inbred mice it is possible to study what would

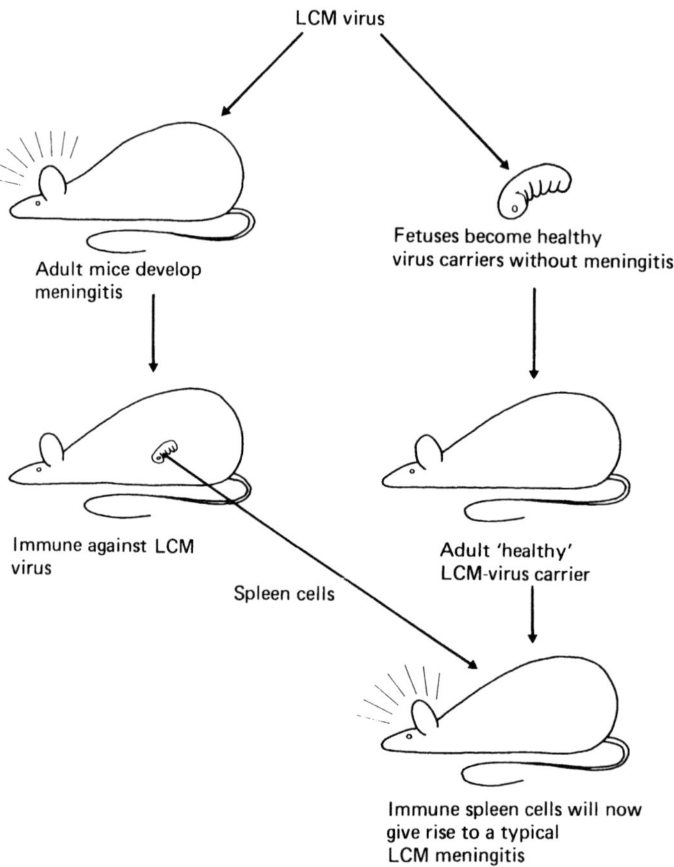



*Figure 8.3* Immune reactions of T lymphocytes do provoke the development of meningitis during LCM virus infection

happen if lymphocytes from LCM immune mice are transferred into these healthy tolerant animals. What occurs in such a case is exemplified in *Figure 8.3*. Previously healthy LCM carriers will now develop a typical meningitis and several of the mice may die. The cells among the transferred lymphocytes, which can produce these consequences can be shown to be immune T lymphocytes. It is thus clear that in this disease it is the reactions of the immune defence against the viral antigens which in fact are producing the classical symptoms of disease. In many infectious diseases it is possible to prove that the major part of the symptoms and damage may be produced by the immune response itself rather than by a direct action of the infecting micro-organism.

Immune tolerance against microbial antigens can also be induced in adult individuals under certain conditions. In man a classical example is the situation with 'old man's friend', i.e. pneumococcal pneumonia of a type mostly seen in elderly men living in social misery. This form of pneumonia originally got its name because of the clinical symptoms that would occur before death. After the introduction of antibiotics the frequency of this disease has been significantly reduced. The underlying basis for the 'old man's friend' syndrome is the fact that the pneumococci have as their principal antigen a polysaccharide which is extremely difficult to metabolize in man. In American investigations it was possible to show that pneumococcal polysaccharide is present in rising concentrations with age in pulmonary tissue in man. In the material studied it could be shown that in men living in socially poor conditions the rise in amount of antigen with time in the lungs occurred much more rapidly due to repeated infections. Antibodies which initially could be produced in high quantities against this antigen did produce immune complexes, but after phagocytosis the polysaccharide would be released from the macrophages or granulocytes, while the antibodies would be degraded. With increasing amounts of antigens in the tissues more and more B lymphocytes would become functionally inactivated, i.e. tolerant. This tolerance would first affect those lymphocytes which could bind avidly but with increasing concentration of antigen functional tolerance will also be induced in B lymphocytes producing antibodies with low avidity for the antigen in question. Finally almost complete tolerance would be produced and a renewed pneumococcal infection could now take the form of 'old man's friend'.

If an antigen is present in a high enough concentration for long enough periods it is thus possible to induce immune tolerance following a state of specific immunity.

## Autoimmunity—a breakage of immune tolerance

Autoimmune reactions frequently arise in situations where immune tolerance in one way or another has been broken. Exceptions do exist however, where tolerance has never been induced in the first place. Beside antigens of type I (*Figure 8.2*) this is also true for minor molecules within our body which do not fulfil the requirements to function as immunogens or tolerogens due to size (chapter 3). However, if such minor molecules, e.g. a corticosteroid is coupled to a large carrier molecule which is immunogenic, an immune response against the small 'self' molecules may be induced. *Figure 8.4* provides examples showing how this may occur if the carrier used is a thymus dependent antigen. Small molecules which are not chemically reactive are thus neither immunogenic nor tolerogenic.

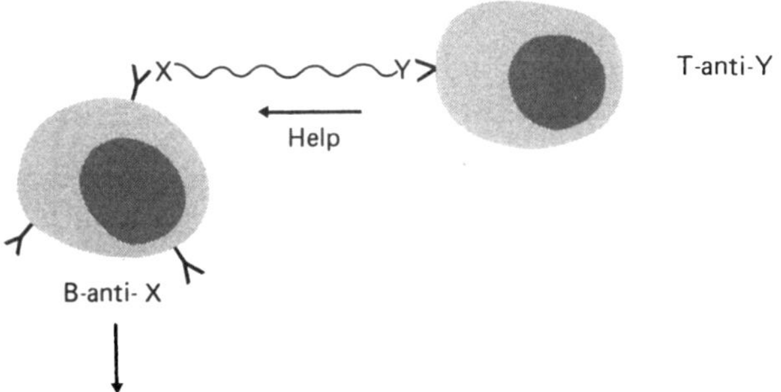


*Figure 8.4* Small molecules within our body may provoke immunity if they are physically coupled together with a foreign antigen. I. The 'self' molecule X of low molecular nature will provoke neither immunity not tolerance in T or B cells. II. If X is now physically linked to foreign antigen Y of thymus dependent nature, T cell and above all B cell immunity can now be produced. Here autoantibodies against X are induced as exemplified

Micro-organisms may have on their surface structures which are identical or cross-reacting with human molecules. This may be exemplified by the appearance of anti-A and anti-B blood group antibodies which appear 'spontaneously' in human beings within the ABO-system (*see* chapter 9). The human being who has blood group A has normally anti-B antibodies in serum. Such antibodies have been produced through the contact with bacterial or other types of microbial antigens of 'B-type'. In chickens, which have a blood group system similar to ABO in man, the corresponding antibodies will not be produced if the animals are brought up in sterile conditions. Blood group AB antigens function according to this scheme as 'self' antigens within group III in man and normally no significant amounts of autoantibodies can be induced against these molecules. As micro-organisms normally have several different kinds of antigenic determinants on their surface the presence of blood group A-like structures on a bacterium does not mean that this bacterium will be more prone to infect human beings having blood group A.

If micro-organisms carry antigenic determinants which also are present in 'self' molecules of type II according to the definition in *Figure 8.2*, this may result in breaking tolerance in various pathways as exemplified in *Figure 8.5*. If the micro-organism can function as a thymus independent antigen this may allow a direct activation of relevant B cells with specificity for a cross-reacting structure without the requirement for helper T cells. Very high concentrations of thymus independent antigens may also, via their capacity to produce polyclonal B cell activation (chapter 6), activate B cells with specificity for 'self' components. A systematic activation of B cells by those polyclonal mechanism can probably only occur in rare septic situations of infectious nature, e.g. by Gram-negative bacteria or severe malaria.

If the cross-reacting structure is present on microbial antigens of a thymus dependent nature a conventional helper T cell activity will now be induced against other determinants on such macromolecules. Through these T lymphocyte reactions help can be transmitted to the B cells with specificity for the cross-reacting structure as exemplified in *Figure 8.5b*. Tissue damage induced by infections or by other ways may also lead to partial denaturation of a type II antigen. This may, as exemplified in *Figure 8.5c*, lead to the production of new antigen groups or fragments against which helper T cell tolerance does not exist. T cell reactions against such new determinants could lead to a subsequent activation of B cells against native determinants still physically linked to the antigen in question. Such a mechanism is considered to underlie the autoantibody production found in certain forms of thyroiditis. As long as the tissue damage is present this may continue to produce partially degenerated antigen thus driving the autoimmune process. High titres of autoantibodies which react locally in the tissue may also generate a very high local concentration of immune complexes. This may, as described in chapter 5, lead to the production of unusual, long-lasting complement complexes in the fluid phase which could cause tissue damage by themselves. An induced autoimmune process can thus, under certain conditions, become self recruiting if its reactions have reached enough local intensity.


**Other predisposing factors for induction of autoimmunity**

In order for autoimmune disease to occur there is often a requirement for predisposing genetic factors. Such genes have been localized both within the HLA and the heavy Ig gene groups (chapter 21). Autoimmunity also has a tendency to appear in situations where a defective handling of immune complexes will occur, frequently in relation to complement deficiencies (chapter 9).

A.

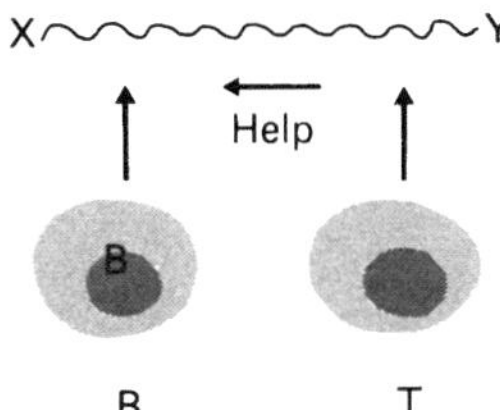



B.

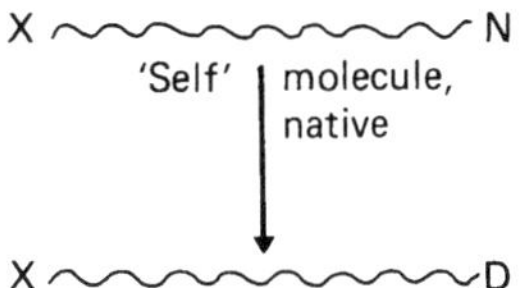



B cells with anti-X- specificity
will be activated via T-helper
cells directed against other
antigenic determinants on
the antigen (here exemplified
by Y)

C.

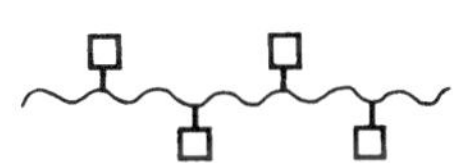



B cells with anti-X-specificity
will be activated by helper
T cells directed against new
antigen determinants of the
antigen (here exemplified as D)

D.

B cells will, regardless of their
fine antigen binding specificity,
be activated by the mitogenic
capacity of the thymus-
independent antigens

*Figure 8.5* Breaking of tolerance against the 'self' component X belonging to the type II 'self' molecules. A. Cross-reacting antigens of thymus independent type (frequently micro-organisms). B. Cross-reacting antigens of thymus dependent type (frequently micro-organisms). C. Partial denaturation of 'self' micromolecules containing the antigen determinant X. D. Polyclonal activation via a high concentration of thymus independent antigens not cross-reacting with X

## Positive autoimmunity?

Autoimmunity may not as such be a negative thing. Autoantibodies against ageing erythrocytes represent one type of antibody which is produced very early in human fetal life and which will continue to be produced during the entire life-span. These antibodies probably have normal positive consequences (leading to a selective elimination of old, probably oxygen-transport-deficient red blood cells) but may under certain conditions, when produced by Gram-negative bacteria, be a cause of pan-agglutination of enzymatically changed erythrocytes.

Our immune defence also uses autoimmune reactions in a positive manner during its

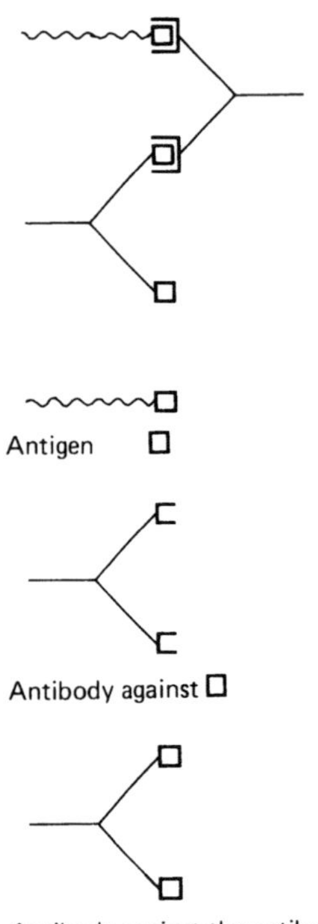


*Figure 8.6* Within our own immune system there are antibodies or antigen binding receptors which may sterically be similar to conventional antigens

own internal regulation. T lymphocytes as already described have a tendency to autoimmunity in their preferential inclusion of 'self' MHC molecules in the complete antigen against which they can react. But there is also with the immune system a specific way of communication between lymphocytes in the form of idiotypic–anti-idiotypic reactions. This network was first described and considered by the Danish immunologist Jerne. He suggested that this potential capacity of a specific communication between lymphocytes in the absence of antigen could serve as a basic and normal foundation for the regulation of the immune system. We now know that the idiotypic network is a reality. In the same manner as we can make antibodies against virtually any kind of antigen (*see* chapter 6) our immune system can also make antibodies against own antibodies and then in particular against antigen-binding areas of these molecules. What is here true for the antigen-binding areas of the immuno-globulins is also true for the corresponding structures of the antigen-binding receptors present on T lymphocytes. We are thus not tolerant to the various parts of our own antibody molecules. This concept also means that we, in the form of anti-idiotypic antibodies/receptors within ourselves, carry, via steric similarities, all the antigenic determinants against which we can make antibodies. It is described in a simplified manner in *Figure 8.6.*

It has now been shown clearly that during conventional immunization with antigens reactions of idiotypic–anti-idiotypic nature are initiated both at the level of antibodies and lymphocytes. Helper T cells with anti-idiotypic specificity have been demonstrated to have the capacity to further enhance the production of antibodies carrying such idiotypic determinants. As there is a statistically proven positive link between idiotypic markers and antigen-binding specificity this frequently means that the specific antibody production against the relevant antigenic determinant is further catalysed by the body making 'more' antigen but now in the form of anti-idiotypic molecules. In a similar manner the opposite reaction may occur, i.e. inhibition induced by other suppressor or killer T cells with specificity for idiotypic determinants. In some experimental systems it has also been possible to completely replace an immunization induced by conventional antigen by using anti-idiotypic antibodies or lymphocytes. Exact details of how this network is contributing to the regulation of the immune system in a positive or negative manner still remains to be discovered. However, it is clear that this immune network does exist and is functioning within our immune system.

## Bibliography


Immunological tolerance (1976). *Br. Med. Bull.*, **32**, No. 2.
MÖLLER, G. (ed.) *Immunol. Rev.*, **43**, 1978; **46**, 1979; **50**, 1980.
JANEWAY, C., SERCARZ, E. and WIGZELL, H. (eds.) (1981). Immunoglobulin idiotypes, *ICN–UCLA. Symp. Mol. Cell. Biol.*, **20**, Academic Press, New York, London.

# Chapter 9

# Immunogenetics

**Rune Grubb and Erna Möller**

Immunogenetics encompasses knowledge about the genetic regulation of the immune response and about marker molecules which can be demonstrated by immunological means and their underlying genetics. The genes coding for various parts of immunoglobulin molecules and their special genetics have already been discussed in chapter 6 and will not be mentioned here. We will above all describe systems which display polymorphism between individuals within the same species, i.e. are allotypic. Among these systems are the blood group systems and their relevance in transfusion and the transplantation antigens and their role during clinical transplantations. The knowledge that the molecules carrying the transplantation antigens also help the T lymphocytes to differentiate self from non-self has already been described in chapter 7. Immunogenetics, although already established by Ehrlich and Landsteiner, is at present in an intense stage of development. Some reasons for the modern interest in immunogenetics are:

(1)   The polymorphism is much greater than we previously could imagine. The reasons for this high degree of polymorphism and its consequences are of interest here.
(2)   There exists a strong positive correlation between certain markers within the HLA system and the likelihood of developing certain important diseases. This may provide a possibility for a deeper insight into the molecular mechanisms underlying these diseases.
(3)   Several clinically important immune reactions are caused by genetically determined allotypes.
(4)   Observations within immunogenetics are relevant to the theories of genetics as a whole.

## Blood groups

### ABO blood groups

Landsteiner detected the ABO groups in 1901 and they are still of dominating importance within clinical blood transfusion. ABO groups and their inheritance pattern can serve as a model system for many allotypes.

The ABO group of a human being as well as other blood group antigens can be determined using agglutination tests. The four well-known groups, A, B, O and AB are determined in the safest manner by exploring both the red blood cells and the serum

**TABLE 9.1. Schematic view of ABO blood groups**

| Blood group | Antigen on red blood cells | Antibody in serum | Approx. frequency in Sweden (%) |
| --- | --- | --- | --- |
| A | A | anti-B | 45 |
| B | B | anti-A | 10 |
| O | — | anti-A + anti-B | 40 |
| AB | A + B | — | 5 |

from the individual. The investigation of the erythrocytes is carried out using known antisera, which contain anti-A or anti-B antibodies respectively and will thus prove the presence or absence of the antigen A and B. The serum of the individual will also be explored using test erythrocytes of known ABO group which can then prove the presence of anti-A or anti-B antibodies in the serum. The groups are defined using an international agreement as indicated in *Table 9.1.*

The main rule during blood transfusion is that the blood donor and the recipient should belong to the same ABO group. A or AB blood must not be transfused into a human being whose serum contains anti-A antibodies or that B or AB blood should be given to an individual having anti-B antibodies. The likely consequence of such a mistake would be a serious and potentially lethal haemolytic transfusion reaction. The previous concept 'universal donor' for people of blood group O and 'universal recipient' for people of group AB has lost much of its relevance as it has been clarified that the antibodies of the donor blood may give rise to haemolysis of a level reaching clinical significance.

A and B antigens are heritable, and unchangeable and can be demonstrated starting from the second fetal month. AB antigens are not only present on red blood cells but can also be found in body fluids and secretions such as saliva, seminal fluid and gastric juice. Thus, approximately 80% of the people belonging to blood group A will secrete the A antigen in a water-soluble form and in relatively high amounts, e.g. in the saliva. These 80% are called secretors of A substance. A substance in solution can be easily demonstrated using the haemagglutination inhibition test. Those people that do not secrete molecules corresponding to the ABO blood group antigens will instead normally secrete Lewis-a-substance (*see below*). As this substance is very stable it is possible, for example, to prove the blood group of someone who has been licking a stamp put on an anonymous letter.

Certain ovarian tumours rich in mucus may contain several grams of blood group substance. The blood group antigens within the ABO and Lewis systems which are present in secretion consist mostly of polysaccharides and only about 25% of the molecules consist of amino acids.

The molecular weight normally exceeds 100 000 but can vary considerably depending on the source of the material from which it has been extracted. Important components in these water-soluble substances, as in many corresponding glycolipids in erythrocyte membranes are galactose, fucose, glucosamine and galactosamine. Antigenic specificity is created by the endgroups of the carbohydrates and their neighbours (*see* chapter 3). Single red blood cells in a person of group AB are equipped with both A and B substances and both types of antigenic determinants can be present on one molecule.

The agglutinating anti-A and anti-B antibodies appear (*Table 9.1*) in a similarly spontaneous manner without any known immunization. The reason that these natural isohaemagglutinins exist, for example against A antigen in individuals of blood group B, is believed to be caused by a cross-reaction by immunization with various bacterial antigens. This high regularity in appearance of antibodies serves as a built-in double control that can be used in ABO blood grouping, i.e. investigating not only the antigens of the red blood cells but also the capacity of the serum to agglutinate red blood cells carrying known blood group antigens. Naturally occurring anti-A and anti-B are normally IgM antibodies but can be of IgG type in particular after immunizing stimuli containing 'true' A substance. Such immunization may occur due to a faulty blood transfusion, injection of preparations containing A substance (which is the case with certain vaccines) or (much more commonly), by pregnancy with an ABO incompatible fetus. Anti-A and anti-B antibodies of IgG class can pass the placenta. If the fetus has the corresponding blood group, presence of IgG antibodies may by passage through the placenta lead to a certain degree of haemolysis of the erythrocytes of the fetus. This normally appears as a slight jaundice during the newborn period but can in rare cases lead to severe disease with symptoms in the child reminiscent of Rh incompatibility (*see below*). Such a danger is greatest in the combination of the mother belonging to group O and the child to group A.

Accuracy in the determination of ABO blood group has been made so high that the investigation can have legal consequences. There exist, however, several possible sources of error which in particular can make themselves noticeable when a large number of people are to be blood grouped or when erythrocytes from sick people are used for testing. Blood group A is not a homogeneous group. It is possible to distinguish subgroups, the most important of which are $A_1$ and $A_2$. $A_2$ is the weak antigen and is, in for example the Swedish population, only present in about 10%. There exist even weaker A antigens but in a frequency which is below one per million. Such weak A antigens may be difficult to prove in particular if they are combined with blood group B. People of blood group $A_2$ or $A_2B$ may sometimes produce an anti-$A_1$ antibody. The subgroups of A do not normally require special consideration during blood transfusion. They may, however, constitute an error during blood grouping.

The genes determining the ABO groups are located on chromosome 9 in one place called the ABO locus. The most important genes are $A_1$, $A_2B$, B and O, where $A_1$ is dominant over $A_2$ and O and $A_2$ over O and B over O. These four genes are multiple alleles which by definition means that they constitute a series of alternative genes on the very same locus, in this case the ABO locus. Every individual has on each gene locus in the autosomes one gene from the mother in one chromosome and one gene from the father in the homologous chromosome. Only two of the genes in a series of multiple alleles can thus be found in a single individual. An individual who has received an $A_1$ gene from the mother and a similar one from the father has the genotype $A_1/A_1$ and the phenotype $A_1$. A person who has received an $A_1$ gene from one parent and an O gene from the other has the genotype $A_1/O$ but has like the previously mentioned individual the phenotype $A_1$. The route of inheritance can be seen from *Table 9.2* in which $A_1$ and $A_2$ have been brought together as A. Exceptions to the rule of inheritance can occur in extremely rare cases whereupon the manifestation of the A or B gene can be suppressed by a suppressor gene present in another gene locus.

It is natural to ask whether the O gene has a gene product of its own. This should mean that O not only means a lack of A and B but does carry a positive feature. Rare human sera may agglutinate O blood groups but not $A_1B$ blood groups. A similar specificity is displayed by serum from eel and from phytohaemagglutinin derived from gorse. Such sera and extracts do also agglutinate $A_2$ as well as $A_2B$ erythrocytes in a

**TABLE 9.2. The correlation between the ABO groups of parents and children**

| Parent combination | Possible groups among children | Excluded groups among children |
|---|---|---|
| O × O | O | A, B, AB |
| O × A | O, A | B, AB |
| O × B | O, B | A, AB |
| O × AB | A, B | O, AB |
| A × A | O, A | B, AB |
| A × B | A, B, AB, O | — |
| A × AB | A, B, AB | O |
| B × B | O, B | A, AB |
| B × AB | A. B. AB | O |
| AB × AB | A, B, AB | O |

strong manner. Their specificity accordingly does not follow the presence of the O gene and the sera are called anti-H sera. H substance is secreted in the saliva in around 80% of the people without relation to their ABO group. It has not been possible to directly prove that any specific product is directly derived from the O gene.

The function of the A and B genes during their biosynthesis of the mucopolysaccharides of blood groups is considered to be that they govern the synthesis of the transferases which add N-acetylgalactosamine for the A gene and D-galactosamine for the B gene to the sugar chain of the H substance (*see Table 3.2*, p. 36).

## Rh factor and its role in blood transfusion and in creating haemolytic disease in neonates

If erythrocytes from rhesus monkeys are injected into experimental animals antibodies will be produced which will agglutinate the erythrocytes from these monkeys. Some of these antibodies also have the capacity to agglutinate red blood cells from approximately 85% of the individuals in a Caucasian population. The Rh factor is the determinant on human red blood cells which will cause such erythrocytes to be agglutinated by anti-Rh antibodies.

Anti-Rh antibodies do not occur in a spontaneous manner, but appear only after specific immunization of Rh-negative individuals. Rh antigen is, as far as we know, only present on red blood cells and the conditions for anti-Rh antibody production are such that Rh-positive erythrocytes will reach the antibody-producing organism within Rh-negative individuals. Such an immunization normally results either from blood transfusion or injection of minor quantities of blood or via transfer of fetal blood during delivery into the circulation of the mother.

If Rh-positive blood is transfused to Rh-negative people anti-Rh antibodies are known to develop in approximately 50% of the cases after one or a few transfusions. The presence of anti-Rh antibodies in an individual will result in haemolytic transfusion reactions if Rh-positive blood is given. It is thus clear that the Rh factor system must be considered in the situation of blood transfusions in the clinic.

In the situation where an Rh-negative mother is pregnant with an Rh-positive fetus this will only result in anti-Rh antibodies in approximately 5% of the pregnancies. If anti-Rh antibodies of IgG-type are present in the mother and the fetus is Rh-positive, it is highly likely that the child will display symptoms of disease. Such symptoms include life-threatening anaemia and jaundice which, in neonates, may give rise to damage of the basal ganglia of the central nervous system. Nucleated red blood cells will appear in the circulating blood which have given the disease its name erythroblastosis. A more modern term is haemolytic disease in newborn or morbus haemolyticus neonatarum. If the disease is particularly severe the fetus may die in the uterus. This will normally occur after the sixth fetal month and the fetus will then frequently display a picture of generalized oedema or hydrops foetalis where, among other things, the liver and spleen are greatly enlarged (erythropoietic organs) and the oedema has smoothed the features of the face (*Figure 9.1*).

The mechanism of the disease is as follows: An Rh-negative woman becomes pregnant with a fetus which has inherited the Rh-antigen from the father. If these Rh-positive erythrocytes reach the antibody producing organs of the woman she may produce anti-Rh antibodies. If the antibodies which are produced belong to the IgG class they can pass through the placenta and the anti-Rh antibodies are thus passively transferred to the fetus. Rh-positive erythrocytes of the fetus will thus be coated on their surface by immunoglobulin from the mother, after which they will be phagocytosed and destroyed. Due to the fact that the greatest danger of immunization during pregnancy is during actual delivery it is almost a rule that the first child will not suffer from this haemolytic disease. Exceptions to this rule will only be noticed if the mother has been previously sensitized either by a missed abortion or by injection of Rh-positive blood.

The treatment of children suffering from morbus haemolyticus neonatarum is to change blood via transfusions. Through such a transfusion the toxic bilirubin that has been created during the abnormally high breakdown rate of the erythrocytes is eliminated and Rh-negative erythrocytes are given. These erythrocytes which will not be influenced by anti-Rh antibodies can take care of the oxygen transport for the fetus during the time it will take for the antibodies transferred from the mother to be broken down in the child. An important part in prophylaxis against haemolytic disease in the newborn is never to transfuse women before or of fertile age with Rh-positive blood unless one has established that the woman is Rh-positive.

It is rare nowadays that exchange blood transfusions have to be made, as the number of cases of haemolytic diseases have been drastically reduced by the introduction of immunological methods which hinder the induction of Rh immunity in women. The underlying principle for this treatment, Rh prophylaxis, is the antibody mediated inhibition of immunity, which has already been described in chapter 6. By transfer of already made human IgG antibodies against Rh factor to an Rh-negative woman after fetal blood has leaked into the circulation of the mother in the context of delivery, abortion or amniocenteses, it is possible to specifically block her immunization against the Rh antigen on the erythrocytes of the fetus.

The protocol for this Rh prophylaxis is as follows: all pregnant women are typed with regard to Rh. If the woman is Rh-negative and she will deliver an Rh-positive child she will receive an injection of IgG antibodies against the Rh factor shortly after giving birth to such a child. Such antibodies have the capacity to specifically inhibit immunization against the Rh-positive erythrocytes of the fetus, which may now be in the circulation of the mother. This means that the next time she becomes pregnant she will not have been immunized against Rh factor and will thus not have IgG antibodies in the circulation, which could pass through the placenta and damage the erythrocytes of the child. This Rh prophylaxis is repeated every single time an Rh-negative woman delivers an Rh-positive child or an Rh-negative woman undergoes abortion or amniocenteses. This propylaxis is highly efficient and it is possible to largely eliminate the genetically determined disease by the help of passive immunity.

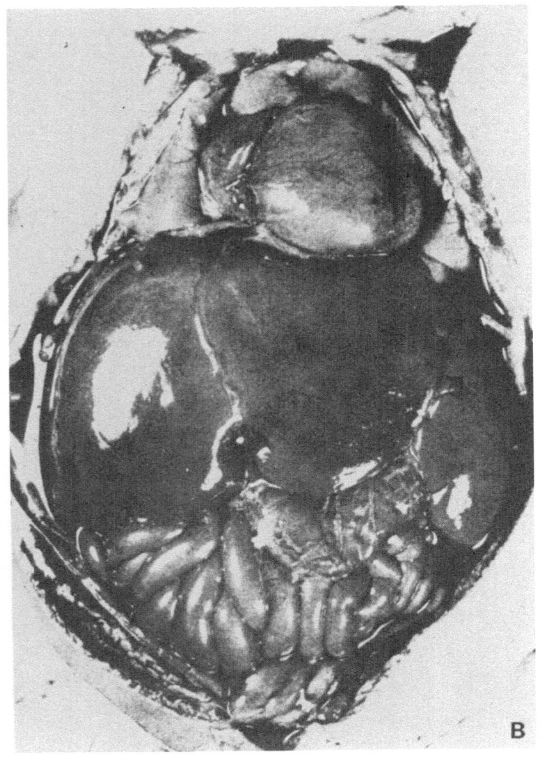
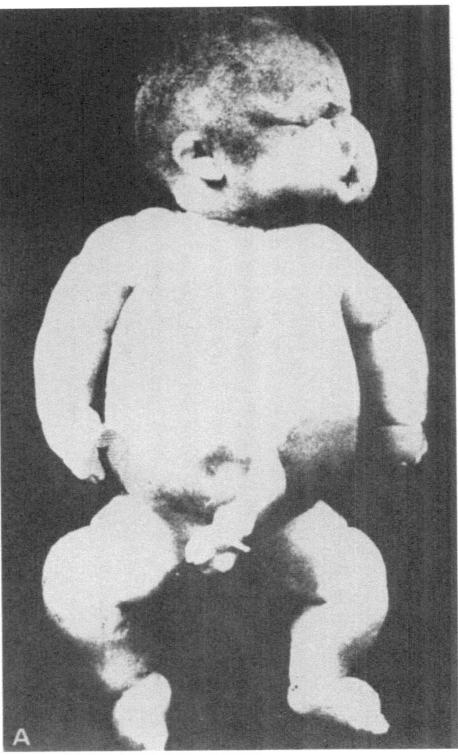

*Figure 9.1* Exterior view and viscera in a child suffering from haemolytic disease caused by Rh incompatibility. (After E. L. Potter (1947), *Rh. Year Book Med. Publ.*)

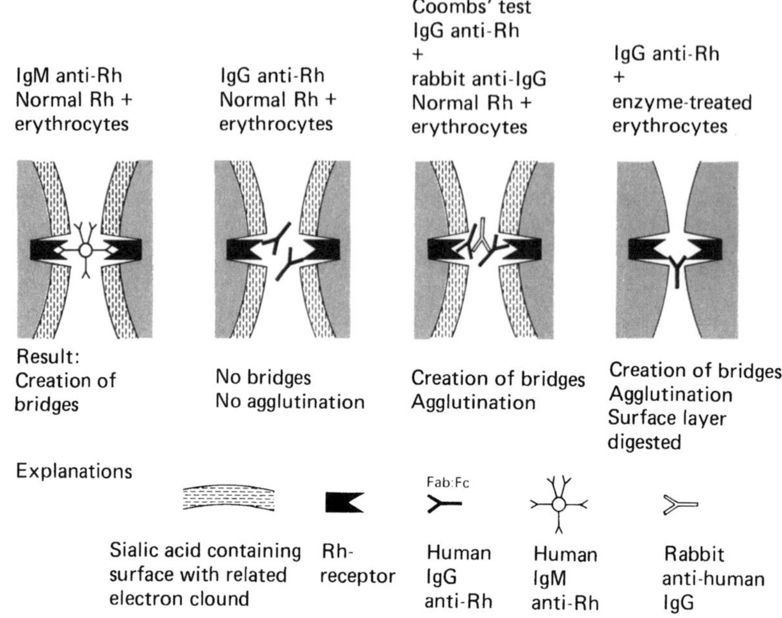



*Figure 9.2* Anti-Rh tests in relation to surface structures on red blood cells

The demonstration of anti-Rh antibodies varies according to the class of the antibodies studied. IgM anti-Rh antibodies are produced early during the immune process. Such anti-Rh antibodies do not have the capacity to pass the placenta and are thus irrelevant for the survival of the child. IgM anti-Rh antibodies are easily demonstrated using agglutination tests in physiological saline. In contrast, IgG anti-Rh antibodies cannot be demonstrated using conventional agglutination tests with physiological saline. This is why such antibodies in earlier literature were called 'incomplete' antibodies. Newer investigations have clarified that the lack of agglutination of Rh-positive antibodies using IgG anti-Rh antibodies in these conditions is due to the fact that the Rh antigens are present below the electrostatic surface of the erythrocytes. Anti-Rh antibodies belonging to the IgM class are able to reach over this distance and make bridges between Rh substances present on two different erythrocytes while the smaller IgG anti-Rh molecules are unable to do this (*see Figure 9.2*). It is of particular importance to be able to demonstrate reliably the presence of IgG anti-Rh antibodies due to their clinical relevance. Special methods have been developed to demonstrate IgG anti-Rh antibodies and the most commonly used are as follows:

(1)    Coomb's test;
(2)    tests using erythrocytes treated with certain enzymes;
(3)    tests using solutions containing certain macromolecules.

In the Coomb's test antibodies against human IgG are used to prove the presence of IgG anti-Rh antibodies. Rabbits are thus immunized against human IgG molecules to obtain such anti-human IgG antibodies. If in a test erythrocytes carry IgG molecules on their surface the additional antibodies against IgG will now cause the creation of bridges between the neighbouring antibody-coated erythrocytes which can then be observed as agglutination (*Figure 9.2*). Note here that the Coomb's test is not in itself uniquely restricted for antibodies of anti-Rh type. The test can of course be used to demonstrate antibodies of other specificities.

The Rh system is considerably more complex than the mere compartmentalization in the Rh-positive and negative individuals. There are more than 25 additional antigens within this genetic system, which can be combined according to the complex. It is a system so complicated that it is fair to say that 'anyone who is not confused is not fully informed'. Certain solid clinical findings are known however. A frequently used nomenclature will consider C, D, E, c and e as symbols for well-established antigens. D represents the classical Rh antigen. If D is present in individuals they are considered Rh-positive and if D is lacking the individual is considered Rh-negative.

The C, D and E antigens are present in various combinations in the immunogen and the common combination CDe and cDE are called with a frequently used nomenclature $R_1$ and $R_2$ respectively. D antigen is present in about 1% of Caucasians in a form called $D^u$ which is more difficult to demonstrate than D. $D^u$ individuals are to be considered Rh-positive both as blood donors and as recipients for blood and women carrying this gene do not require anti-Rh prophylaxis after delivery. Antibodies produced against any of the above-mentioned Rh antigens may however give rise both to transfusion reactions as well as haemolytic diseases in the newborn. Haemolytic disease based on Rh incompatibility can thus occur in the newborn even in situations where the mother and child are both classified as being Rh-positive. However, anti-D reactions are much more common and important than the reactions against all the other factors combined. For unknown reasons anti-e-specific antibodies are a relatively frequent finding in the form of autoantibodies in acquired haemolytic anaemia. The knowledge about various factors within the Rh systems is also important in forensic medicine and in the determination of paternity.

## Other blood group systems

Many additional blood group systems exist where variants are so frequent within a population that these systems are important in identification situations (*see Table 9.3*). From this table it can be seen that five of the ten systems mentioned carry family names, i.e. the name of the person in whose serum the antibody allowing a definition of this antigen system was first found. The systems can be separated from each other by classical inheritance analysis. As seen from the table in six of the systems the chromosome carrying the structural genes for this system have been determined.

The antigenic differences in most blood group systems outside ABO and Rh can, in

**TABLE 9.3. Important blood group systems**

| | System | Frequently used connotations | Governing chromosome |
|---|---|---|---|
| 1. | ABO | | 9 |
| 2. | Rh | CcDdEe | 1 |
| 3. | MNS | | 2 |
| 4. | P | | 6 |
| 5. | Kell | K | |
| 6. | Lewis | Le | |
| 7. | Lutheran | Lu | |
| 8. | Duffy | Fy | 1 |
| 9. | Kidd | Jk | |
| 10. | Xg | | X |

situations of repeated transfusion, in some cases give rise to transfusion complications. Likewise, incompatibility between fetus and mother may also in rare cases lead to haemolytic disease in the newborn and particularly in the Kell-positive child–Kell-negative mother. Blood group antigens can also be linked to certain diseases. Thus, the Kell-types in cases of chronic granulomatosis are frequently aberrant from the norm both at the level of erythrocytes and leucocytes. It is also likely that the antigen Fy(a) within the Duffy system serves as a specific cell surface receptor on the erythrocyte for plasmodia of one particular malarial species.

The discovery of Xg meant an important new structural gene was located on the X chromosomes and serving as a useful X chromosome marker. It is thus logical that the frequency of individuals being positive to the Xg antigen is larger among women with their two X chromosomes than among men, the figure being 98% as compared to 62% amongst men. The beautiful exception is women with the Turner syndrome, XO, which are positive for the Xg antigen in the same proportion as men.

Outside the large blood group systems there exist several types of private antigenic systems and also a similar number of public systems. Private systems are only seen in certain isolated families and may be encountered in the population in a frequency ranging from one out of 500–10 000 individuals. Public antigen systems, in contrast, are represented in 99.9% of all individuals. The public antigen I here attracts special interest as it serves as a target antigen for the great majroty of cold agglutinins. Antigen I is reduced during certain types of leukaemias and can also be broken away from the blood cells by enzymes from certain microbes belonging to the *Mycoplasma* species.


## Transplantation antigens

Blood group compatibility is of relevance during blood transfusion. As previously mentioned, transplantation of tissue or nucleated cells from one individual to another will frequently lead to a rejection of the foreign tissue. The recipient of a transplant then normally reacts immunologically against foreign antigens present on the donor cells. Such cell-mediated immune reactions directed against foreign transplantation antigens within the species can be very strong. This can be exemplified by the fact that approximately 5–10% of all the T cells in a given individual may be capable of reacting against foreign transplantation antigens present in the tissues of a single foreign donor.

The strong transplantation antigens or, as they are also known, the major histocompatibility complex antigens were first discovered in mice some 50 years ago. In the mouse the system is called H-2. This system expressed a high degree of polymorphism in various inbred strains of mice and also later in individual 'wild' mice. It was later discovered that all species have a similar extremely polymorphic system of genes which decide the structure of the MHC antigens of that species. The MHC antigens which constitute one of the basic structures for what the immune system will consider as 'self' or 'non-self', are from the point of biochemistry cell surface molecules which are glycoprotein in nature. The reason for the very strong immune reaction against foreign transplants was for a long time unclear. In 1974, however, the discovery was made that mice immunized against LCM (Lymphocytic Choriomeningitis) virus develop cytotoxic T cells which could kill virus-infected cells *in vitro*. The new finding was that the cytotoxic effect was directed against virus antigens seen in the context of self-MHC antigens. Using special inbred strains of mice which only differed with regard to isolated genes within the MHC region, it was possible to prove that the effector cells and the target cells normally required one or more class I MHC antigens in common to function in such systems. Cytotoxic T cells recognize as previously mentioned foreign antigen (= x) together with certain 'self' antigens. Or in other words, the cytotoxic specificity of the T cells is thus normally comprised of both x and 'self' MHC. This MHC restriction is thus a common feature for both helper and killer T cells, as previously mentioned in chapter 7. As stated there, helper T cells frequently recognize foreign antigen determinants together with the class II MHC antigens, while cytolytic T cells normally see such determinants in the context of class I 'self' MHC structures.

This MHC specificity with regard to the antigen-binding receptors of the T cells also explains the strong reaction against foreign MHC antigens in conventional transplantation immunology. Foreign transplanted cells are thus recognized as foreign in the very same manner as would 'self' cells infected with viruses. Later it was also found (*see* chapter 7) that the immunological repertoire, i.e. the collection of different specificities found in the T cell population within one individual, will in part be determined by the unique constitution of transplantation antigens of that individual.

Most of our knowledge about transplantation antigens and their biological functions has come from experimental investigations carried out in mice. If skin is transplanted between H-2 incompatible mice, it is normally rejected within 10–11 days. If however donor and recipient mice carry the same H-2 antigens rejection may occur within 20–200 days. That rejection still takes place depends on the fact that there exist, besides MHC antigens, many weak transplantation antigen systems. Genes coding for such weak transplantation antigens are present in approximately 30 different loci, one of which is localized to the Y chromosome (H-Y).

**The H-2 system of the mouse**

The H-2 system of the mouse is localized to chromosome 17 which contains genes determining several different kinds of transplantation antigens. Today, many different genes are known within this region (*Figure 9.3*).

Genes within the H-2-K, D and L loci govern the creation of the 'classical' transplantation antigens present on nearly all nucleated cells, i.e. the class I antigens. These antigens show a large degree of polymorphism between various inbred strains of mice. Closely connected to the H-2 region, there are also additional genes (Qa and TL) the products of which have a chemical structure in part analogous to the class I antigens but with a somewhat smaller degree of polymorphism. Qa and TL antigens do not exist on all nucleated cells, and are normally only present on certain cells at a given stage of differentiation, i.e. they are differentiation antigens. Experiments using hybrid DNA technology to measure the number of structural genes which may determine the production of various class I-like molecules have produced numbers well above 15 which suggests that there are several yet not defined H-2 or H-2-like genes and corresponding antigens.

All class I molecules consist of two chains, one large polypeptide chain which passes through the cell membrane and a small chain which is called $\beta_2$-microglobulin. The gene for $\beta_2$-microglobulin is not linked to the H-2-region. All H-2-K-, D, and L-antigens like the differentiation antigens Qa and TL would seem to contain $\beta_2$m as a constant chain. The variability between different H-2 antigens would thus consist of differences in the structure of only the large chain. The chemical structure is simplified and expressed in *Figure 9.4*. The large chain can be subdivided into three parts, two of which (part 2 and part 3) contain a disulphide bridge. Part 3, closest to the cell membranes, shows an amino acid sequence very similar to that of $\beta_2$m. The general construction of

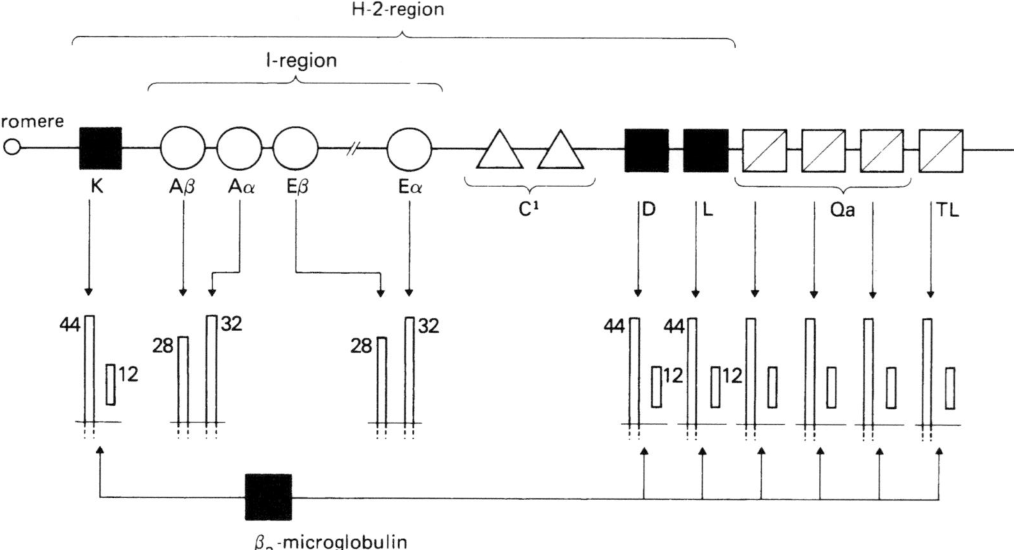



*Figure 9.3* Schematic description of the H-2 region in mouse. K, D and L loci determine the classical transplantation antigens (class I). Qa and Tl loci also govern synthesis of class I molecules containing one polymorphic large chain and a little invariable chain called $\beta2$ microglobulin. The large chain is determined by genes within the H-2 region whilst the gene for $\beta2$ microglobulin is present on another chromosome pair. The loci of the I region will determine the production of class II molecules, so called Ia antigens. They consist of two chains named $\alpha$ and $\beta$. Genes for both $\alpha$- and $\beta$-chains are localized in the I region. The figures denote the molecular weight of the chains $\times 10^3$

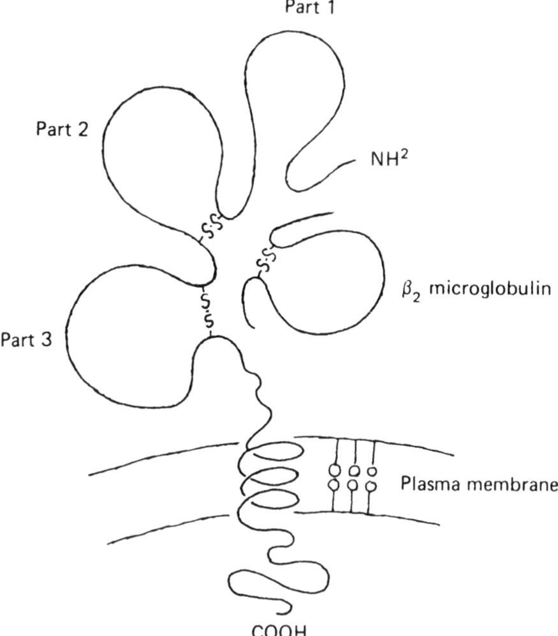


*Figure 9.4* Schematic picture of the chemical construction of class I molecules. The large chain has approximately 270 amino acids extracellularly, which can be subdivided into three regions. Region 2 and 3 contain disulphide bridges. The domain 1 and 2 will display homology with each other whilst part 3 and the small non-covalently associated $\beta2$ microglobulin chain are homologous to the constant domains of immunoglobulin molecules. Polymorphism with the species occurs predominantly in part 1 and 2. The chain contains, in addition, a transmembranous part containing predominantly hydrophobic amino acids and an intracellular part with hydrophilic amino acids

the molecules also displays great similarities with the domain construction of the immunoglobulin molecules. It has been suggested that part 3, $\beta_2$m and constant parts in light and heavy chain immunoglobulins may all be derived from a common ancestor gene.

Other types of genes are present in the I region which today are comprised of at least two loci. They govern the production of Ia antigens (I region associated), which are predominantly present on antigen-presenting monocytes/macrophages and B lymphocytes. These antigens constitute the class II type of MHC antigens and have a chemical structure which differs from that of class I. Class II antigens have two polypeptide chains ($\alpha$ and $\beta$). The molecular weight is approximately 32 000 for the $\alpha$-chain and approximately 28 000 for the $\beta$ chain. The differences in molecular weight are mainly ascribed to different content of carbohydrate side chains. Both chains pass through the cell membrane. The best defined antigens are the I-A and I-E Ia antigens. The relative position of the Ia genes can be seen in *Figure 9.3*.

The similarity to immunoglobulins is also valid for the class II MHC molecules. This would indicate that the genes for immunoglobulins, $\beta_2$-microglobulins, class I and class II antigens all have a common origin. This is exemplified in *Figure 9.5* by the similarity

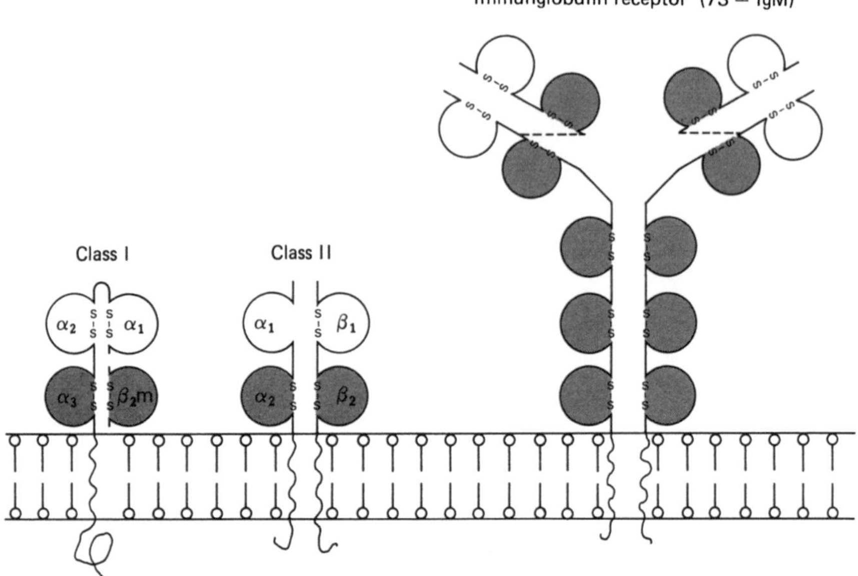


*Figure 9.5* Schematic drawing of the membrane orientation of class I and class II and immunoglobulin receptor molecules. Grey areas show homologous domains indicating common phylogenetic origin. (From Hood, L. *et al.* (1983), *Ann. Rev. Immunol.*, **1**)

in chemical composition between the transplantation antigens of class I and II and immunoglobulin molecules of B cell origin. Both class I and class II molecules contain constant parts in their primary structure and most likely even their three-dimensional structure is homologous with the constant part of the light and heavy chains of the immunoglobulin molecules. In addition there are also certain sequence similarities between the structural parts 1 and 2 of the class I heavy chain which have also been demonstrated in the variable regions of class II and which make it very likely that the two types of cell surface molecules indeed have a common genetic origin and a similar biological function. The similarities between the build-up of the antibody molecules and of the MHC antigens are striking and strengthen the hypothesis that perhaps all foreign determinants in order to be able to function as immunogens for immuno-competent T cells must have an ability to associate with one or other of the 'self' MHC molecules. If the primary function within the immune system of the strong trans-plantation antigen molecules is in fact to bind peptide fragments, their antibody-like chemical structure would make sense. It should be pointed out, however, that very little is known about how this postulated chemical association may occur. Another problem is also to understand how an individual with the limited polymorphism within the 'self' MHC molecules can still express and create an effective association with so many different antigenic structures.

The variability of transplantation antigens carried by different individuals is very high and thus different individuals are likely to have unique immune systems with different repertoires. In this manner the possibility within the species that an almost infinite immune repertoire can be created even if single individuals may lack reactivity against certain antigenic determinants.

## IR genes

At the beginning of the 1960s, it was noted that certain animals would fail to respond either against some antigens containing few antigenic determinants or when immunized with low doses of certain antigens. This lack of immune activity could, in particular, be shown to be valid for the production of IgG antibodies and development of delayed-type hypersensitivity, i.e. this defect seemed to be T cell dependent. Upon immunization using inbred strains of mice it was discovered that a particular mouse strain was able to react against a certain antigen but not against a second one whilst in another inbred strain of mice the response pattern was the opposite. This proved that this particular lack of immunological reactivity was genetically determined and also that this defect was specific, i.e. only involved a reaction against certain determinants. Various breeding experiments including F1 hybrid mice and backcrosses demonstrated that the immunological reactivity normally was dominant and that it was determined by one or more linked genes, i.e. genes localized to one chromosome pair.

It was soon shown that the genes governing this kind of immunological reactivity were linked to the MHC system. A more detailed analysis demonstrated that the genes governing this specific immunological reactivity were normally localized to the region between the H-2-K and D loci. This chromosomal region was thus called the I region. Because this specific immunological defect involved the T lymphocytes, it was also suggested at the time that the IR genes could be the structural genes for the antigen-specific T cell receptor.

An immunologist who has shown that there are structural genes which determine specific reactivity within a certain genetic region, and who can use inbred strains of mice which only differ with regard to that genetic region, will naturally try to produce antibodies against the products of these genes in order to characterize the polymorphic feature which distinguishes the two inbred strains of mice. Many immunologists believed that it should be possible to produce antibodies against specific T cell receptors in this way and thereby illuminate their chemical structure or nature. It was quite easy to produce antibodies against products encoded by genes within the I region. These antibodies did not react as expected with T cells but rather with B lymphocytes, macrophages and monocytes.

These antisera did in fact represent the first antibodies experimentally used against MHC products which were not classical antigens of the type H-2-K or D. In fact these antisera detected what we now call class II antigens, but they were first called I region associated antigens (Ia antigens). The essential role of these molecules in the development of T cell reactions has already been described in this book in detail. As to their chemistry, the class II antigens are determined by two MHC genes, namely those that determine the structure of the $\alpha$ and $\beta$ chains respectively. An important part of our knowledge about the biological function of these class II molecules came from studies showing that in certain specific cases two mouse strains which both lacked specific reactivity against a certain antigenic determinant could upon breeding give rise to an $F_1$ hybrid which did react against the very same antigenic structure. It was then possible to prove both biologically and chemically that one parental strain may have one gene to produce an $\alpha$ chain but could lack the corresponding gene for the $\beta$ chain for a particular class II MHC molecule and thus fail to produce the adequate antigens. If such a mouse was bred with another strain of mice with a reciprocal defect the progeny $F_1$ hybrid mouse was now able to produce a complete molecule of that particular class II and also respond to the relevant antigen.

T helper cells and T cells responsible for delayed-type hypersensitivity reactions, predominantly recognize foreign antigens together with syngenic 'self' class II molecules. The lack of reactivity against a certain antigen determinant may here be due to the absence of a particular class II MHC structure with capacity to bind or associate with this determinant, thus failing to create an immunogenic complex for the T cell system. Alternatively, the immune system may lack immunocompetent T cells capable of reaction with the created ('self' + X) complex. One can say in a symbolic manner that either the foot does not fit the shoe, or the shoe does not fit the foot. In both cases, however, there is a lack of interaction between antigen-presenting cell and immuno-competent T cells and thus no initiation of the complex circuits subsequent to T cell activation.

It is today considered that both the chemical nature and the immune function of class I and class II MHC structures, in principle, are very similar. This would then mean that a lack of activation of T helper cells may depend on an IR gene defect within the I region (class II) but a similar specific immune defect can also sometimes be localized to class I determining loci governing for instance the development of cytotoxic T cells.

**The MLC reaction**

An important part of the current knowledge about the relevance of major transplantation antigens with regard to the internal regulation of immune reactions, originates from investigations using transplantation immune systems. In the beginning of the 1960s, it was shown that a surprisingly large fraction of immunocompetent T lymphocytes participate in the reaction against a transplanted allograft. Superficially this would seem to indicate that the T cells are preoccupied with reactions against foreign tissue, but it was clear that this could not be their primary function within the body. If lymphocytes from an individual are mixed with lymphocytes from another individual of the same species, a reaction normally occurs *in vitro* which is called MLC (Mixed Lymphocyte Culture) reaction. It is a typical T cell reaction where clonal proliferation, differentiation and development of T effector cells will occur within a few days. The dominant stimulatory structures here are foreign, antigen-presenting cells and their class II antigens (e.g. HLA-D in humans), which will stimulate T helper cells to proliferate and excrete lymphokines which in turn may then cause the differentiation of other specific T cells. Among these cells are the cytotoxic cells which predominantly react against foreign class I antigens. This means that in an immune reaction against foreign tissue, a similar compartmentalization exists within the T cell system as in the normal immune reaction, i.e. T helper cells recognize predominantly class II antigens and T cytotoxic cells normally recognize class I antigens.

Using new methods for the cultivation of lymphocytes for prolonged periods of time *in vitro*, it has been possible to produce pure individual clones of alloreactive T lymphocytes. When studying the specificity of such clones demonstrating allo-reactivity, it has also been possible to demonstrate that many of these clones can recognize 'self' targets modified by various means. This supports the view that the strong alloreactivity is in fact an expression of a potential cross-reaction between the given transplanted foreign tissue and 'self' tissue modified by various means.

**The HLA system**

The MHC system of the human is called HLA (HLA = Human Leucocyte antigen-group A). Since this nomenclature was accepted it has been shown that the antigens are

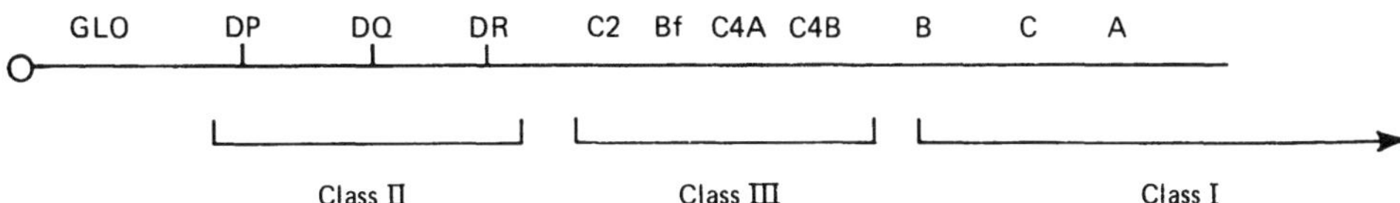



*Figure 9.6* Schematic diagram of the organization of MHC class I, II and III genes on the short arm of chromosome number 6. The GLO locus is located centromeric to DP. Information from hybrid DNA experimentation has shown that the DP locus contains two distinct genes for $\alpha$ chains and two for $\beta$ chains. However, one of the $\alpha$ genes seems to be non-functional, and therefore it is not known whether more than one DP gene product is expressed from each haplotype. The DQ locus contains two $\alpha$ and two $\beta$ genes, but it is yet unknown whether more than one DQ antigen can be expressed. The DR locus contains only one $\alpha$ gene, which is non-variant and a varying number of $\beta$ genes in different haplotypes. Therefore, the expression of DR molecules is not yet resolved. The polymorphic class I genes are referred to as A, B and C. Additional class I genes exist, most probably located telomeric to HLA-A, but are still only incompletely characterized. The equivalent of Qa and TL antigens probably exist in the human as well as in the mouse. The MHC-linked class III genes encode complement factors C2, C4 (all chains) and factor B of the properdin system. Their order is indicated but the definite orientation between HLA-B and DR remains to be established. Very recent information indicates that the basic genetic structure of the mouse H-2 and the human HLA region is similar. This also implies that the locus corresponding to DP in the human might exist also in the mouse (see *Immunol. Rev.* **84**, 1985).

present on many (maybe all) nucleated cells meaning that this connotation in fact is inadequate. The structure of the genes known to govern the human class I and II antigens can be seen in *Figure 9.6*. Within the HLA-A, B and C loci there are genes which determine the class I molecules A, B and C while DR, DQ and DP determine the production of class II antigens. As in the mouse the class I antigens are present on all nucleated cells whereas class II antigens are predominantly expressed on antigen-presenting cells such as macrophages, monocytes and the Langerhans cells in the skin. In addition, class II antigens are present on B lymphocytes and some of these cells may also have an antigen-presenting function for T cells. Activated T lymphocytes in the human can also express class II antigens.

It is important to realize that there are also many weak transplantation antigen systems in man, but that they have so far been difficult to define. This means that transplantation of tissue between HLA-identical individuals normally will not result in the survival of the transplant unless the recipient is treated with immunosuppressive drugs.

To each HLA locus there are many alternative genes (alleles). These genes appear as multiple alleles with one allele present in each locus on the chromosome in a pair. Thus each person has two alleles belonging to the A locus, two to the B locus, two to the C locus and so on. The combination of genes present in one of the two chromosomes is called haplotype. Every individual carries a combination of HLA antigens present in the haplotype from the respective parent. The inheritance of HLA antigens can be seen from *Figure 9.7*. Two haplotypes of the father are called a and b and those of the mother c and d respectively. Children will inherit one relevant chromosome from the father and the other from the mother. The possible combination of these haplotypes in the children will thus become ac, ad, bc and bd. As four different combinations of haplotypes can exist in the children, statistically speaking 25% of all children are HLA-identical. The individual frequencies of alleles within the different loci of the HLA region in a given population is seen in *Table 9.4*.

All HLA genes are expressed in a dominant manner meaning that is one individual with regard to the A locus has the allele 1 on one chromosome and 2 on the other, the

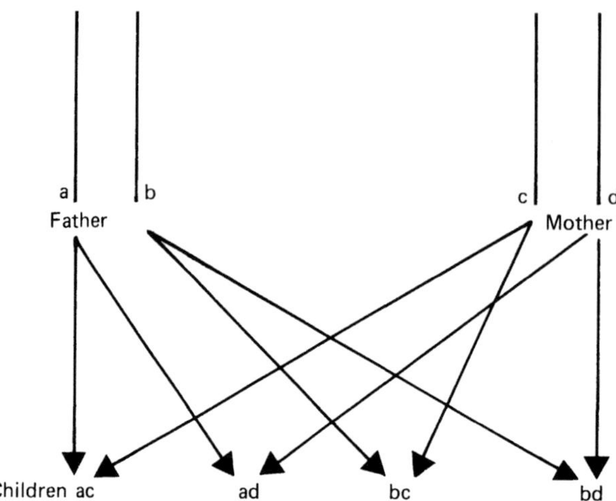


*Figure 9.7* The inheritance pattern of HLA antigens. Each child inherits one chromosome from either parent. The number of possible combinations amongst the children is four. Thus 25% of all siblings are HLA identical

**TABLE 9.4. Alleles within the HLA region A, B, C and D/DR loci**

Alleles are divided in gene frequency from high to low:

A locus: A2, 3, 1, 9, 11, 28, 29, 32, 31, 25, 26, 30, 33, 34 ... blank 0.01
B locus: B7, 12, 8, 15, 40, 35, 27, 5, 17, 18, 21, 22, 37, 16 ... blank 0.01
C locus: Cw7, w3, w4; w1, w6, w5, w2 ... blank 0.20
DR locus: DR2, 7, 3, 2, 1, 4, 5, 6, 8, w9, w10 ... 0.10

These frequencies are valid for Caucasians. Blank 0.01 means that the gene frequency of unknown A alleles is approximately 1%. Many B alleles are not any longer considered to be homogeneous. Thus for instance B5 has been subdivided into Bw51 and 52, B40 into Bw60 and w61 and so on. W means that the figure is temporary (w = workshop). D locus products are determined by cell-mediated reactions (MLC), DR with serological methods.

antigens A1 and A2 will simultaneously be present on all nucleated cells in that individual. Another individual may have the antigens A3, A9, a third A11, A28 and so on. The possible number of HLA phenotypes in the human species is, even with today's somewhat incomplete knowledge about the genetics of this region, more than 10 billion. It is thus extremely rare to find unrelated individuals carrying the same HLA antigen composition.

The inheritance of individual HLA-A and B antigens can be illustrated by one family (*Table 9.5*). On the cells of the father the four individual HLA antigens A1, 2, B7 and B8 were determined serologically. The combination of HLA antigens which can be determined by the use of a serological test is called an HLA phenotype. The cells of the mother were killed by antibodies directed against antigens A2 and 3 and B7 and 12 which thus constitute the HLA phenotype of the mother. From the table it can be seen that child 1 inherited antigens A1 and 3, B7 and 8, child 2 inherited antigens A2 and B7 and 12 and so on. The antigens A1 and B8 were present in the father and not in the mother. It can be seen that child 1 and 4 inherited the antigens A1 and B8 together. One of the haplotypes in the father thus contained the alleles A1 and B8. The child who did not inherit A1, B8 from the father has instead inherited the antigens A2, B7. The

**TABLE 9.5. HLA phenotypes and genotypes in parents and children in a family**

|         | *Phenotype* | *Genotype* | *Chromosome combination* |
|---------|-------------|------------|--------------------------|
| Father  | A1, 2 B7, 8 | A1B8/A2B7  | ab |
| Mother  | A2, 3 B7, 12 | A2B12/13B7 | cd |
| Child 1 | A1, 3 B7, 8 | A1B8/A3B7  | ad |
| Child 2 | A2, B7, 12  | A2B12/A2B7 | bc |
| Child 3 | A2, 3 B7    | A2B7/A3B7  | bd |
| Child 4 | A1, 2 B8, 12 | A1B8/A2B12 | ac |
| Child 5 | A2, 3 B7    | A2B7/A3B7  | bd |

haplotypes of the father with regard to HLA are thus A1B8/A2B7. This combination of two haplotypes is called an HLA genotype. In the same manner it can be seen that child 2, 4 and 6 has inherited the haplotype A2B12 from the mother. The remaining children have inherited the haplotype A3B7. Child numbers 3 and 5 are thus HLA identical. These children have only three HLA-A and B antigens in their phenotype but judging from the inheritance scheme it can be seen that the children have both inherited B7 from the mother and father and are thus homozygous for this gene. In the same manner it can be seen that child number 2 is homozygous for the gene A2. HLA genotypes and homozygocity are thus determined using family investigations in the above related manner. Because of the extreme polymorphism within the HLA system and a dominant inheritance, the HLA determinations are of great importance in the determination of fatherhood.

## Determination of HLA-A, -B and -C class I antigens

Antibodies against foreign HLA antigens are not present naturally but some individuals will become immunized against HLA antigens and will then produce antibodies useful for the determination of HLA antigens. Among these individuals there are patients who have received many blood transfusions, people who have received transplants of foreign organs and women who have delivered many children. The most frequently used source is antibodies from multiparous women and such sera contain antibodies against few HLA antigens and are more easily made monospecific by absorptions. When determining HLA-A, -B and -C antigens a blood sample is taken from the patient. The lymphocytes from the blood are purified and the suspension of these cells is mixed with antibodies against A1 in one tube, A2 in a second tube and so on. Determination of these HLA antigens is normally carried out using a cytotoxic method. Addition of complement will, in the presence of antibodies reacting with the cells, lead to lysis of the cells. Addition of stains distinguishing dead from living cells will facilitate the reading of the cytotoxic effect using a microscope. Because of the great number of alleles within the HLA system and because one normally will use two distinct antisera for each antigen, single HLA determinations will be comparatively time- and labour-consuming. Approximately 100 microscopical readings are necessary for the determination of the HLA composition of one single individual.

## Linkage disequilibrium

A special feature of the genetics of HLA is the fact that alleles belonging to different loci frequently exist together in one haplotype much more frequently than one would expect as judged from the individual frequency of the respective genes. This phenomenon is called linkage disequilibrium. Thus for instance allele A1 occurs together with the alleles C7, B8 and DR3 more than 50 times more frequently than one would expect on one and the same haplotype. Other examples of such haplotypes expressing linkage disequilibrium are A3 C7 B7 DR2 and A2 C5 B12 DR7. The explanation for the occurrence of this linkage disequilibrium is unknown. It is however likely that this gene combination carries certain selective survival values. It is plausible that this is because two gene products linked together on that chromosome stretch can collaborate in a positive way during certain situations in life. The phenomenon of linkage disequilibrium is also of great relevance for the understanding of the association between the inheritance of certain specific HLA antigens and disease, and this will be discussed in detail in chapter 14. Linkage disequilibrium also exists for the Rh system and for the genetic systems of immunoglobulins.

## Additional genes within the HLA system

As can be seen in *Figure 9.6*, the HLA system also contains genes for certain complement factors, such as C2, C4 and factor B in the properdin system. These genes are sometimes called class III. Some of these genes were discovered in patients expressing a certain disease related to a defect with regard to a particular complement factor. Analysis of HLA antigens and of complement levels within families have clearly indicated the genetic linkage between certain complement deficiencies and HLA genes. The existence of recombinations within haplotypes have led to a further localization within the HLA system. A C-2 factor defect has been described in individuals with HLA haplotype A25 C-B18 DR2 and probably depends on a mutation affecting an individual with this HLA chromosome many years ago and that C'2 deficient individuals are homozygous for this haplotype.

## The genetics and biological function of the MHC molecule

As already mentioned with regard to the genes of the H-2 system, direct chemical and genetic investigations have shown that class I and II antigens have great similarities to immunoglobulins. It is also clear that there exist great similarities between class I and II MHC antigens of mouse and man indicating that the genes have been stable for a long time during phylogeny. The organization of the DNA segments determining class I and II molecules is now well-known. The separate parts (the domain-like structures) of these proteins are determined by isolated exon DNA segments separated from the next exon by intron DNA. With regard to the heavy chain of the class I molecule, there accordingly exists three exon DNA segments for the three domains of that chain which is extracellular with an additional exon part for the transmembranous area of the molecule and one or more exon DNA segments for the intracellular parts of that chain. The genomic organization of the MHC class I and II genes is therefore similar for the genes coding for the immunoglobulins. The polymorphism between different class I and II molecules however is only apparent when considering the species as a unity, while the variability of the immunoglobulin genes for the major part can be found in the DNA of a single individual.

Previous discoveries concerning the biological function of class I and II antigens in mice have also been verified to be true for the HLA system in man. This would mean that virtually all T cell-specific immune reactions in man are probably to a major degree determined by MHC gene products. This should also mean that in man as in mice certain specific immunological reactivities may be governed by MHC genes in a decisive manner. A very important part of clinical immunology in this area will deal with associations between the presence of a particular HLA antigen and disease. In the same manner as IR genes in mice will govern immunological reactivity in the murine T cells, the HLA genes will do the same in man. Wrong or erroneous immune reactions may lead to disease. If a virus-infected cell in the body cannot be eliminated in an adequate manner, or if an erroneous immune reaction is initiated against a 'self' component which has been changed, this may lead to tissue damage. In line with such arguments, it has been possible to prove that many autoimmune diseases which afflict human beings, such as juvenile diabetes, multiple sclerosis, rheumatoid arthritis and so on, will occur in individuals with a high frequency only if they carry certain HLA genes. This will be discussed in detail in chapter 14.

**The MHC antigens (molecules displaying 'a Dr Jekyll and Mr Hyde' behaviour?)**

Molecules which were first described as transplantation antigens, i.e. inducing a very strong immune reaction against allografts, are now known to have a function within our body. This function is central both with regard to activation as well as regulation of specific immune reactions. When the chemical structure was clarified, it was realized that MHC antigens have great similarities with those of immunoglobulins and a common phylogenetic origin was suggested. An antibody-like molecule should have a biological function which may involve 'binding' of foreign or 'self' substances. This leads to the concept that the primary immunological role of these molecules was to bind foreign antigenic fragments to create a complex which could be recognized by the immunocompetent T cells recognizing 'self' plus X in the same manner as they could recognize a foreign transplanted cell. This would thus put a dual feature on the transplantation antigens also making them antibody-like. This antibody-like function would make it possible for the MHC antigens to create an immunogenic complex with foreign substances ('self' + X) whereupon they change the function to become the real 'antigens' for specific T cells in our own body.

# Bibliography

GILES, R. C. and CAPRA, O. D. (1985). Structure, function and genetics of human class II molecules. *Adv. Immunol.*
HOOD, L., STEINMETZ, M. and MALISSEN, B. (1983). *Ann. Rev. Immunol.* **1**, 529
MÖLLER, G. (ed.) (1978). Acquisition of the T cell repertoire. *Immunol. Rev.*, **45**
MÖLLER, G. (ed.) (1985). Molecular genetics of HLA class I and II MHC antigens. *Immunol. Rev.*, **84**
MÖLLER, G. (ed.) (1985). Molecular genetics of class III MHC antigens. *Immunol. Rev.*, **86**
SOLHEIM, B., FERRONE, S. and MÖLLER, E. (eds.) (1985). *Structure and function of class II MHC antigens*. Springer Verlag, Munich (in press)

# Chapter 10

# Tumour immunology

Hans Olov Sjögren

A solid basis for tumour immunology was created in the 1950s, when it was shown, using inbred strains of animals, that animals could frequently be immunized against their own tumour whilst tolerating skin transplants from animals of the same strain. Such tumour-associated specific immune reactions have later been shown in many experimental animal systems using tumours generated by various means. In situations where inbred strains of animals have been lacking, it is considerably more difficult to prove conclusively the specificity of a demonstrated immune reaction. Tumour immune mechanisms will thus predominantly be discussed using as a basis animal experimental systems where adequately inbred strains of animals are available.

## Tumour antigens

### Definition of TAA and TAM

It is important to distinguish between tumour-associated antigens (TAA) and tumour-associated molecules (TAM). The term TAA refers to molecules that are immunogenic in the original host of the tumour and that in a qualitative or possibly quantitative manner are associated with tumour cells and not with normal cells. Tumour-associated molecules (TAM) are not necessarily immunogenic in the original host but can be demonstrated using for instance antibodies produced in other strains of animal species. The surface antigens of the cells, i.e. the antigens which are present exposed on the plasma membranes, have mostly been studied but many examples also exist demonstrating an intracellular localization of TAA.

### Different major groups of TAA

It is possible to separate three main groups of TAA. One group consists of individually unique membrane molecules different for different tumours even if they have been produced using the same carcinogenic agent in the same individual. Another group is constituted by the virus-related antigens. They may consist of virus particle-associated antigens which in certain tumour types can be found associated with the cell membrane. In other systems the TAAs will only be expressed by tumour cells transformed by the virus in question. In both situations the specificity of the TAA is determined by the virus and the antigens are normally common for all tumours produced by the same virus. A third antigen group consists of the embryonic or oncofetal antigens which normally exist in an individual during a certain embryonic developmental stage but which will later disappear but may return in parallel with neoplastic transformation.

## Experimental tumours

Chemically-induced experimental tumours were the first tumours demonstrated to contain individually unique surface antigens (*Table 10.1*). Later embryonic antigens have also been demonstrated in such tumours. These latter antigens could be tissue type-specific but are often expressed in several different embryonic organs.

Tumours induced with viruses often have several virus-determined antigens. These are, as mentioned, common for all tumours induced by the same virus. This is true even if the tumours are produced in different animal species. Tumours produced by DNA viruses such as polyoma, SV40 or adenovirus have intranuclear T antigens, which are characteristic for the virus type but which are absent in the virus particles themselves. In addition, there are membrane antigens which are characteristic for tumours induced with the respective virus type. Distinct from the membrane-associated antigens, T antigens are also demonstrable in virus-infected normal cells even if such cells will not be transformed into malignancy. Tumours induced by RNA virus such as leukaemia or sarcoma virus in mice are also associated with several different virus determined antigens. Among these are several virion antigens localized to the cell surface as well as to the cytoplasm. It has also been possible to prove the existence of two types of membrane antigens non-identical with known virion antigens. One is present both in tumour cells and virus-infected normal cells, whilst the other can only be found in tumour cells. Virion antigens can also be demonstrated in chemically induced tumours in mice and of course in different types of cells which have been infected with the respective virus. This property can be used as a marker indicating virus infection but can also cause complications in the analysis of the antigenicity of a given tumour. In addition to these virus-related antigens there are in virally induced tumour cells embryonic antigens and also individually unique antigens demonstrable on the cell membrane.

Spontaneous tumours in experimental animals, i.e. tumours arising in ageing individuals without known exposure to carcinogens are characterized by individually unique antigens and by common embryonic antigens as well. But in a high

**TABLE 10.1. Survey of TAA**

| Tumour type | Tumour associated antigens (TAA) | | | |
|---|---|---|---|---|
| | Individually unique | Common for a group of tumours | | |
| | | Virus determinant antigens | Embryonic antigens | |
| | | | Common for different organs | Tissue-type specific |
| Experimental | | | | |
|   Chemically induced | + | | + | + |
|   Virus induced | + | + | + | |
|   Spontaneous | + | | | + |
| Human | + | + or − | | + |

proportion of such spontaneous tumours it is impossible to demonstrate any TAA. Tumours induced purposely, for example by chemical means, also have widely varying amounts of antigens and several examples also exist of experimentally induced tumours lacking detectable TAA. It is not clear if this is a matter of qualitative differences or mere quantitative variations. On the other hand, it is noteworthy that new antigens are indeed demonstrable on the great majority of tumours. It is possible that such antigens are part of membrane disturbances linked to decisive steps in the malignant transformation.

Tumour cells may also lack antigens which the corresponding normal adult cells express. One such example is fibronectin, which is associated with the membrane of normal fibroblasts but which will disappear in parallel to neoplastic transformation of such cells. Also during serial passage of tumour cells in inbred strains or in tissue culture, dramatic losses or reductions in the concentration of certain normal antigens and TAA may be seen. Certain tumour-associated antigens will also be expressed at lower concentrations on the cell surface if the tumour cells are exposed *in vitro* to strong antisera directed against such TAA.

## Human tumours

When studying human tumours one frequently finds tissue type-specific antigens which for some tumours have been shown to be of embryonic type. Such antigens are thus common for tumours of the same tissue, for instance different kinds of tumours of the intestine. Analogous antigens have also been demonstrated in melanomas, urine bladder carcinomas, mammary carcinoma and sarcomas. In Burkitt's lymphoma there are several different types of antigens determined by the Epstein–Barr virus (EBV) which is also present within such tumour cells. There is also suggestive evidence for the presence of individually unique TAA in human tumours although this is technically more difficult to prove. Several cellular components in the form of TAM are present in increased amounts in tumour cells. Presence of such components can sometimes be measured using sensitive immunological techniques and these structures are therefore called tumour-associated antigens. This is however misleading as they are normally not recognized as antigens within the individual in which the tumour arises. However, such quantitative differences between tumour cells and normal cells can be highly valuable and interesting both from a theoretical and practical view. For diagnosis, these quantitative differences can serve as an equally good basis as TAA molecules. They can also constitute target structures for certain immunotherapeutic measures (*see* chapter 15).

## Induction of tumour immunity

Immunization against TAA can result in the inhibition of tumour growth *in vivo*. Thus, in animal experiments it has been possible to prove that immunity against certain tumour-associated antigens will cause rejection of tumours carrying such antigens. This form of immunity is of special interest both with regard to the antigens and the immunization procedures which will induce such specific tumour resistance. It is possible to induce this immunity by transplanting live tumour cells followed by resection of the tumour, or by repeated inoculations of tumour cells inactivated in various ways, for instance by irradiation, treatment with mitomycin C or lyophilization. The strongest rejection reactions induced are normally found against the tumour which has been used as immunogen or in the case of viral tumours against tumours induced by the same virus type. The immunity is thus in such situations directed against individually unique antigens or against common virus-related antigens. Immunization against embryonic antigens normally results in a much weaker reaction frequently consisting of initial inhibition of growth of the tumour graft, but fails to cause a complete rejection. The same has frequently been found for tumour-associated antigens with tissue type-specificity.

Animals which have developed a primary tumour which has then been resected normally display resistance against subsequent transplantations of the same tumour. Surprisingly, animals which may carry an intermediately sized but progressively growing tumour are often at the same time able to reject a new transplant of the same tumour if it is applied on a site different to that of the original tumour. This phenomenon has been called concomitant immunity.

## Immunological surveillance

Theories discussing the fact that the immune defence may normally be able to inhibit the appearance of tumours by rejection of malignant cells before they have proliferated to recognizable size have existed for a long time (Ehrlich 1908; Thomas 1959; Burnet 1970). A prime case referred to in support of such a surveillance is the polyoma virus system in mice. Infection by this tumour virus will cause tumour development only if the infection occurs in newborn mice, while adult mice will fail to develop tumours subsequent to virus infections. In both cases infectious virus is rapidly eliminated.

In adult mice which lack T lymphocytes, such polyoma virus infection, however, will lead to tumour development. The development of tumours can be inhibited by the transfer of normal mature T lymphocytes during the latency period even if this occurs at a time when all infectious polyoma virus has been eliminated by induced antiviral antibodies. In this case, the T cell system functions as an efficient barrier against the outgrowth of visible tumours by eliminating the tumour cells. However, a similar deficiency in the T cell function in certain other tumour-induction systems will not result in an increased incidence of tumours. It would thus seem clear that a T cell-mediated immune defence does not serve as a general efficient surveillance mechanism against tumour development.

It is possible that other parts of the immune machinery being relatively T cell independent, may have the ability to carry out such an immunological surveillance. A certain support for the assumption that the NK cell system may have such an ability has been found in experiments using mice:

(1)  Using genetically different strains of mice a strong positive correlation has been found between NK activity *in vitro* against a particular tumour and the capacity to reject small tumour cell inocula of the same tumour *in vivo*.
(2)  The passive transfer of NK cells is often efficient in protecting against grafted tumour cells of NK sensitive type.
(3)  Thymectomized and lethally irradiated $F_1$-hybrid mice which have been repopulated with bone marrow cells from low or high NK parental strains will inhibit tumour outgrowth in the same manner as the respective bone marrow donor.
(4)  A mutation in one inbred strain of mice, the beige mutation, will have as a consequence a relatively selective defect in NK activity and in such mice the growth and ability to metastasize of NK susceptible tumour cells is clearly enhanced.

None of the above mentioned indications prove that NK cells carry a surveillance function but they point to the possibility that such cells may do so under certain circumstances. It is especially important to prove whether during the primary induction of tumours in an individual, the relative NK levels in such an individual influence the danger of developing a tumour or not. Such data are still, however, largely lacking.

In man two observations exist which fit the concept of immunological surveillance. For instance a highly increased frequency of primary lymphoid tumours, Kaposi's sarcoma and skin cancer exist in patients who have either acquired immunodeficiency disorders or are undergoing immunosuppressive therapy in conjunction with organ transplantation or autoimmune diseases. An increased cancer frequency of similar type of tumours also exists in various types of hereditary immunodeficiency disorders. It can be argued, however, that in the first systems the increased tumour incidence may depend on the presence of a virus inducing the acquired immunodeficiency or the carcinogenic effect of the immunosuppressive therapy. In individuals with inheritable immunodeficiency disorders, one can also argue that there is a linked hereditary disposition for tumours being a parallel phenomenon rather than a result of immunodeficiency.


## Mechanisms by which tumours may avoid the rejection reaction

The paradoxical fact that the majority of the experimentally induced tumours will grow despite their ability to induce an easily demonstrable transplantation immunity, indicates that mechanisms must exist allowing the tumour cells to avoid the cytotoxic effect of tumour immune mechanisms.

An important point is probably that the specific immune defence requires a certain critical level of antigen before being initiated. This would automatically mean that a tumour cell population has already achieved an initial size when the adoptive immune system starts to recognize it as being present. If the proliferative capacity of the tumour cells is larger than the rate of increase of the immune rejection mechanism, this may allow progressive tumour growth to occur. Such a situation also explains the phenomenon of concomitant immunity where a large solid tumour will grow more rapidly than the rate of elimination by immune mechanisms, whereas a small number of transplanted tumour cells of the same type can be more easily attacked. Concomitant immunity may also partially explain why the majority of the tumour cells seeded out from the original tumour will fail to establish viable metastasis. Other important mechanisms which will decrease the capacity to reject tumours *in vitro* can exist of both antigen-specific and non-specific nature (*Table 10.2*).


**TABLE 10.2. Mechanisms allowing tumour cells to avoid rejection reactions**

(1)  The membrane antigens can be covered by certain membrane-associated substances (sialomucin).
(2)  Increased concentration of certain inhibitory $\alpha$ globulins.
(3)  Suppressive effects of tumour-associated substances ($\alpha$ fetoprotein).
(4)  Appearance of non-specific suppressor cells.
(5)  Appearance of specific suppressor cells.
(6)  Blocking of cell-mediated reactivity via antigen–antibody complexes, soluble antigens and certain antibody types.
(7)  Antigen modulation.
(8)  Tumour heterogeneity allowing progressive enrichment for tumour cells with lower antigenicity.

Sialomucin exists as a glycocalyx around certain tumour cell types and can then conceal membrane antigens. The treatment of such cells with the enzyme neuraminidase will lead to an exposure of the cell membrane whereby the immunogenicity may drastically increase. Injection of neuraminidase into certain experimental tumours may thus lead to a regression of the inoculated tumour followed by rejection of untreated tumours of the cell line growing elsewhere in the body.

In individuals carrying large tumours, a general depression of the immune reactivity often exists. This may be linked to the increase of certain $\alpha$-globulins known to have a non-specific suppressive effect on immunological reactivity. In such individuals one can also frequently prove the appearance of suppressor cells of a non-T origin with a non-specific inhibitory impact on lymphocyte functions. It is of interest that $\alpha$-fetoprotein which is a fetal protein, but which also can be produced by certain primary liver cancer cells, can have a direct immunosuppressive effect on T cell functions. Besides these non-specific mechanisms there may also exist a specific suppression of immunity against tumour antigens in the tumour-bearing host. One reason for this is the creation of suppressor T cells, but tumour carriers may also have circulating complexes of tumour antigens together with antibodies. Such immune complexes can block the cytotoxic effect of effector T cells as well as of K cells.

In certain mouse leukaemias it has been possible to prove antigenic modulation where leukaemia cells exposed to antibodies against membrane-associated tumour antigens will be changed in such a way that these antigens drastically decrease in concentration. This will render the leukaemia cells insensitive to the cytotoxic effect of the tumour antibodies. It is possible that this phenomenon could be of importance for the survival of certain tumour types *in vivo*.


## Possibilities of increasing immune reactivity against tumours

Two principal ways exist through which immune reactivity can be increased. One may either try to increase the efficiency of the effector cells and their mechanisms, or decrease suppressor mechanisms. Active or passive immunization belongs to the first category and is efficient in individuals not already carrying a growing tumour. 'Immunization' with two to three inoculations of $1-10 \times 10^6$ tumour cells which have been irradiated or treated with mitomycin will in many tumour systems lead to a resistance against subsequent viable tumour cell transplants of the same tumour line. These specific effects can also frequently be further emphasized by parallel immunization with certain immunostimulatory agents such as BCG or other bacterial products.

However, this method has proved relatively inefficient when dealing with already growing tumours. There may be several reasons for this but suppressor mechanisms seem to be of dominating importance in such situations. Measures to counteract the suppressor mechanisms are thus central if one would like to achieve rejection of already established tumours. In order to selectively decrease the activity of T suppressor cells it is possible to use their relative radiation sensitivity and also their high susceptibility to low doses of cyclophosphamide. In the mouse the presence of a selective surface marker (the I–J antigens) may make them susceptible to the corresponding antiserum in the presence of complement. It has been possible in certain mouse tumour models to completely inhibit tumour growth by such manipulations of suppressor T cells.

It is likely that the possibilities of allowing T cells to grow *in vitro* will have a future importance in tumour immunology. When TAA has been chemically characterized it may thus be possible *in vitro* to expand the corresponding effector cells which can then be brought back to the tumour bearer to analyse the relative capacity to influence the growth of the tumour. T cell hybridomas which produce lymphokines of various types will also become available. Their potential as a tool to manipulate immune reactivity *in vivo* is yet only partially understood but is very promising. The possibilities of directing the immune reactivity via the use of anti-idiotypic antibodies (chapter 8) is also of great interest in tumour systems.

Exogenous histamine will activate T suppressor cells under *in vitro* conditions. It has been shown to occur through histamine $H_2$ receptors and $H_2$ antagonists can inhibit this activation. Efficient ways to use such antagonists to manipulate the immune reactivity *in vivo* has not yet been established.

Besides the antigen-specific suppressor activity, as already mentioned there also exists in tumour bearers a non-specific suppression which to a great extent is mediated via prostaglandins, in particular $PGE_2$. This effect can under certain *in vitro* conditions be inhibited using prostaglandin inhibitors such as indomethacin. The capacity of such inhibitors to function *in vivo* with regard to human immune reactivity has still not been clarified.

The possibilities of using antibodies against TAA with specific Ig class and in an amount large enough to affect tumour growth, has been dramatically increased due to the development of monoclonal antibodies and hybridoma techniques. It has still however proved difficult to produce antibodies against the individually unique TAAs within the same animal species in contrast to the abundance of antibodies against TAM which will be produced when immunization across species barriers are carried out.

## Analogy between cancer in man and in experimental animals

One should expect that the same common principles valid for a number of different mammals would also be true for man but with significant differences in certain details. The fundamental question is of course the presence or absence of TAA being immunogenic in the particular tumour patient. In man such a question must currently be studied in patients with regard to specific reactivity against their own tumour cells. Many types of immune reactivities against tumour cells which seem to be tissue-specific do exist. It is here important to clarify whether such reactions merely mean an autoimmune reaction against organ-specific normal cellular components with no rejection capacity *in vivo*. It is also of great importance to be able to chemically identify TAA in man in order to allow sharp analysis to be performed *in vivo* to support possible immunotherapeutic attempts. It is likely that a very important tool for such characterization will be provided by monoclonal antibodies.

## Bibliography

SELA, M. (ed.) (1979). *The Antigens*. Academic Press, New York.

# Chapter 11

# Host defence against infections

Lars Å Hanson

Man is exposed to numerous micro-organisms of various species. Some normally colonize the throat or colon. The *normal flora* cover a spectrum, from some strictly anaerobic intestinal bacteria totally unable to infect, to others which have the capacity to invade man and cause infection and disease. The property of producing disease in a host is called *pathogenicity*. The term *virulence* is used as a measure of the degree of pathogenicity for a certain type or strain of micro-organism. Whether a micro-organism succeeds in inducing disease or not depends, on the one hand, on its virulence, and on the other, on the efficiency of the host to defend against that micro-organism. Often there is a balance between the disease-producing capacity of the micro-organism and the defence of the host (*Figure 11.1*). We can have potentially pathogenic bacteria, such as staphylococci or meningococci, surviving in our throats without us being sick. If the sensitive balance between the micro-organism and the host is disturbed, the situation may quickly change to the advantage of one or the other. On the one hand the milieu can become disagreeable for the micro-organism so that it cannot survive. On the other hand the defence of the host can decrease, e.g. through malnutrition or disease, so that the micro-organism can surmount the defence and invade the individual with infection as a result. Furthermore the defence is not equally effective at all sites and a micro-organism which normally cannot cause infection via the skin, respiratory tract or intestinal tract, can cause a severe infection if it is introduced into the meninges or into a joint. Whether an infection appears or not depends on *the relationship between the host and the micro-organism* in each case.

The capacity to defend itself against the attacks of infectious agents is developed early in the phylogeny of the organism. Higher species have more complex tissues to defend. Multiple, differentiated and co-operating host defence mechanisms have developed to fight potentially dangerous micro-organisms.

Host defence is composed of several non-specific factors (*Table 11.1*) and of the specific immune defence mediated via humoral antibodies (chapters 2 and 6) and T lymphocytes (chapter 7).

## Non-specific host defence

After contact with an infectious micro-organism protection (*immunity*) develops against later infections with the same micro-organism via the specific immune response (*Table 11.1*). But already at the first infection, before the acquired immune defence has had time to develop, there is a non-specific congenital defence against infection, often

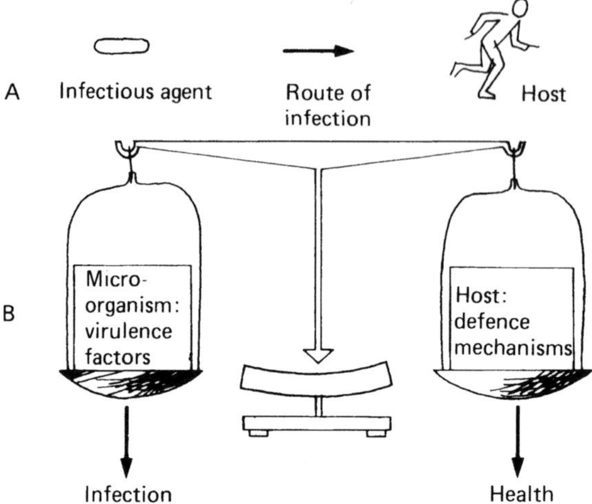



*Figure 11.1* A. Infectious agents reach the host, man, via various
routes of infection. B. By means of its virulence factors the micro-
organism can cause infection if it is not countered by the various
defence mechanisms of the host

called '*natural* resistance'. This natural resistance is the result of several not yet fully
defined cooperative factors.

**Genetic factors**

Genetically-based non-specific host defence plays an important role in protection
against infections. This is especially evident from the striking difference between
sensitivity to infections among different species. While *Corynebacterium diphtheriae*
causes a severe infection in man, it is apathogenic for rats. In the same way
*Mycobacterium leprae* and meningococci can cause disease in man, but as far as we
know not in any other species. These bacteria have specialized in man as the host
organism and have adapted themselves to human tissues. The specificity is probably
often due to the fact that the bacteria as a first step in the infection attach to receptors
on epithelial cells in mucous membranes. *E. coli* bacteria causing renal infections as a
rule bind to a special glycolipid receptor on the urinary tract epithelium. This

**TABLE 11.1. Host defence**

*A. Non-specific host defence*
(1)   Genetic factors
(2)   Mechanical and chemical factors
(3)   Age, hormone balance, nutritional status
(4)   Lactoferrin
(5)   Interferon
(6)   The inflammatory response
(7)   Phagocytosis

*B. Specific immunity against infection*
(1)   Immunity mediated via humoral antibodies
(2)   Cell-mediated immunity

glycolipid is part of the blood group system P; those who belong to blood group $P_1$ more often have recurrent renal infections, pyelonephritis, than those who belong to $P_2$ and probably have less of the receptor on their urinary tract epithelium. Pneumococci which cause middle ear infections attach to another carbohydrate-containing receptor on the epithelial cells of the throat.

Within the same species genetic differences in resistance against infections have been observed. Sheep in Algeria are more resistant to anthrax than sheep in Europe. The greater susceptibility to tuberculosis in negroes and Indians compared with Caucasians is another well-known example. These differences can be difficult to evaluate because of variations in living conditions, hygiene and nutrition, which are also of importance for the sensitivity to infections.

Genetic differences in defence against infections can also be traced in the family. The risk of a sibling to a child with tuberculosis developing turberculosis is three times higher for an identical twin compared with a non-identical twin, or other sibling.

The increased resistance to malaria caused by *Plasmodium falciparum* in individuals with sickle-cell anaemia or $\beta$-thalassaemia are further examples of genetically based resistance against an infection. These patients have abnormal haemoglobins depending on congenital defects in the haemoglobin synthesis and abnormalities which presumably result in the appearance of free radicals (*see below*) which are toxic to the malaria parasite. Red blood cells from individuals of the Duffy phenotype Fy(a-b-) are resistant to malaria. Probably the Duffy determinant on the cell surface is required for the malaria merozoites to invade.


**Mechanical and chemical factors**

Undamaged *skin and mucous membranes* are a mechanical hindrance for most micro-organisms to enter tissues. The cilia of epithelial cells in the respiratory tract transporting foreign material up towards the throat are supported by the *coughing* mechanism. The secretion from the sweat glands and sebaceous glands of the skin support host defence through the bactericidal activity of *fatty acids*. The mucous membranes of the eyes, respiratory tract, intestinal tract and the genitourinary tract are covered by *mucus* secretions which also are bactericidal because they contain *lysozyme*, an enzyme which can degrade glycopeptides of Gram-positive bacteria. The *acidity* of the skin and especially of the gastric juice protects against micro-organisms. Most micro-organisms, with the exception of mycobacteria, are killed by the acidity of the stomach.


**Age, hormones and nutrition**

Resistance to infections is influenced by such factors as the age of the host as well as its nutritional situation and hormonal balance. It is well-known that an infection in a fetus or a neonate can be much more serious and different from that seen in the adult with the same infectious agent. Rubella (German measles) in the adult is a very mild disease. Infection in the fetus can cause severe disease with brain damage, heart malformation and defects in vision and hearing. The increased sensitivity to infections in the fetus and newborn has a complex background depending on certain ot the components in the host defence still being incompletely developed at birth. Thus the complement activity is half that of the adult and the specific immunity is also not comparable with that of the adult. In old age defence against infections is again decreasing in connection with the physiological ageing of the tissues, which also includes the lymphoid tissues. This may cause less efficient immune defence with lower IgM and T cell levels.

Changes in hormone balance can also explain age-related variations in host defence. Gonococcal infection in the vagina is practically only seen in small girls. This is believed to be dependent on the fact that the secretion of the girl's vagina is not acidic as that of the adult. The lower oestrogen levels in the child result in less glycogen and therefore less acid metabolites in the child's vagina. The importance of hormones for the host defence is also illustrated by the increased frequency of skin infections and tuberculosis in patients with diabetes mellitus (deficiency in insulin) and occurrence of mycotic infections, especially *Candida*, in individuals with hypoparathyroidism. An increased sensitivity to infections has also been noted in individuals with decreased cortisone production (Addison's disease), or an increased cortisone level (endogenous in Cushing's disease or exogenous when given therapeutically).

Proper nutrition is important for competent host defence. Malnutrition increases the risk of infections, for example tuberculosis. This is mainly caused by an impaired cell-mediated immunity, but phagocytosis and other defence factors can also be impaired.

An increased risk of infection can also be due to exhaustion or a decreased body temperature. Hens which normally are resistant to anthrax can be made receptive by decreasing the body temperature. For certain infections an increased temperature can add to the host defence by decreasing microbial replication. Temperatures of 40–42°C can kill gonococci causing arthritis or the treponema in neurosyphilis. The fact that lepra almost only involves superficial parts of the body may be because *Mycobacterium leprae* cannot survive the higher temperatures in deeper tissues. There is no evidence that exposure to cold weather increases the risk of attracting a 'common cold'.


**Lactoferrin**

Iron is a necessary growth factor for most aerobic bacteria, except lactobacilli. The bacteria produce iron-binding proteins, ferromyns, which bind iron, but lactoferrin, a protein found in all exocrine secretions, binds iron in competition with the ferromyns. Lactoferrin is therefore bacteriostatic for *E. coli* bacteria. The host protects itself by a decreased uptake of iron from the intestine and deposits iron in depots during an infection. The ensuing 'infection anaemia' is part of host defence and should not be treated if the infection is not under control. Parenteral injections of iron preparations in infected neonates have led to acute life-threatening sepsis. Lactoferrin is also important for the function of phagocytes as further developed below.


**Interferon**

It was reported in 1803 that measles could modify the course of smallpox. It was later noted that vaccination against measles often prevented a successful ensuing smallpox vaccination. This is probably explained by the first virus infection inducing production of interferon, preventing the second virus infection. Interferon, which was discovered in 1957, is an important factor in the non-specific defence against virus infections.

Interferon is produced by different cell types including leucocytes, fibroblasts and epithelial cells in different tissues. The production is induced by viruses, probably all types of viruses, but also by other organisms such as rickettsiae, mycoplasma, protozoa and some bacteria multiplying in the cytoplasm of cells. Polynucleotides, certain plastic polymers and endotoxin can induce production of interferon and cortisone can inhibit the production.

Interferon, which is biologically characterized via its virus-inhibiting activity, is really a group of proteins. Three subgroups of interferons have been identified: α *interferon*, or leucocyte interferon, which is produced by NK-like lymphocytes; β *interferon* produced by fibroblasts; γ *interferon*, or immune interferon which is produced by antigen or mitogen-stimulated T lymphocytes. A relation between γ interferon and the lymphokine MAF has been suggested. The amino acid sequence is known for several α and one β interferon. The molecular weight is around 20 000.

All viruses are more or less sensitive to interferon. A mechanism for the antiviral effect of interferon is that translation of virus-specific mRNA on the ribosomes of the host cell is inhibited. As a result the reproduction of the virus is blocked. The importance of interferon in host defence is related to its rapid appearance during an infection, before the specific immune defence. The antiviral effect is enhanced by fever. Interferon produced by virus-induced human leucocytes has a prophylactic effect on rhinovirus infections and seems to have therapeutic effects on herpes zoster and recurrent herpes keratitis. Larger amounts of interferon can now be produced by bacteria by means of hybrid DNA technology. Different interferon inducers have been tested but have been too toxic for human use.

Interferon is active against certain tumours such as osteogenic sarcoma and larynx papilloma. This may depend on interferon increasing the levels of NK cells which are cytotoxic for tumour cells. Interferon also inhibits cell division and may decrease transplant rejection, antibody production and the development of delayed hyper-sensitivity reactions. Macrophages and prostaglandin synthesis are stimulated.

**The inflammatory response**

Bacteria infecting a wound have managed to pass through the first line of defence consisting of skin and mucous membranes. A second line of defence is established by the *inflammatory response*. An inflammatory reaction may arise from tissue damage caused by infecting bacteria and their products, as well as by physical and chemical factors (heat, ionizing irradiation, toxic substances, mechanical trauma, etc.). Immediately after the damage vasoconstriction occurs but this is quickly followed by vaso-dilatation and an increased flow of blood. Certain neuropeptides from sensory nerves, called substance P, probably play an important role in the vasodilatation. Substance P also mediates the pain. Prostaglandins are formed and cause vasodilatation, leukotrienes increase vascular permeability.

The increased blood flow results in the *redness* and *heat* which characterize the inflammatory reaction in the damaged tissue. The increased vascular permeability causes the *swelling*, oedema, through the extravasation of fluid. The lymph flow is increased simultaneously. The tissue damage also causes production of tissue thrombokinase, which makes fibrin from plasma fibrinogen. The network of fibrin in the damaged tissue prevents the spread of the infection by blocking the lymph vessels left open after the damage, offering a route of spread for the bacteria. The bacteria release components which attract neutrophilic granulocytes to the damaged tissue (*Figure 11.2*). This is called *chemotaxis*. Some complement factors, especially C5a and leucotriene B4 are also chemotactic for the polymorphonuclear (PMN) leucocytes. A few hours after the extravasation of the granulocytes from the blood, mononuclear cells such as monocytes and lymphocytes follow. The monocytes develop into macrophages and dominate together with the lymphocytes and plasma cells the later stages of resolution, as well as the cell pattern in chronic infections, such as tuberculosis.

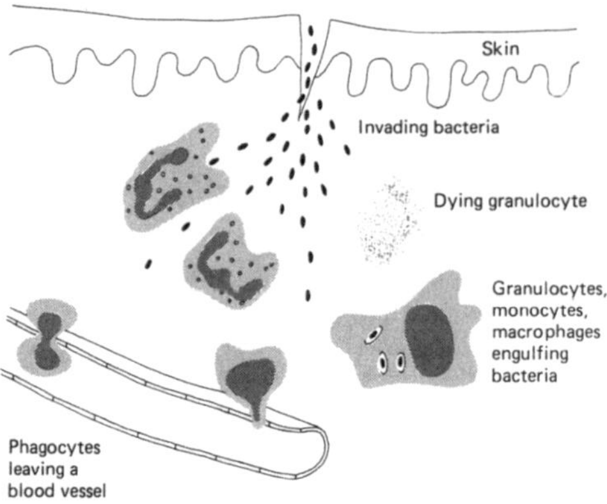


*Figure 11.2* Phagocytosis of bacteria in a non-immune individual. Bacteria infecting the host wound will be met by phagocytes, first granulocytes and later macrophages. If this defence is insufficient the bacteria may spread further via blood and lymph vessels

Granulocytes and macrophages play a very important role in the defence against infection functioning as phagocytes. Phagocytosis is described in detail below.

The inflammatory response is released especially via enzymes from the lysosomes or damaged cells, but several other substances such as histamine released from mast cells in the damaged tissue, also play a role. The granules of the PMNs contain a number of different tissue-damaging and pathogenic components, especially enzymes (acid proteases, glucoronidases, esterases, cathepsin, peroxidases, lysozyme and alkaline phosphatase), but also chemotactic substances. Of great importance is the reduction of $O_2$ to free superoxide and hydroxyl radicals in the cell membrane of activated phagocytes. These very reactive *free radicals* play a major role in the development of the inflammation. The phagocytes are clearly an important prerequisite for the development of the inflammatory response. The chemotactic factors produced by the complement system, activated by antibodies in the area, or via the alternative pathway are important for the appearance of the granulocytes in the damaged tissue. The complement system probably also adds to the inflammatory reaction via the increased vascular permeability caused by the anaphylatoxins releasing histamine. On the one hand, inflammatory reactions are part of our host defence by limiting and fighting infections and through the oedema diluting toxic bacterial products. On the other hand, before the lymph vessels have been blocked by fibrin, they may provide an open route for spreading the infection, further supported by the oedema. Furthermore, the inflammation adds to tissue damage in many instances, especially in chronic infections such as tuberculosis (*see below*, page 144).

### Phagocytosis

By 1880 Metchinkoff had discovered that certain cells had the capacity to engulf foreign material. Phagocytosis (from the Greek fagein = eat; kytos = cell, cavity) was defined as an important part of the defence against infecting micro-organisms. The phagocytosing system consists of the *polymorphonuclear leucocytes or granulocytes* in the blood and cells in the *reticuloendothelial* system (RES), now more often called the mononuclear phagocyte system (MPS). The MPS consists of *macrophages* in various tissues. They are found in the blood as *monocytes* and in the central nervous system as *microglia*. They are found as sinus-lining cells in the liver, Kupffer cells, and in the lymph sinuses of the spleen and lymph glands, as well as in the blood sinuses of the bone marrow. The lungs are rich in macrophages. The phagocytic cells, *histiocytes*, found especially in connective tissue and lymphoid organs, are also included in the MPS, or RES.

On contact between the phagocyte and invading bacteria a depression is formed on the phagocyte by means of the microfilament consisting of actin and myosin under the cell membrane. The bacteria are quickly enclosed so that they are found in a cavity surrounded by a membrane, a 'phagosome' in the phagocyte (*Figure 11.3A* and *B*). The granules found in polymorphonuclear granulocytes as well as macrophages contain as mentioned above a number of different enzymes and correspond to the lysosomes of other cells. Such granules are gathered around the phagosome and empty their contents in them, usually resulting in the degradation of the bacteria in the phagosome.

Phagocytosis increases the oxidative metabolism of the cell, producing energy. The strongest antimicrobial activity in the phagocyte is most probably mediated via oxygen-dependent systems, especially the free superoxides and hydroxyl radicals produced when oxygen is reduced. Hydrogen peroxide together with myeloperoxidase, halogens and thiocyanates add to the antimicrobial activity. Several non-oxygen-dependent systems also participate:

(1) reduced pH due to the lactic acid produced during the increased metabolism;
(2) lysozyme splitting glycosidic linkages. Few bacteria are sensitive before they have been affected by hydrogen peroxide, or antibody plus complement;
(3) basic proteins which probably damage the permeability barrier of bacteria;
(4) lactoferrin which under certain circumstances can kill bacteria, but probably plays its major role by increasing the adherence of the phagocytes;
(5) proteolytic enzymes including elastase and collagenase activate the complement factors C3 and C5 to C3a and C5a.

Macrophages have smaller and fewer granules in their cytoplasm than granulocytes. They are also said to lack basic proteins, lactoferrin and the enzymes that participate in the oxidative metabolism. The active free oxygen radicals can be produced without enzymes.

The neutrophilic granulocytes which are first found at the site of infection (*Figure 11.2*) try to engulf and kill the infecting bacteria. These phagocytes which produce the *pus* during, for example staphylococal infection, die in large numbers after a few hours. The granulocytes are followed by monocytes which develop into macrophages and continue to phagocytose bacteria, dead and dying granulocytes and damaged tissue. The bacteria that are engulfed by the macrophages are also degraded, but part of the material remains in an immunogenic form. Macrophages transport this immunogenic material to the lymph glands, spleen and other lymphoid tissues in the body where the specific immune response is induced. A factor produced by the macrophages during this process, lymphocyte activating factor (LAF) or interleukin-1, seems to be a major *pyrogen* causing fever, which may add to the host defence.

If the infection is not stopped in spite of the local inflammatory response, the infecting bacteria are spread, often via the lymph vessels to the local lymph glands. They function as a filter where the bacteria meet a new barrier of phagocytic cells. On continued spread to the blood the bacteria are caught by a similar filter mechanism in

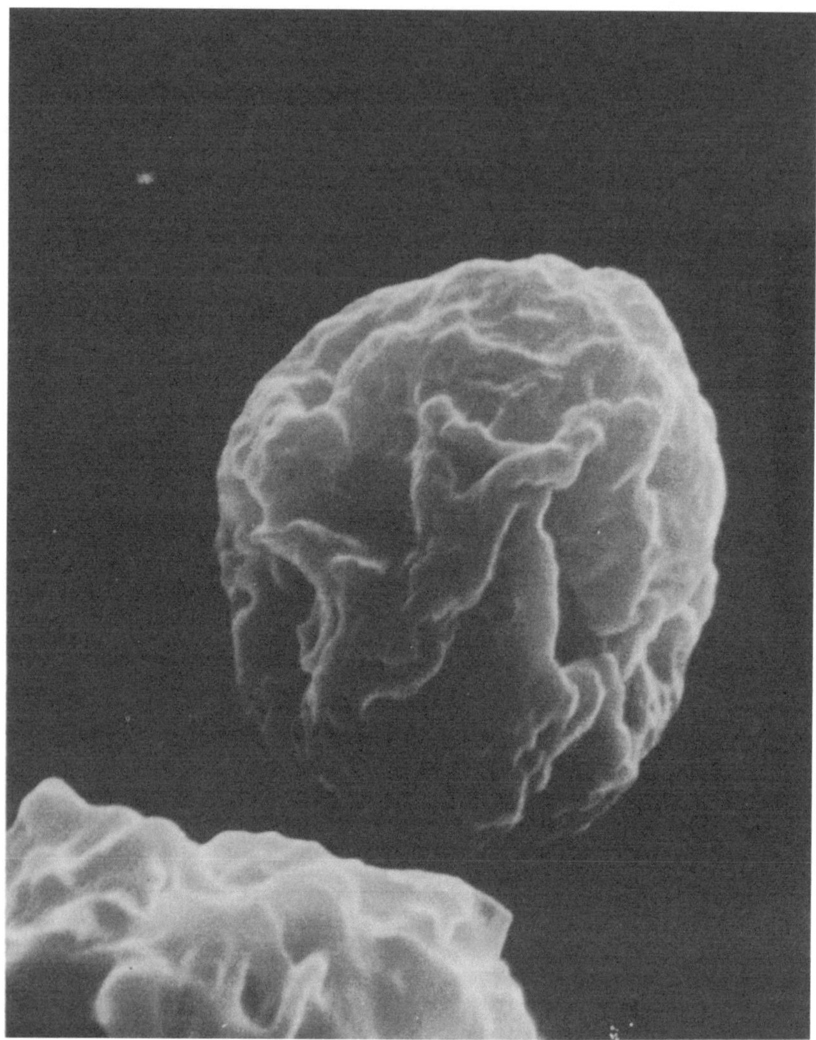

*Figure 11.3* A. Scanning electron microscopy of blood leucocytes fixed in suspension, most probably granulocytes (Magnification  × 20 000).

the spleen and liver. RES cells there as well as in other tissues in the body usually manage to quickly eliminate the bacteria from the blood, if they are not so virulent that they can manage to multiply faster than they are eliminated. The blood granulocytes seem to play a minor role for the elimination of the bacteria from the blood. Granulocytes that have engulfed bacteria are caught in capillaries especially in the lung, where they are eliminated by the local macrophages.

Bacteria of low virulence such as *Staphylococcus epidermidis* are easily engulfed and killed by phagocytes (*Figure 11.4A*), while other have virulence factors making them resistant to phagocytosis and intracellular killing. The presence of such virulence factors enhances their possibility to survive the host defence. Pneumococci have a

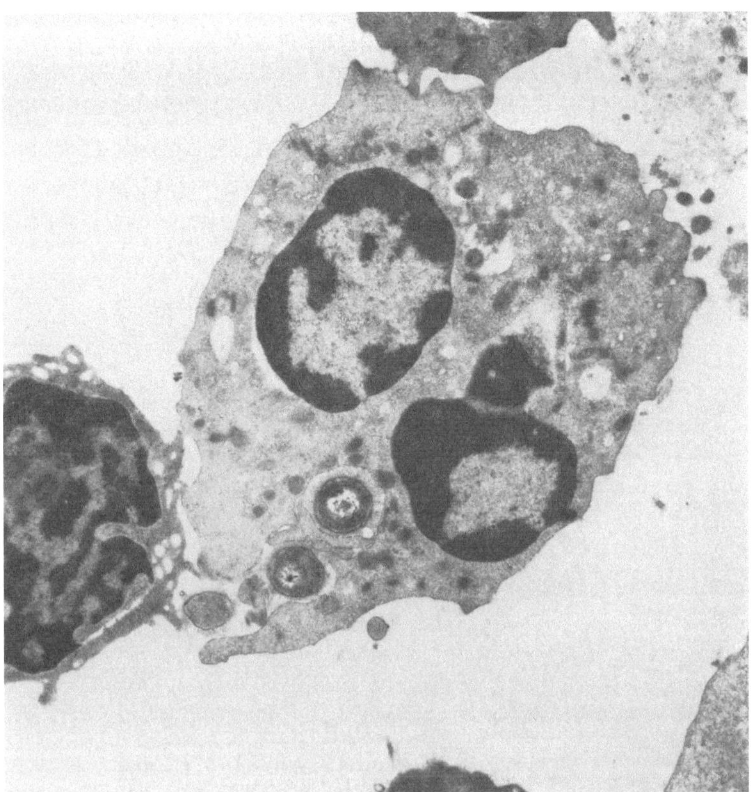

*Figure 11.3* B. Transmission electron microscopy of granulocyte engulfing three bacteria in the lower left corner close to the dark lymphocyte. One of the bacteria is already enclosed in a phagosome. Granules are gathering around the phagosome to empty their bactericidal content into the phagosome (magnification × 20 300). (Photo: S. Olling and C. Svalander, Göteborg)

polysaccharide capsule which hampers or prevents phagocytosis (*Figure 11.4B*). Other virulent bacteria produce substances toxic for granulocytes, leucocidines. Staphylococcal leucocidine decreases the glycolysis of granulocytes and makes them empty their granules outside the cell membrane and not in the phagosomes. Streptolysin O from streptococci and α toxin from staphylococci kill granulocytes by damaging the membranes of the lysosomes of the granulocytes so that the active enzymes are released into the cytoplasm. This may explain why some staphylococci can survive in phagocytes (*Figure 11.4D*). Bacteria of several other species can also survive after phagocytosis and in some cases even multiply in the phagocytic cells. Intracellular parasites like salmonella and mycobacteria are examples of such virulent micro-organisms (*Figure 11.4E*).

Viruses are engulfed by granulocytes and macrophages as well. Granulocytes usually do not seem to be able to inactivate virus. In contrast monocytes and macrophages play a major role in the defence against virus infections, but only after activation via T cell lymphokines or immune complexes and C3b. Phagocytes which do not manage to inactivate an engulfed virus may spread it to other sites in the body.

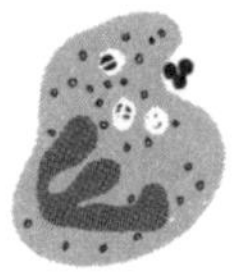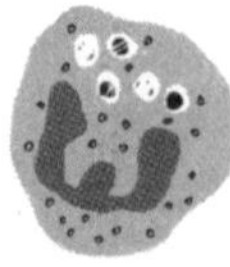

A  Phagocytosis of *Staphylococcus albus*

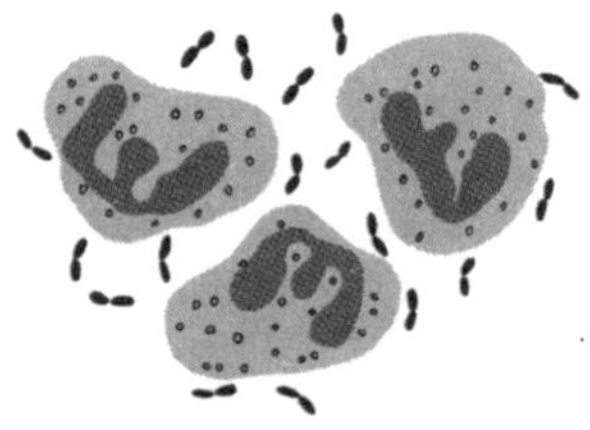

B  Encapsulated pneumococci are not engulfed
in the absence of antibodies

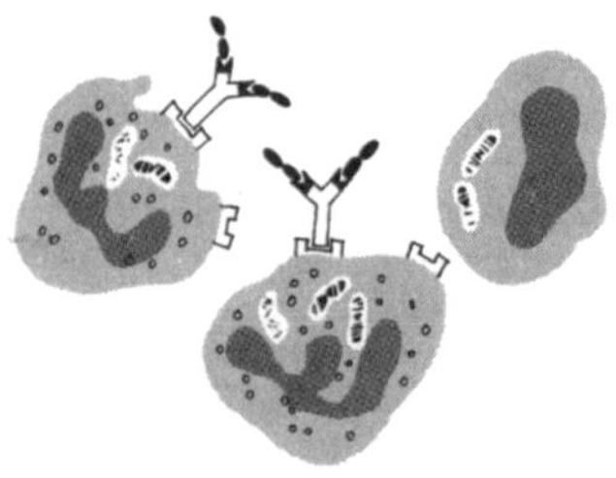

C  Encapsulated pneumococci are engulfed in
the presence of antibodies

*Figure 11.4* A. *Staphylococcus albus* (*epidermidis*) is easily engulfed and killed by phagocytes since it is of low virulence. The phagocytes empty their granules into the phagosome enclosing the engulfed bacteria. The bacteria are killed and degraded.
B. A carbohydrate capsule is a major virulence factor for pneumococci since it prevents phagocytosis. The bacteria are found outside the phagocytes in the absence of antibodies.
C. In an immune individual opsonic antibodies make it possible for the phagocytes to engulf and destroy the pneumococci.

The inflammatory response and phagocytosis have been discussed here as non-specific mechanisms, but these processes occur also in the absence of a specific immune response against the invading micro-organism. Mostly the defence against infection occurs as a close cooperation between non-specific and specific components. The fluid that comes out into the tissues, following the increased vascular permeability during inflammation, often contains specific antibodies which can play a major role in the defence as further discussed below. Phagocytosis is faster and more efficient in the presence of antibodies. The antibodies, which in this function are called *opsonins*, attach the bacteria to phagocytes via receptors for the Fc-portion of the antibodies. In addition there are C3b receptors on the phagocytes making complement activation support the phagocytosis by stabilizing the coupling between the bacteria and the phagocyte. Encapsulated pneumococci which can resist phagocytosis are easily engulfed and killed by phagocytes in the presence of antibodies against the capsule (*Figure 11.4C*). In the acute phase of an infection caused by bacteria an acute phase

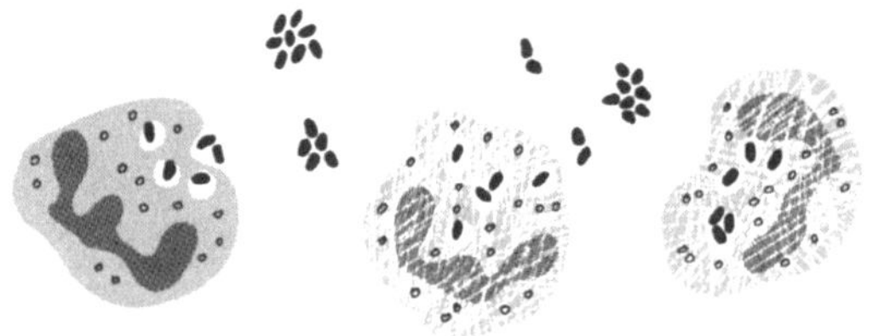

D  Phagocytosis of *Staphylococcus aureus*

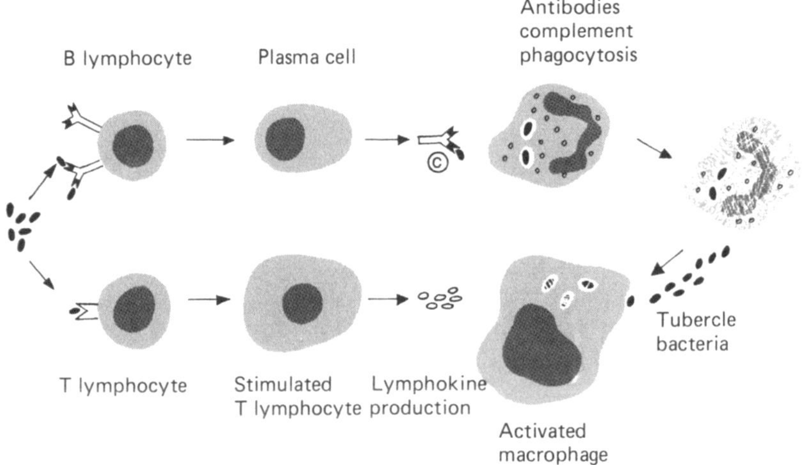



E  Phagocytosis of tubercle
   bacteria

*Figure 11.4* D. *Staphylococcus aureus* is taken up by phagocytes, but one of the virulence factors of these bacteria, the staphylococcal leucocidin, makes the granulocytes unable to kill since the granules will not empty themselves in the phagosome. Therefore many of the staphylococci survive intracellularly.
E. *Mycobacterium tuberculosis* can be engulfed by granulocytes, but survives even if antibodies and complement add to the phagocytosis. Only if the bacteria are engulfed by macrophages activated by lymphokines from specifically stimulated T lymphocytes are the bacteria killed

protein, C-reactive protein (CRP), is produced which seems to have opsonic activity. The antibodies also add to a more efficient phagocytosis via chemotaxis and immune adherence induced by the activated complement system. The aggregated granulocytes fight the infection both via phagocytosis and the inflammatory reaction they help to release (*Figure 11.5*).

Phagocytosis is more efficient in the presence of antibodies, but also in the absence of antibodies, macrophages are more efficient in an immune than a non-immune individual. The reason for this activation is that the macrophages are non-specifically stimulated via lymphokines from antigen stimulated T lymphocytes in the immune individual. The inflammatory response and phagocytosis appear faster and more efficient in an immune than in a non-immune individual, and this may be of critical importance for the outcome of an infection.

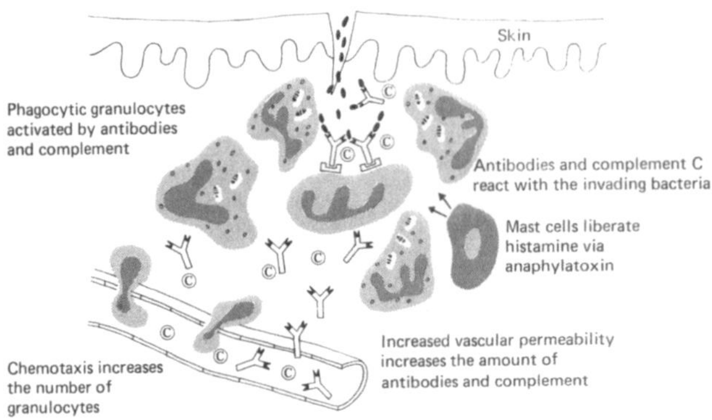


*Figure 11.5* Phagocytosis of bacteria in an immune individual. As in a non-immune host the bacteria are met with granulocytes, but in the immune host these cells are more numerous and phagocytosis is more efficient. This is due to the presence of opsonic antibodies directed against the bacteria and the effects of the activated complement system

# Specific immunity against infections

The immunity acquired via the specific immune response during an infection is mediated by B lymphocytes producing humoral antibodies and by cytotoxic and lymphokine producing T lymphocytes.

## Immunity mediated by humoral antibodies

The importance of the protective capacity of antibodies varies for different kinds of infections. They are not of the same decisive significance during tuberculosis, or mycotic infections as they are in individuals with tetanus, pneumococcal pneumonia or poliomyelitis.

### Bacterial infections

The efficiency of the antibody response in protection against an infection is influenced both by the virulence of the infecting micro-organism and the type of antibody response. All the symptoms in diphtheria and tetanus are caused by the exotoxins of the bacteria and the homologous antibodies neutralizing the toxins can totally prevent disease. This was shown by von Behring and Kitasato in the 1890s. Such antibodies, called antitoxins, must neutralize the toxin before it has reached the tissue it binds to. Antibodies are also produced against toxins from other bacteria such as streptococci and staphylococci. These antitoxins can probably influence the course of infections with such bacteria, but not in the same manner as in tetanus and diphtheria, because streptococci and staphylococci produce significant virulence factors other than toxins.

Antibodies of the IgG class are the most efficient at neutralizing toxins. Very small amounts of antibodies are sufficient for neutralization of many toxins. Approximately 0.1 $\mu$g of diphtheria antitoxin per ml of serum can protect against diphtheria in man. With diphtheria vaccine much higher antibody concentrations are produced. Due to the formation of memory cells during the primary antibody response, revaccination against diphtheria will, many years later, result in a secondary antibody response with large amounts of antibodies being quickly produced.

Antibodies add to the defence against bacterial infections via their agglutinating capacity. *Agglutination*, which is much more efficiently brought about by the large polyvalent IgM antibody than the smaller bivalent IgG antibodies, makes the aggregated bacteria more easy to engulf. In the presence of complement these antibodies may also induce bacteriolysis (*see* chapter 5). IgM antibodies are more efficient in this capacity since only a single IgM antibody is necessary, but several IgG antibodies are required per bacterial cell to activate the complement. Some Gram-negative bacteria of rather low virulence are sensitive to this bacteriolysis.

The *stimulating effect on phagocytosis* by antibodies is, as previously mentioned, very important for defence against bacterial infections. The most important antibody function may be to enhance the efficiency of phagocytosis. Virulent bacteria often have the capacity to resist phagocytosis. What makes *Haemophilus influenzae* and pneumococci virulent seems to be primarily their carbohydrate capsule, which decreases or prevents phagocytosis. The opsonic antibodies which protect against infections with these micro-organisms are mainly directed against the capsule and facilitate phagocytosis by utilizing the Fc and C3b receptors of the phagocytes (*Figure 11.4B* and *C*). Virulent anthrax bacteria have a capsule, but strains lacking a capsule can also be of high virulence. Antibodies against the capsules of these bacteria are not protective, since the virulence of the anthrax bacteria is determined by characteristics other than production of a capsule.

The capacity to survive intracellularly after phagocytosis is more decisive for the virulence of a bacterium than the capacity to resist phagocytosis. *Staphylococcus epidermidis*, which usually is apathogenic, is easily engulfed and killed. *Staphylococcus aureus*, which is pathogenic, is also engulfed but can survive in the phagocyte (*Figure 11.4A* and *D*). Virulent strains of salmonella and mycobacteria can even multiply in phagocytes (*Figure 11.4E*). Bacteria surviving in phagocytes are protected against antibodies which are only found extracellularly.

Various exocrine secretions such as tear fluid, saliva, nasal and bronchial secretion, the secretions of the urogenital organs and the gastrointestinal tract contain antibodies, mainly in the form of secretory IgA. These antibodies, which are locally produced, have a stable structure resisting the varying milieu of different secretions. They consist of IgA dimers together with two extra polypeptide chains, the J chain and the secretory component (*Figure 11.6A* and chapter 2). Secretory IgA antibodies are found in the secretions but also in the mucus layer on most mucous membranes. These antibodies function primarily by binding and aggregating micro-organisms, hindering their contact with the mucous membrane, thus preventing invasion and establishment of infection. In this way they can protect against infections with, for example, *Shigella* and *E. coli* bacteria. Binding cholera bacteria, the secretory IgA antibodies can prevent them from reaching the mucous membrane. In addition the antibodies bind the cholera toxin so that it cannot bind to its ganglioside receptors on the intestinal epithelium, protecting the immune individual against cholera.

Secretory IgA antibodies dominate among the immunoglobulins in human milk. It is striking that many of these secretory IgA antibodies produced locally in the mammary gland are directed against intestinal bacteria. This is explained by the fact that antigens present in the gut are taken up by the special aggregates of lymphocytes, the Peyer's patches, found in the small intestine. The antigens are processed by macrophages presenting the antigen to the lymphoid cells in the Peyer's patches. Many of these cells are committed to IgA production and leave the patches via the lymph and the blood

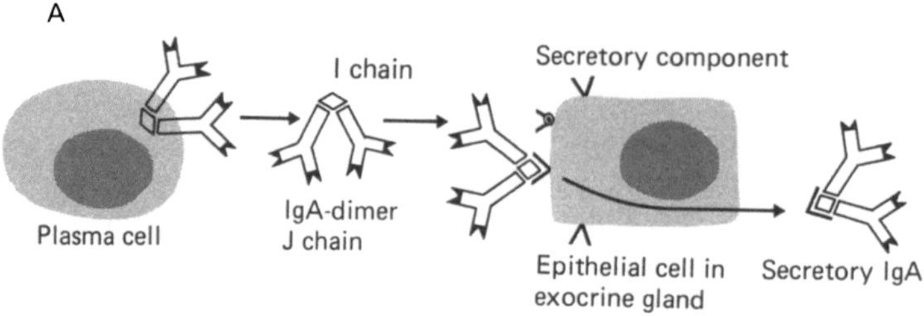


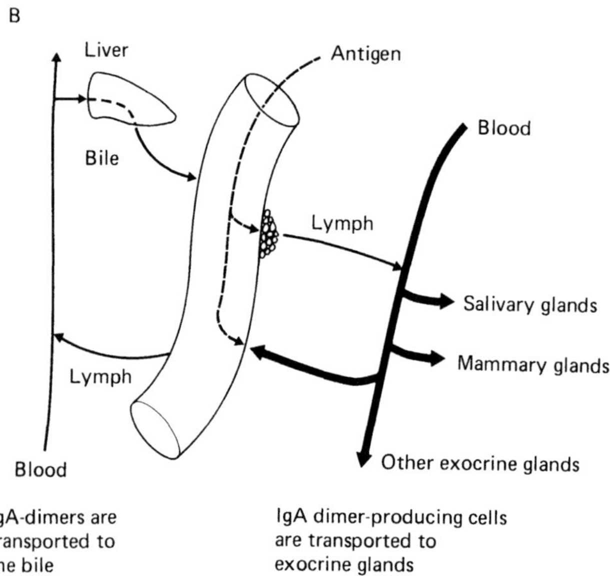


*Figure 11.6* A. Production of secretory IgA antibodies. Plasma cells producing IgA dimers with J chain are found close to the basal portion of epithelial cells in exocrine glands in the respiratory tract, the digestive tract, the genitourinary tract as well as salivary, lacrimal and mammary glands. The J chain acts as a ligand for the secretory component found in the cell membrane of the epithelial cells, functioning as a receptor transporting the completed secretory IgA molecule through the epithelial cell out on the mucous membrane.
B. Antigens in the gut are presented to lymphocytes in the Peyer's patches. The committed lymphocytes migrate via the lymph and blood to exocrine glands (right part of the picture) where secretory IgA is produced as demonstrated in A. The left part of the figure demonstrates how IgA dimers, mainly from the IgA production in the gut, may reach the blood via lymph vessels. These IgA dimers are selectively taken up in the liver and are found as secretory IgA in the bile. This provides approximately 75% of the secretory IgA in the gut of the rat, but only a small proportion in man

which reaches the exocrine glands such as the tear glands, salivary glands and the mammary glands, as well as the exocrine glands of the respiratory and intestinal tracts where the local production of secretory IgA antibodies takes place (*Figure 11.6B*). In this way the secretory IgA antibodies against the intestinal micro-organisms are found in various exocrine secretions, including the milk. This is called the enteromammaric link. As a result the breast-fed baby is protected on its intestinal mucosa against those micro-organisms which have passed through the mother's intestine and to which the infant most probably is also exposed. The milk has huge amounts of such antibodies which play a major role in the defence especially against intestinal infections, but possibly also against respiratory tract infections and otitis media. Exocrine secretions contain several other host defence factors in addition to secretory IgA, for example lactoferrin. This iron-binding protein functions in synergy with secretory IgA antibodies against iron-binding proteins, which anaerobic bacteria use to obtain the iron required for their growth.

The protective capacity of antibodies in bacterial infections is clearly illustrated by the recurrent purulent bacterial infections, otitis media, sinusitis, pneumonia, meningitis, etc., occurring in individuals with antibody-deficiency syndromes (*see* chapter 13).


*Viral infections*

Humoral antibodies can provide immunity against viral infections. This is illustrated by the prevention of measles and epidemic hepatitis resulting from injection of immunoglobulin containing antibodies against the measles and hepatitis A virus. This is not true for all virus infections. Furthermore the antibodies can only bind the virus as long as it is available on mucous membranes or in the blood during the viraemia stage. The antibodies prevent the virus from penetrating the host cells. Intracellular virus is protected against antibodies, which do not penetrate living cells. On the other hand viral antigen can be found on the surface of infected cells and virus antibodies together with complement may lyse such cells. Since the virus then becomes exposed it may be neutralized by antibodies.

A virus is efficiently neutralized by circulating IgG antibodies, but IgM antibodies also have this function. The first four complement factors improve this neutralizing effect. Virus infecting via mucous membranes in the respiratory or gastrointestinal tract mainly meet secretory IgA antibodies, which may prevent infection by binding and neutralizing the virus. This is true for polio, myxo-, paramyxo- and rhinoviruses. If the virus still manages to infect the host tissues, an inflammatory reaction appears adding to the defence by increased vascular permeability, resulting in the appearance of IgG and IgM antibodies from the blood.

Very small amounts of antibodies may be sufficient to prevent further virus infections. Only a few million antibody molecules per ml blood are required to protect against poliomyelitis. The infant is immune up to the age of six to eight months against several viral infections because of the transplacentally transported IgG antibodies from the mother, although they have a half-life of only three weeks (*see* chapter 2). Viral infections in deeper tissues and a virus reappearing several times during life may induce lifelong immunity. This is due to the immunological memory of the immune response and also the fact that repeated exposures to the same virus keeps up the immunity.

The antibody response during a first virus exposure is often too slow to prevent the infection from being established with clinical symptoms as a result. Interferon, which appears faster, is important in this situation. Initially during the course of a primary influenza virus infection, interferon plays a major role, but at a later stage IgM and finally secretory IgA antibodies appear and fight the infection. In the already immune individual the virus may at best be stopped by the secretory IgA antibodies before it has reached the mucous membranes. Antibody-dependent cell-mediated cytotoxicity with human K cells (chapter 7) has been demonstrated for measles virus infected cells. It is not yet clear if this mechanism plays a significant role in defence against infections.

### Other infections

Humoral antibodies appear during mycotic, protozoal and helminthic infections. Protective capacity has not been demonstrated for antibodies against *fungi*, but antibodies against *Candida* and *Aspergillus* seem to produce tissue-damaging immune complexes under certain conditions (chapters 16 and 19). Antibodies against a number of other fungi like *Micropolyspora, Thermoactinomyces, Coniosporium, Penicillium, Alternaria, Cladosporium* and *Botrytis* are actually also claimed to cause lung diseases via such mechanisms (chapter 19).

Antibodies against *protozoa* such as *Toxoplasma* and malaria plasmodia can protect and there is much interest in developing vaccines against these parasites. Antibodies against an antigen on sporozoites can prevent this form of the parasite from reaching the liver cells where they move to develop into merozoites after the mosquito bite. In the next phase, when the merozoites infect erythrocytes antibodies have again been found to protect. Certain antigens from the merozoites as well as from late schizonts can induce such protective antibodies. Finally the spread of malaria can be hindered by antibodies against gametocytes, the form which infects mosquitoes biting infected humans, starting the cycle over again. Even if there is a good chance of producing vaccines on the basis of this knowledge it should be added that antigen variation and immunosuppressive effects of the parasite complicate the matter.

In leishmaniasis and trypanosomiasis there is also an immunodepressive effect and trypanosoma can, in addition, through continuous changes of their surface antigens in some 20 variants avoid the attacks of the host immune response. This may be the reason why the antibody response against this parasite does not seem to protect.

*Entamoeba histolytica* seems to resist elimination by the antibody response by becoming resistant to complement-mediated lysis. In contrast hydatid cysts caused by *Echinococcus granulosus* were destroyed by injection of immune serum from an infected individual, a measure that seems to be simpler than surgical resection.

Large amounts of IgE antibodies are formed and eosinophilia appears during *helminthic infections*. IgE antibodies induce specific chemotaxis for eosinophils and a tissue reaction depending on local release of mediators including histamine, prostaglandins and leukotrienes from mast cells (immediate hypersensitivity reaction, *see further* chapters 16 and 17). T lymphocyte-dependent mast cells aggregate in large numbers during parasite infestations in the intestinal mucosa. It is still not quite clear to what extent mast cells, IgE antibodies and eosinophils can protect against different helminthic infections.

IgG antibody-dependent cytotoxicity of eosinophilic granulocytes has been demonstrated against *Schistosoma mansoni* and may be an important defence mechanism. Eosinophils kill parasites especially via the eosinophil cationic protein (ECP). Also the major basic protein (MBP) participates together with the hydrogen peroxide system. It is interesting that the effect of the eosinophils is blocked by antigen–antibody complexes in a similar way as has been suggested for blocking of tumour immunity.

IgE and IgG mediated macrophage activity has also been demonstrated against *Schistosoma* and *Toxoplasma*. It has been suggested that first IgG and later IgE mediated antibody dependent cell-mediated cytotoxicity (ADCC) can protect against *Schistosoma*.

During microfilaraemia, a special form of filariasis, a suppressed antibody response can be seen. This immunosuppression seems to depend on an increased level of T suppressor cells induced by the parasite. This has been noticed in infections with *Naegleria fowleri* as well, resulting in a deadly infection.

**Cell-mediated immunity**

The role of cell-mediated immunity in defence against infections has long been an enigma. It is clear that it plays an important role in infections with intracellular parasites such as viruses, certain bacteria, fungi and protozoa. Severe, often lethal infections with such agents occur in individuals with deficiencies in cell-mediated immunity (*see further* chapter 13 on immunodeficiency). With increased knowledge about cell-mediated immunity we can start to understand how this defence mechanism functions.

Antigen stimulated T lymphocytes become cytotoxic to cells with the antigen on the surface, but T lymphocytes also produce substances, lymphokines, some of which are chemotactic and activating for macrophages (chapter 7). These functions of stimulated T lymphocytes are probably very important in the defence against intracellular parasites which humoral antibodies cannot reach, or which are resistant against antibody-mediated defence. Antibodies do not provide any protection against bacteria belonging to *Salmonella, Listeria, Brucella* or *Mycobacterium*. As illustrated in *Figure 11.4E*, mycobacteria survive the attack of antibodies and complement and phagocytic granulocytes, but are engulfed and efficiently killed by macrophages which are activated by T lymphocytes specific for mycobacterial antigens.

The first step is the specific immune reaction between the T lymphocytes and the mycobacteria. In the second step lymphokines produced by the specifically activated T lymphocytes stimulate the macrophages which non-specifically engulf and kill micro-organisms in the surrounding tissues. Exposure of an experimental animal immune to mycobacteria to these micro-organisms results in activation of these macrophages, protecting it also, for instance, against *Listeria*. These activated macrophages are most probably an important defence mechanism against viruses, fungi and protozoa as well. Immunity against *Leishmania tropica* depends on cell-mediated immunity in the human. Activated T lymphocytes can destroy *Schistosoma mansoni* parasites.

In viral infections two other functions of antigen-stimulated T lymphocytes are important. The interferon production of lymphocytes should play an important role, since interferon protects against several viral infections. Furthermore stimulated T lymphocytes are cytotoxic which permits them to attack virus infected cells carrying viral antigens on their surface. They can lyse these target cells, exposing the virus to humoral antibodies and neutralization. Virus-specific T lymphocytes have been demonstrated already within a few days of a viral infection. Such lymphocytes then seem to be able to destroy virus infected cells before the virus has started to propagate and spread.

An immune response including T lymphocytes develops during infections with various micro-organisms such as bacteria, viruses and fungi. Injection in the skin of antigen from the micro-organism produces a typical inflammation; a delayed hypersensitivity reaction which depends on the effect of the lymphokines released from the specifically stimulated lymphocytes (chapters 16 and 17). If a protein preparation from mycobacteria, tuberculin, is injected into the skin of an individual who has had tuberculosis, he will, within approximately 24 hours have a typical erythema and induration in the skin which becomes maximal in about 48 to 72 hours. This individual is 'tuberculin-positive' (colour plate 1C, after p. 198). If an individual who has not previously been positive to tuberculin develops such a reaction, it usually means that he has been exposed to tuberculosis. Therefore tuberculin testing can be used diagnostically to detect tuberculosis. The positive tuberculin reaction can be due to an active infection or an already healed process. Tuberculin hypersensitivity also appears after vaccination against tuberculosis with BCG vaccine (chapter 12). In a previously vaccinated individual it cannot be decided if the tuberculin sensitivity is a result of vaccination or of infection. Tuberculin testing is used in vaccinated individuals to detect those who lack tuberculin hypersensitivity and therefore should be vaccinated. The tuberculin reaction is no absolute indicator of the degree of immunity against tuberculosis, but only shows a certain parallelism. In the single individual the presence of a positive tuberculin reaction only suggests that he may be immune against tuberculosis. It has not been possible to show that tuberculin sensitivity as such adds to the defence against tuberculosis. The delayed hypersensitivity reactions appearing after several other infections can also be used diagnostically. Tests corresponding to the tuberculin test have been developed for brucellosis, lepra, several mycotic infections and some viral infections. *In vitro* tests in the form of lymphocyte stimulation with microbial antigens can also be used (*see further* Appendix 2).


## Host defence can cause tissue damage

A functioning defence against infections is necessary for survival, but at the same time it is dangerous and can cause tissue damage. There are numerous examples of deleterious effects of the host defence. In fact a considerable share of the symptoms of many infections are caused by the host defence. Certain micro-organisms, such as *Mycobacterium leprae* or lymphocytic choriomeningitis virus, seem quite harmless on their own and the symptoms and complications caused by infections with these agents are to a large extent induced by the host defence trying to eliminate them.

Antibody-mediated immune reactions cause a tissue damaging inflammation by complement activation. Complexes produced between IgG antibodies and antigens from viruses (e.g. hepatitis virus), bacteria (*Treponema pallidum*) or parasites (*Schistosoma mansoni*) can cause vasculitis, nephritis and other immune complex diseases (*see further* chapters 16 and 19). Complement activation by such complexes and by the alternative pathway is found in the two life-threatening forms of dengue fever, the shock syndrome and haemorrhagic fever.

Complement activation especially by the alternative pathway caused by products from bacterial plaque on teeth is an important cause of the inflammation in the supportive tissues of the teeth including the bone, resulting in the very common periodontitis, which may cause loss of teeth.

A deficient T lymphocyte control of antibody production, together with a deficient killing and elimination of growing micro-organisms may be the reason for increased antibody production with immune complex formation as a result. This may occur in patients with erythema nodosum peprosum where large numbers of bacteria and antibodies are found in the skin together with signs of complement activation resulting in an Arthus' reaction (chapter 19). The mechanism behind subacute sclerosing panencephalitis (SSPE) may be similar. This lethal progressive dementia arises several years after acute measles or rubella and has been suggested to depend on the formation of complexes between antibodies and viral antigens remaining in the brain because of a deficient cell-mediated immunity not capable of elimination.

Virus infected host cells with viral antigens in the cell wall can stimulate virus specific T lymphocytes which then may support B lymphocytes to produce autoantibodies (cf. chapter 21). This may explain the autoantibody production often occurring during influenza, hepatitis and coxsackie infections. Autoimmunity is also seen in chronic bacterial infections such as syphilis, tuberculosis and leprosy. The tissue damage in chronic Chagas' disease, caused by *Trypanosoma cruzi*, may depend on autoreactive T lymphocytes induced against *T. cruzi* antigens cross-reacting with human tissue.

Injection of mycobacteria in the skin of a non-immune animal causes a limited local reaction whereas a much more extensive reaction with local necrosis (Koch's phenomenom) appears in an immune animal. A strong T lymphocyte mediated delayed hypersensitivity can on tuberculin testing cause a severe reaction with local necrosis and general symptoms with fever and malaise. The severe nerve damage seen in the tuberculoid form of leprosy, especially in the acute lepra reaction, is thought to depend on a strong cell-mediated immune reaction which also engages autologous tissues. The attack of the defence against the Schwann's cells, which often contain lepra bacteria, plays a major role in this sequence of events. In experimental infections with lymphocytic choriomeningitis virus, insignificant cell damage and symptoms occur if the animal does not have T lymphocytes directed against the virus. If such cells are injected into the experimental animal an immunological reaction is obtained destroying virus infected cells. As part of the host defence, the T lymphocytes kill the virus infected cells in the central nervous system, cells which cannot be regenerated. It is probable that such a mechanism can be involved in the pathogenesis of post-infection encephalitis that may appear after, for example measles and varicellae.

During chronic infections such as osteomyelitis, tuberculosis and leprosy, a complication called *amyloidosis* occasionally occurs. It depends on the deposition in parenchymal organs such as liver, spleen and kidneys of a homogeneous, hyaline extracellular substance, amyloid. Its fibrillar structure is visible on electron microscopy. It consists of a protein called AA and another still unknown high molecular weight protein. Amyloidosis appears not only secondary to infections, but also in patients with rheumatoid arthritis, ankylosing spondylitis and malignant tumours. Primary amyloidosis is seen in different forms and consists primarily of the variable part of L chains together with the same high molecular weight protein as in secondary amyloidosis. In multiple myeloma and Waldenström's disease a similar amyloid may occur as in primary amyloidosis. The pathogenesis is unknown but chronic stimulation of experimental animals with endotoxin or casein may give rise to amyloid deposits.

## Bibliography

BIENENSTOCK, J. (ed.) (1984). *Immunology of the Lung and Upper Respiratory Tract*. McGraw-Hill, New York.
EDEBO, L. B., ENERBÄCK, L. and STENDAHL, O. I. (eds.) (1981). Endocytosis and exocytosis in host defence. *Monogr. Allergy*, 17.
HANSON, L. Å., KALLOS, P. and WESTPHAL, O. (eds.) (1983). Host parasite relationships in Gram-negative infections. *Progr. Allergy*, 33.
HANSON, L. Å. and BRANDTZAEG, P. (1980). Secretory antibody systems. In *Immunologic Disorders in Infants and Children*, 2nd edn, Ed. by Stiehm, E. R. and Fulginiti, V. A. W. B. Saunders, Philadelphia.
KALLOS, P. (ed.) (1982). Immunity and concomitant immunity in infectious diseases. *Progr. Allergy*, 31.
LIEW, F. Y. (1982). Regulation of delayed type hypersensitivity to pathogens and alloantigens. *Immunology Today*, **3**, 18.

# Chapter 12

# Immunoprophylaxis—immunoglobulins, vaccines

**Erling Norrby**

Immunological reactions are important for the recovery from an infection and for the development of protection against a new infection. The degree and duration of the protection against a reinfection can vary depending on how extensively the infection is spread in the host. In many cases the protection is lifelong. It is important to distinguish between protection against renewed disease and protection against renewed infection. The infectious agent causes a reinfection, but this will be limited and does not cause any obvious symptoms. This renewed infection stimulates the immune response, enhancing the protection. Certain infectious agents can avoid the specific immune response either by having the capacity to change their surface antigens (such as influenza virus) or by appearing in a number of different stable antigenic varieties. Whereas *active immunization* through vaccination can induce lasting immunity, the injection of antibodies from another individual, *passive immunization*, will only protect temporarily. It can, however, be of great value to passively protect individuals with a decreased capacity to produce antibodies. All immunoprophylaxis, whether active or passive, is specific against certain infectious agents. By the use of polyvalent preparations the protection induced can be broadened.

## Passive immunization

An important source of protection for the newborn is the passive immunization resulting from the transfer of maternal IgG antibodies via the placenta. In other mammalian species, like the cow and pig, no immunoglobulins are transferred via the placenta, only via the milk. In these species the colostrum immunoglobulins are resorbed within the first one to two days after birth and appear as immunoglobulins in the blood of the offspring. In man there is a very limited uptake of antibodies from the milk and this takes place only during the first few days of life. Instead the dominating secretory IgA antibody fraction of the human milk remains on the mucous membranes where the antibodies prevent micro-organisms from coming into contact with the host.

The passively transferred specific maternal IgG antibodies protect efficiently against virus infections such as measles and poliomyelitis. Antitoxic antibodies against diphtheria and tetanus are also transferred. In this way the neonate is protected against neonatal tetanus if the mother has been vaccinated. The duration of the protection relates to the level of circulating antibodies in the mother. Measles antibodies of maternal origin may in some cases prevent the effective vaccination with a live measles virus vaccine up to 14 months of age. This is important to consider when determining

**TABLE 12.1. Vaccination calendar***

| | *Children under school age* |
|---|---|
| Tetanus–diphtheria | Three doses starting as 2–3 months of age and with 4–6 weeks' interval between the doses |
| Poliomyelitis I | At 9–10 months of age |
| Poliomyelitis II | At 10–11 months of age |
| Poliomyelitis III | At 18 months of age |
| Measles, mumps, rubella | At 18 months of age |
| Poliomyelitis IV | At about 6 years of age |
| | *Children of school age* |
| Tetanus–diphtheria | At 11 years of age |
| Measles, mumps, rubella | At 12–13 years of age |
| Tuberculosis | Only tuberculin-negative at 15 years of age |
| | *Adult* |
| Rubella | Post partum (seronegative primipara) and in risk groups, during anticonception treatment |

* There are large variations between vaccination programmes in different countries. This is the scheme recommended in Sweden, where inactivated polio vaccine is used. Oral polio vaccination is often given with DTP I, DTP II and at 18 months and 4–6 years.

the proper time of administration of live vaccines. Usually the infant is protected during the first six to eight months against measles infection. The maternal IgG antibodies do not prevent local infections on mucous membranes, or infections where cell-mediated immunity is of major importance.

For passive immunoprophylaxis or immunotherapy either heterologous hyper-immune serum or homologous human antibodies in the form of immunoglobulin preparations are used.

*Heterologous hyperimmune serum* from horse, cow or other animal species is used for protection against botulism, gas gangrene and snake poison and in developing countries also against tetanus and rabies. One advantage of the use of these hyperimmune preparations from heterologous donors is their high level of specific antibodies. A decisive drawback is their heterologous origin, which often causes dangerous side effects in the form of serum sickness. Because of this risk homologous preparations or active immunization is preferred. If a heterologous immune serum must be used, it should be taken from an animal species to which the recipient has not previously been immunized. It is likely that in the future heterologous hyperimmune sera can be replaced by hybridoma-produced monoclonal antibodies. *Homologous human antibodies* are mostly used in the form of purified IgG from pools of normal blood plasma. According to recommendations by WHO such preparations are called immunoglobulins. Specific preparations enriched in antibodies against one infectious agent are designated, for example, immunoglobulin against rubella or hepatitis B. Plasma from normal individuals is occasionally used for passive immunoprophylaxis. Serum from an individual recovering from a certain infection can be employed for enhanced protection against the specific infectious agent. The risk of transfer of infectious agents such as non-A, non-B hepatitis virus with plasma or serum should be considered.

Passive immunization by intravenous injection provides immediate protection. If the preparation is given intramuscularly approximately 20–40% of the dose is found in the circulation within two to three days. Active immunization does not induce adequate protection for several days. Because the half-life of IgG is three weeks (less for heterologous immunoglobulin) the effect of the passively transferred immunity is of little duration. The duration depends on the amount of immunoglobulin given and the content of the specific antibodies in the preparation. Optimally the protection lasts for some months.

The content of antibodies against different micro-organisms varies between individuals reflecting experiences of infections and capacity to mobilize humoral immune responses. Plasma to be used for an immunoglobulin preparation is therefore pooled from large numbers of individuals of different origin. In industrialized countries it may in some cases be necessary to import plasma in order to guarantee the presence of antibodies, for instance, against hepatitis A.

Immunoglobulin for intramuscular use is usually available as a 16.5% solution. These preparations often contain IgG polymers which may cause side effects especially in hypogammaglobulinaemia patients. They must be given intramuscularly since the risk of side effects is greater after intravenous administration. Special preparations for intravenous use are now available. These are usually freeze-dried and dissolved to an IgG conc. ixration of 5–10%. Immunoglobulin preparations are given either to patients with antibody deficiency syndromes as described in chapter 13 or prophylactically in the following situations:

*Measles* After exposure of an infant without protection against measles, immunoglobulin may be used. The amount of immunoglobulin given can be adjusted either to completely suppress or to mitigate the infection. A small modifying dose of immunoglobulin permits a mild infection, frequently inducing an immune response that provides lasting immunity. The immunoglobulin should be given within at least five to six days of the exposure. To ascertain lasting protection, an immunoglobulin dose totally protecting against the infection can be given with live measles vaccine administered six months later.

*Hepatitis A* The protective capacity of passive immunization against epidemic hepatitis is good. Immunoglobulin should be given to contacts of hepatitis patients and to travellers to countries where the risk of infection is significant. The long incubation period of this disease also gives an opportunity of passive immunization after exposure. Still it is urgent that immunoprophylaxis is given as soon as possible.

Specific immunoglobulin is mainly used against the following infections.

*Varicellae* To prevent severe infections in the neonatal period or to individuals with impaired host defence such as tumour patients undergoing immunosuppressive and/or cytotoxic treatment. This immunoglobulin preparation is made from convalescent serum from patients with herpes zoster.

*Other herpes infections* Preparations of immunoglobulin against herpes simplex virus and cytomegalovirus are being tested.

*Hepatitis B* To protect individuals likely to be exposed to this infection, such as hospital staff working with drug addicts or renal transplantation.

*Rabies* Given in combination with vaccination to attain immediate protection.

*Tetanus* To prevent or reduce the effect of the tetanus toxin.

*Rh prophylaxis*    This immunoglobulin with high levels of anti-D is given to prevent Rh immunization in an Rh-negative woman with an Rh-positive fetus, or in connection with an erroneous transfusion of Rh-positive blood to an Rh-negative individual (chapters 6 and 9).


## Active immunization

### Definitions

Towards the end of the eighteenth century, Jenner developed a method for prophylaxis against smallpox which, at that time, was one of the most severe infectious diseases. This happened half a century before Pasteur discovered the nature of infectious agents and before the concept of immunity existed. Jenner noted that individuals who, after contact with sick cattle, had attracted cowpox (which is a mild disease in man) acquired protection against the severe disease smallpox. He found that the cowpox infection could be transferred experimentally from cattle to man and further from man to man. Obviously the infectious agent of cowpox induced immunity against smallpox. Since the infectious agent originated from the cow (cow = vacca in Latin) it was called vaccine. This term is now generally used for all preparations employed for active immunization.

Two kinds of vaccines—inactivated and live—are being used. *Inactivated vaccines* either consist of whole killed micro-organisms, of isolated antigens of varying purity, or of detoxified toxin. *Live vaccines* contain infectious agents of selected strains with decreased pathogenicity. They function by causing a mild or symptom-free infection, which leaves immunity similar to that arising from the disease caused by a virulent strain.


### Inactivated vaccines

*General principles*

Immunization with these products results in the formation of antibodies. Cell-mediated immunity usually does not arise. Admixture of adjuvant may lead to induction of this type of immunity as well. Inactivated vaccines are usually given parenterally, but local application on mucous membranes has also been tried. Lasting local immunity has not been attained. Parenterally given vaccine induces production of circulating antibodies. The level of these antibodies depends on the amount of antigen in the preparation and the immunization schedule employed. Repeated injections at varying time intervals are usually required for the booster effect to result in a high antibody level. An exception may be vaccines composed of polysaccharide antigens which are only slowly degraded in the host.

The effect of an inactivated vaccine is primarily to induce immunity which prevents the spread of the infectious agent or its toxins from the primary site of infection. Efficient immunization may also induce a local protection on mucous membranes. The effect of the inactivated polio vaccine can be used as an example. With the immunization schedule employed for instance in Sweden, higher levels of circulating antibodies are attained than after a natural infection. Some of these IgG antibodies will appear on mucous membranes and in addition there is an induction of secretory IgA antibodies. This prevents the appearance of reinfections. The duration of the protection is related to the level of circulating antibodies. With the presently available inactivated polio vaccine lifelong protection seems to result from four injections. The use of new vaccines with a higher antigen content in which one or two injections may be sufficient, are currently being tested. In this situation it does not seem that a continuous exposure to antigen is necessary to give lasting protection.

The ideal inactivated vaccine should contain purified isolated antigens inducing efficient immunity. Elimination of irrelevant antigens reduces the competition with the important immunogens and eliminates them as causes of side effects such as allergy. Only a few currently available inactivated vaccines have accomplished this. Most vaccines contain whole infectious agents destroyed by various treatments. In addition to the microbial antigens there are often components from the substrate, for instance cell residues and antibiotics in virus vaccines. Preservatives may also be present.

The inactivating treatment is critical since it is a delicate task to selectively destroy the infectious capacity while keeping the immunogenic properties intact. In the early phase of vaccine development, crude measures like heating or treatment with phenol or merthiolate were used. Treatment with formalin has also been applied extensively. Lately other procedures with a more direct effect on the genetic material such as treatment with beta-propiolactone or hydroxylamine have been tried. Inactivated vaccines used today are mostly produced with methods developed before the time of molecular microbiology. Often the essential antigens in the vaccines have not been fully defined. This is especially true for certain bacterial vaccines.

Inactivated vaccine preparations must be controlled as to their harmlessness and efficiency. The inactivation of all infectious agents, the absence of impurities with other infectious or inactivated micro-organisms, as well as the content of potentially harmful components such as preservatives and foreign proteins must be controlled. As a verification of the potency of a preparation, the content of relevant antigens is usually employed. This content is compared with a standard preparation which has been proved to immunize humans.

The effect of an inactivated vaccine can be studied by determination of specific circulating antibodies appearing after immunization. The levels of antitoxins, or neutralizing antibodies against a virus can be measured. The most critical measure of efficiency is to determine the capacity of the vaccine to prevent the appearance of disease after natural exposure in large groups of completely vaccinated individuals.

Hypersensitivity reactions are the most common type of side effects of vaccines. They can be directed against foreign proteins, or remaining antibiotics in the preparation. An intradermal prick test (*see* chapter 17) can be performed to control the tendency to react before the vaccination. If a reaction occurs, but the vaccination is regarded as necessary, a small repeated dose of the vaccine can be tried using intervals of a week. It is important that the possibility of treating anaphylactic shock is available when vaccinating.

*Bacterial vaccines*

Toxoids, i.e. detoxified toxins, have been produced for immunization against *diphtheria* and *tetanus*. The extracellular toxins are purified by eliminating the bacteria from the culture. A chemically and immunologically homogeneous toxin can be obtained and detoxified by treatment with formalin without any essential loss of the immunogenicity. Currently used vaccines consist of semipurified products. Both toxoids are included in the triple vaccine (DTP: diphtheria, tetanus, pertussis; *see below*). Preparations only containing diphtheria and/or tetanus toxoid are used for booster immunization and also for primary immunization if the pertussis component is to be avoided. The DT vaccine often contain aluminium phosphate as an adjuvant.

Another type of inactivated bacterial vaccine consists of *polysaccharide antigens*, such as capsular material from *pneumococci* and *meningococci*. Purified polysaccharide capsules from pneumococci were already used during the 1930s but interest in them disappeared after the discovery of penicillin. There is a need for these vaccines, however, especially in elderly people and also in splenectomized individuals who run a large risk of attracting severe, even lethal pneumococcal infections. A vaccine composed of 12–14 of the most common pneumococcal capsules out of the 84 known serotypes is now available.

There are also vaccines against meningococcus type A and C whereas no useful vaccine against type B has yet been prepared. Purified polysaccharides are poor immunogens and frequently even function as tolerogens. There is also a deficient antibody response before the age of two presumably due to a poor production of IgG2 antibodies. Attaching the polysaccharides to protein carriers opens possibilities for the development of a new generation of polysaccharide vaccines.

A satisfactory and presumably long-lasting immunity is produced by the available bacterial polysaccharide vaccines, often after a single dose. This may be due to the inefficiency of the host in degrading these substances.

A number of inactivated bacterial vaccines containing killed intact micro-organisms are now being used. The vaccine against *pertussis* is given separately or included in the DTP vaccine. In the latter mixed preparation *Bordetella pertussis* functions as an adjuvant similar to mycobacteria. Carefully controlled field trials have shown that the vaccine is protective. Some recent preparations have shown less efficient protective capacity and complications causing brain damage have occurred in rare cases. In recent years there has been a resistance in some countries against the use of this vaccine. As a result there has been a resurgence in the number of pertussis cases. New pertussis vaccines are being developed, especially based on the pertussis toxin.

Inactivated *typhoid vaccine* consists of whole killed bacteria. Heat treatment or acetone inactivation is usually employed. The problem with typhoid vaccination is that the parenteral immunization should be required to produce local immunity in the gut. The protection obtained with the available vaccines in field trials has varied strikingly but usually figures around 70% are given. Since the vaccine often produces local side effects, probably Arthus' type, and gives limited protection it should only be used in well-defined situations. The protective capacity of *paratyphoid vaccines* which are similar to the available typhoid vaccines, is so poor that they are rarely used.

The *cholera vaccine* offers problems similar to those of the typhoid vaccine. The protective capacity of parenteral immunization with heat-killed bacteria against a local bacterial infection in the gut has generally been assumed to be rather limited and of short duration. The cholera toxin producing the symptoms of cholera has been identified and characterized as to its structure during the last few years. The non-toxic binding portion of the toxin has been found to be immunogenic and induces immunity which is enhanced by the presence of lipopolysaccharide antigen from the bacteria. Such combined vaccines are being tested.

### Virus vaccines

A number of different killed virus vaccines have been produced. Of major importance are the vaccines against rabies, influenza and poliomyelitis. Formalin killed vaccines against measles and mumps have caused problems since the employed inactivation procedures have destroyed certain critical antigens. Similar problems have occurred during the development of a formalin killed vaccine against respiratory syncytial (RS) virus and parainfluenza virus. Reactions of the Arthus' type have appeared in the lungs of vaccinated individuals exposed to wild virus.

*Rabies vaccine*    This was first developed by Pasteur who used attenuated virus from rabbit brain. Now killed vaccines are used instead. Virus cultivated in human diploid cells are good immunogens. This vaccine should be used prophylactically in selected cases, only where there is a high risk of exposure. Inactivated rabies vaccine is also used for immunization of humans who are suspected of having been exposed to the virus. The problem is that in previously non-immunized individuals there is a very slow increase in the antibody levels so that the infecting virus may not be neutralized before it has become inaccessible because of intra-axonal localization. The most important measures to stop rabies infection is therefore local revision of the infected wound and immediate injection of immunoglobulin with high levels of antibodies against rabies virus.

*Influenza vaccines*    These have been used since the Second World War. The virus is cultivated in the allantois of embryonated eggs. After purification and concentration the virus is inactivated with formalin. The effect of the inactivated influenza vaccine depends on a number of factors. Of major importance is the capacity of these viruses to gradually change the character of their surface antigens. Because of this virus strains to be used for the vaccine preparation must be selected every year. The objective is that the antigens of the vaccine virus should be as similar as possible to the virus that is expected to circulate in the community during the forthcoming season. Of major importance from an epidemiological point of view are the different subtypes of influenza virus type A. The vaccines often also contain strains of type B virus. This type has a lesser tendency to change its antigenic character and also causes more limited epidemics.

The vaccine is usually given as a parenteral injection. This should not be expected to give an efficient immunity in the respiratory tract, but because of the previous sensitization with similar antigens via natural infections a protective effect is obtained. This effect is estimated to vary between 40–80%. The large variations depend on differences in the similarity of the used vaccine strain and the circulating wild virus. To immunize more efficiently against new antigenic determinants two injections with one month's interval may be used.

The influenza vaccine has a relatively limited use in its present form. If an expected epidemic is due to a totally new variant of the virus and causes severe disease, it may be reasonable to vaccinate large parts of the population. In this situation small children can also be vaccinated, but generally young children should not be immunized against influenza, since the disease is usually milder in children than adults. Furthermore the children should acquire their initial immunity against influenza infections through natural exposure.

*Inactivated polio vaccine*    This is produced by formalin treatment. Sweden, Holland and Finland are among the few countries in the world that have continued to use only inactivated polio vaccine. Most other countries where polio vaccination is performed have turned to live vaccine. The vaccination programmes with the inactivated vaccine have been very successful in eliminating not only poliomyelitis, but also the polio virus from the society. This suggests as mentioned above that the parenterally given vaccine also induces a certain mucosal immunity, preventing or restricting virus replication in the gut.

Since polio virus no longer circulates in the society subchronic infections are rare and the only way to become immune is by vaccination. In this situation it is very important that there is complete coverage with the vaccine. Continuous follow-up of the population suggests that a long-lasting immunity has been obtained and that further boosters are unnecessary.

*Other inactivated vaccines*   A formalin killed vaccine which can protect against *tick-borne encephalitis* is available. It is used only to protect individuals with a high risk of exposure. A vaccine against *hepatitis B* virus has recently been introduced. Since this virus cannot be propagated in tissue cultures, serum from carriers of chronic hepatitis B virus infection is used as a source of the antigen for the vaccine production. The vaccine contains parts of the virus membrane. These purified products are inactivated with formalin for safety. The preparation should only be used for immunization of people with increased risk of exposure.

*Future inactivated vaccines*   Herpes simplex virus vaccines similar to the previously mentioned influenza vaccine have been produced.

Modern biotechnology has opened totally new possibilities for the production of vaccines. Genes directing the production of critical surface structures of viruses have been introduced in bacteria. Antigens from foot-and-mouth disease virus, influenza virus and hepatitis B virus have been produced in this way. In the systems employed there is no glucosylation, but antigen activity has been demonstrated in the produced proteins. Successful expression of genes for virus surface antigens has also been obtained in yeast and mammalian tissue culture cells. Another projected possibility for preparation of vaccines is the synthesis of polypeptides of 6-20 amino acids. These polypeptides have been selected to represent exposed parts of viral surface proteins. Somewhat unexpectedly it has been found that such polypeptides can induce formation of antibodies which can react with the intact protein. It is possible that future vaccines can be made chemically homogeneous and be produced without the cultivation of any micro-organism. Finally it should be added that protective antibodies against bacterial polysaccharides have been produced by means of anti-idiotypic antibodies in animal models. It seems quite realistic that vaccines may be produced using this principle.

## Live vaccines
*General principles*

The principle behind the use of live vaccines is to produce a mild infection in the host. In connection with this infection relatively large amounts of immunogens are produced and the immunity induced shows many similarities with that resulting from a natural infection. The infectious agent used must be attenuated so that it does not cause any, or only mild, symptoms. The possible reactions caused by the vaccine must always be compared with those occurring after a natural infection. In the evaluation of live vaccines one must differentiate expected and acceptable vaccine reactions from side effects. In individuals with deficient cell-mediated immunity live vaccines can cause very severe, at times lethal, infections (*see* chapter 13).

A special type of live vaccine is used in the USA to prevent respiratory tract infections caused by adenovirus. The vaccine consists of regular wild virus contained in a capsule which dissolves in the intestine after oral ingestion. A symptomless gut infection follows. The infection does not spread to the respiratory tract, but the immune response induced gives future protection against infections in the respiratory tract.

The first live vaccine developed had a natural background. As mentioned earlier Jenner noticed that the pox virus infecting cows could induce immunity against the smallpox virus in man. Yellow fever, measles, mumps and rubella vaccines were developed by repeated passages of virus in cell cultures of animal origin. The viruses were modified in their capacity to cause disease in man. More recently genetic methods have been used to produce modified vaccine strains of viruses. Temperature sensitive mutants have been produced, primarily of various respiratory tract viruses. The objective is that these mutants should be able to propagate well at 32–33 °C, but not at 37°C, and that therefore when applied in the airways they can only cause a limited infection. So far, however, no useful vaccine strains have been developed by this approach.

The major problem has been that when the infectious agent propagates in the host in several consecutive generations, there is the possibility for mutational reversion of the virus to its wild form. The problem of the genetic instability of the virus is especially evident if it has the capacity to spread from the vaccinee to other individuals in the surrounding area. Such a spread does not occur with, for example yellow fever, measles, mumps and rubella virus vaccines, but does occur with the live polio vaccine. Using genetic engineering hopefully more stable live vaccines (for instance against poliomyelitis) will become available.

Live vaccines are relatively easy to administer and can in some instances give immunity of a very long duration with only one injection. Several live vaccines are given in repeated doses at intervals. The live polio vaccine is given in three consecutive oral immunizations at monthly intervals. The reason is that the three types of live polio virus included in the vaccine have a tendency to compete with each other when replicating in the gut. This interference results in one type dominating during the first immunization and another type during the next immunization, etc. Interference phenomena are important to take into consideration when several live virus vaccines are used in a short period of time and also because of the risk of competition between a vaccine virus and naturally circulating wild viruses. In general, the interval between two immunizations of live vaccines should be at least four weeks. It has been found, however, that live measles, rubella and mumps can be given simultaneously with responses against all three vaccines equal to those which would occur if they had been given separately.

Interference between vaccine virus and wild virus has caused great problems with the use of live polio vaccine in developing countries. In such areas often only about 50% of the vaccines become seropositive. Another problem in developing countries concerns the stability of some of the live virus vaccines. The use of lyophilized products kept at $+4\,^{\circ}\mathrm{C}$ provides the possibility of successful vaccination in 90–100% of the vaccinees. Unfortunately there are often great problems maintaining an effective cold chain from the producer to the vaccinee.

The presence of circulating antibodies can prevent a live vaccine from inducing an immune response. A live vaccine should therefore not be given to a person who can be expected to have antibodies, either due to placental transfer of maternal antibodies in a young infant, or originating from recently given immunoglobulin, or blood transfusion. Some live vaccines should therefore not be used before the age of 14 months. By necessity such vaccines may need to be given earlier in developing countries.

Live vaccines are controlled in a number of ways. The presence of a sufficient amount of infectious material is determined. For virus vaccines the dose usually varies between $10^3$ and $10^5$ infectious units. The degree of attenuation of the used vaccine strain is mostly defined by the determination of certain genetic markers. For several live vaccine strains no useful markers are available. Finally the vaccine must not be contaminated with irrelevant micro-organisms, and should be checked for purity.

### Bacterial vaccines

Among live bacterial vaccines *BGG* (Bact. Calmette–Guerin), or the Calmette vaccine, is the only one of interest in human medicine. This vaccine consists of an attenuated variant of bovine mycobacteria, which has been produced by long-term cultures on a special growth inhibiting medium. Field trials in Great Britain and Scandinavia have shown the vaccine to be protective in about 80% of vaccinees. Less clear-cut results have been obtained in countries where related saprophytic mycobacteria commonly occur.

The parenteral vaccination with the BCG vaccine causes a local usually limited inflammatory reaction. Occasionally the local reaction can be more extensive and with some preparation osteitis has occurred. Therefore vaccination of neonates, for instance in Sweden, has been stopped and only children who are still tuberculin-negative at the age of 13–14 are given BCG vaccination.

A new type of *typhoid vaccine* has been produced in Switzerland. The vaccine strain is a mutant which cannot survive in the intestine due to a metabolic deficiency. Still it seems to provide good immunity.


*Virus vaccines*

A number of effective live virus vaccines are available. Six of them will be discussed in detail. The vaccine against *smallpox* eliminated this disease which for thousands of years had been the cause of severe epidemics in man. Vaccine virus replicates in the epidermis. At times the vaccination could cause severe complications. It caused fatal disease in infants with severe combined immunodeficiency. In patients with eczema generalized skin infections could result. Post-vaccinal encephalitis also occurred occasionally. It probably had an immunopathological background since it appeared about a week after the normal vaccine reaction had started to disappear and was characterized by demyelinization and absence of infectious virus.

The efficiency of the vaccine was well illustrated by WHO during the last decades in a programme for global eradication of smallpox. Three circumstances made this programme possible and successful. Firstly there is only one antigen type of the virus and the vaccine protected efficiently against this type. Secondly the virus only caused acute infection. The virus did not remain in the organism and did not reappear in active form. The third condition was that there was no reservoir for the virus among animals. In 1978 the last case of smallpox was seen and in 1980 the Earth was declared free of smallpox.

*The yellow fever vaccine*   This is made from an attenuated virus strain, designated 17D. The vaccine very rarely causes any side effects and it gives a very long-lasting immunity. One injection protects for at least ten years.

*Live polio vaccine*   This is used to a large extent world-wide. The strains included in the vaccine today are mainly those introduced by Sabin in 1960. The vaccine is given orally and causes a symptomless intestinal infection followed by excretion of the vaccine virus. The vaccine which contains all three virus types is given three times at monthly intervals. In a successfully vaccinated individual lifelong immunity is expected to occur, providing that no other enteroviruses have interfered preventing one or all of the three vaccine type strains from inducing immunity. The genetic instability of the vaccine virus has caused some problems. In careful follow-up studies in the USA it has been noted that cases of paralysis occur once per 3.2 million distributed vaccine doses. These cases appear in the vaccinee or in non-immune individuals infected with the virus excreted by a vaccinee. During 1969–1980, 102 vaccine associated cases of poliomyelitis were reported in the USA. Twenty-five of these were healthy vaccinees, 65 were healthy contacts and 12 were individuals with a previously unknown immunodeficiency. Currently there are more cases of poliomyelitis caused by the vaccine virus in the USA than by the wild virus. This is primarily an expression of the fact that the vaccination programme has been so efficient that wild virus infections have been virtually eliminated. The few vaccine associated cases of paralysis are a problem, which can only be eliminated by changing the character of the virus included in the vaccine. Protection after vaccination with a live virus is good and there should be an especially good local immunity in the intestine. The duration of this immunity may be limited and asymptomatic reinfections may occur some years after the vaccination.

*Live measles vaccine*    In the beginning of the 1960s Enders developed a live vaccine by adapting the virus to growth in chicken embryo cultures. The vaccine strain gave some reactions with fever and exanthema but with the further attenuated vaccine strains used today reactions after vaccination are negligible. A slight increase in temperature and occasionally a discrete exanthema can appear but the symptoms do not usually influence the activities of the vaccinated child.

Vaccination can be performed as late as five days after exposure to wild measles virus. The mild vaccine virus infection can then replace the normal measles infection.

Vaccinated individuals do not excrete virus. Side effects after the vaccination are rare. There has been a careful evaluation of the appearance of complications from the central nervous system. The frequency of acute encephalitis is only about 1 case per million vaccinated, as compared with 1 case per 1000 patients with measles.

The more severe but very rare late complication to natural measles, SSPE (subacute sclerosing panencephalitis), is reduced by a factor of at least five to ten with the use of live vaccine. The protective capacity of the vaccine in field trials has exceeded 90% in several studies.

Failing protection after vaccination can have several causes. In some cases the propagation of the vaccine virus has been hindered by the presence of low levels of antibodies either of maternal origin, or from previously given immunoglobulin. In other cases the vaccination has not functioned since the vaccine was not stored properly. This is a common cause of vaccination failure in developing countries. A vaccine with better heat stability is presently being tested. Another special problem in developing countries is that measles causes a very severe infection during the first year of life. If possible vaccination therefore should be given by the age of six to nine months and a renewed vaccination at the age of one and a half years. There is currently no information stating that more than one vaccination is required in industrialized countries. Still, in Sweden two immunizations are given in the combined live measles, mumps, and rubella vaccine with one dose at one and a half years of age and the other at 12–13 years of age.

*Live mumps vaccine*    The vaccine is produced in chicken embryo cultures. It causes an infection which is not spread from the vaccinee. Complications are rare. The antibody response after vaccination is much lower than after natural infection, but seems to be of long duration. More than 90% of the vaccinees are protected.

*Live rubella vaccine*    This vaccine is used to protect against infection of the fetus during the first trimester of pregnancy. The target group of this vaccine therefore is females of child-bearing age. Immunization can be performed as mentioned at one and a half and 12–13 years of age. Vaccination of older females should be done during contraception treatment for at least two months so that the vaccine virus cannot be transferred to the fetus causing congenital damage, although the risk for this seems to be negligible judging from available data. Just like the natural infection caused by wild virus, the vaccine reaction is mild, but occasional cases of arthralgia are seen. The vaccine infection is not spread from the vaccinee. The duration of the protection is probably long-lasting, although local reinfections in the respiratory tract can occur as soon as 6–12 months after vaccination.

*Live vaccines for the future*   These will probably mainly include products aiming at protection against respiratory tract infections caused, for instance, by influenza, parainfluenza and RS (respiratory syncytial) virus. Live influenza vaccines have been tested in field trials but no virus strain with a suitable degree of attenuation and genetic stability has yet been found. The problem concerning the RS virus infections can be seen during the first year of life. It is therefore difficult to select the best time for administration of this live virus vaccine. Live vaccines against varicella and cyto-megalovirus infections are currently being tested. Severe primary infections apparently can be avoided, but even vaccine virus strains cause latent infections.

## Bibliography

FULGINITI, V. A. (1982). Immunizations: Current controversies. *J. Pediat.*, **101**, 487.
NORRBY, E. (1983). Viral vaccines; the use of currently available products and future developments. *Archives Virology*, **76**, 163.
SELBY, P. (ed.) (1976). *Influenza: Virus Vaccines and Strategy.* Academic Press, London.
VOLLER, A. and FRIEDMAN, H. (eds.) (1978). *New Trends and Developments in Vaccines.* MTP Press Ltd, Lancaster, England.

# Chapter 13

# Deficiencies in host defence

**Lars Å. Hanson**

In 1952 Bruton described a boy who had repeated severe bacterial infections and who lacked the gammaglobulin fraction in serum on electrophoresis. His serum also lacked antibodies. Bruton called the syndrome 'agammaglobulinaemia'.

Many other cases with different types of deficiencies in host defence have now been described. Most, but not all immunodeficiency syndromes are rare. It is important to find these patients because many of them can be successfully treated. Furthermore these 'experiments of nature' with different deficiencies in the immune response contribute significantly to our present knowledge about the various components in the immune response and their importance for the host defence against infections. Observations made in patients with immunodeficiencies have given support to the concept that the immune response can be crudely divided into two systems:

(1) immunity mediated via humoral antibodies produced by antigen-stimulated B lymphocytes developing into plasma cells, and
(2) immunity mediated by antigen-stimulated T lymphocytes which develop into cytotoxic T cells and T cells involved in delayed hypersensitivity producing lymphokines.

Bruton's case of 'agammaglobulinaemia' illustrates a deficiency in the production of the humoral antibodies. The deficiency indicated by A in *Figure 13.1* can be located at different levels from the bursa equivalent down to the plasma cell, but also in T helper and suppressor cells (*Table 13.1*, Part I). Furthermore there are deficiencies at different levels of the cell-mediated immune system indicated as B in *Figure 13.1* and summarized in Part II in *Table 13.1*. Combined deficiencies including antibody-mediated as well as cell-mediated immunity are found in various forms and are indicated by C in *Figure 13.1* and summarized in Part III, *Table 13.1*. Patients with deficiencies in leucocytes and complement demonstrate the important role of these non-specific components in the defence against infections (Part IV in *Table 13.1*).

There are many and varied forms of deficiencies in the host defence. The schematic outline in *Figure 13.1* gives a rough and simplified presentation of the most important among at least 23 types now known, several of which have subgroups.

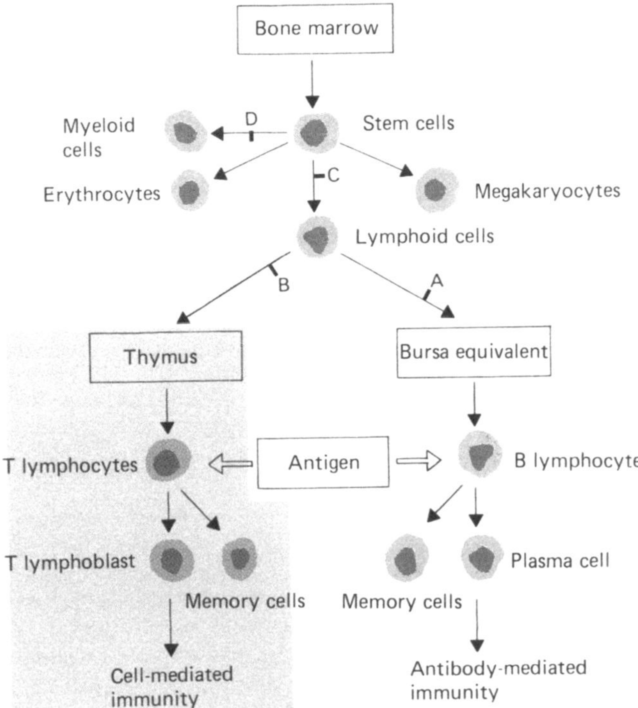


*Figure 13.1* The same diagram of the lymphoid system as presented in chapters 1 and 7, here with approximate localizations of various deficiencies in host defence. A, the deficiencies in antibody production; B, in cell-mediated immune reactions; C, combined deficiencies in both of these effector mechanisms; D, indicates abnormalities in phagocytes

## Deficiencies in immunity mediated by humoral antibodies: hypogammaglobulinaemia–antibody deficiency syndromes

In individuals with deficiencies in the production of the three dominating immunoglobulin classes IgG, IgM and IgA, there is often a lack of the gammaglobulin fraction in serum analysed with electrophoresis. Quantification of the immunoglobulins (Appendix 2) usually demonstrates small amounts of immunoglobulins. *Hypogammaglobulinaemia* is therefore often a better designation than agammaglobulinaemia. The designation *antibody deficiency syndrome* is also useful.

### Physiological hypogammaglobulinaemia

The active transport of maternal IgG via the placenta results in a higher serum IgG concentration in the full term newborn than in the mother, but the neonate lacks or has very little IgA and IgM. The transferred maternal IgG is catabolized with a half-life of three weeks and the infant's IgG serum level drops to approximately 3–5 g/l at three to

**TABLE 13.1. Deficiencies in host defence**

I. *Deficiencies in immunity mediated by humoral antibodies: Hypogammaglobulinaemia–antibody deficiency syndrome*
  (1) Physiological hypogammaglobulinaemia
  (2) Transient hypogammaglobulinaemia
  (3) Infantile X-linked agammaglobulinaemia (Bruton)
  (4) Common variable immunodeficiency
  (5) Acquired, secondary hypogammaglobulinaemia
    (a) Impaired differentiation (intrauterine rubella infection)
    (b) Increased losses (via kidneys, intestine or burns)
    (c) Abnormal production (leukaemia, myeloma, immunosuppression, malnutrition)
  (6) Selective immunoglobulin deficiency

II. *Deficiencies in cell-mediated immunity*
  (1) Congenital deficiency with thymus hypoplasia and hypoparathyroidism (Di George); chronic mucocutaneous candidiasis
  (2) Acquired deficiencies in AIDS (acquired immunodeficiency syndrome), Hodgkin's disease, sarcoidosis, certain infections, malnutrition and after immunosuppression

III. *Deficiencies in immunity mediated by humoral antibodies and cell-mediated immunity*
  (1) Severe combined immunodeficiency (SCID)
  (2) Reticular cell dysgenesis
  (3) Bare lymphocyte syndrome
  (4) Ataxia–telangiectasia
  (5) Wiskott–Aldrich's syndrome

IV. *Deficiencies in non-specific host defence*
  (1) Granulocyte abnormalities
    (a) Agranulocytosis and granulocytopenia (several forms); Autosomal recessive (Kostmann); autosomal dominant (Hitzig); Cyclic agranulocytosis; agranulocytosis +dysgammaglobulinaemia; acquired toxic or allergic agranulocytosis
    (b) Chronic granulomatous disease
    (c) Chediak–Higashi syndrome
  (2) Complement deficiencies

four months of age (cf. *Figure 2.7*, p. 29). Because of the IgG antibody production of the infant the level increases slowly thereafter. IgG1 and IgG3 antibodies are produced at a higher rate than IgG2 and IgG4 during the first two years of life. During the neonatal period an efficient IgM antibody response is mounted against the many antigens to which the newborn is exposed.

The physiological hypogammaglobulinaemia is not accompanied by any clinically noticeable sensitivity to infections, even if bacterial sepsis/meningitis (often due to Gram-negative organisms) show an aggregation in the neonatal period. This has been connected with the fact that only IgG antibodies are transplacentally transferred, whereas IgM antibodies which provide most of the bactericidal activity against Gram-negative bacteria increase during the first weeks of life.

Premature babies have an increased risk of infections. This is probably due to a number of defence factors which are not yet fully developed. For instance the serum IgG level increases with fetal age and can therefore be low in premature babies. The capacity to produce IgM is clearly decreased in the premature infant of gestational age below 33 weeks.

## Transient hypogammaglobulinaemia

In a few infants the antibody production is delayed. The IgG level in these infants may drop to about 1 g/l where it remains for several months. During this period they show an increased risk of infections with repeated bacterial purulent infections in the skin, respiratory tract and meninges. The delayed antibody production usually starts at approximately one to two years of age and they then normalize. The cause of this abnormality in antibody production is unknown.

## Infantile X-linked agammaglobulinaemia (Bruton)

Pronounced antibody deficiency appears in two forms; either as an *X-linked recessively inherited* disease, or as '*variable immunodeficiency*'. Both forms are characterized by genetically based abnormalities of the antibody production. The lowest serum immunoglobulin levels are found in patients with the sex-linked form (I (3) in *Table 13.1*).

*Histological picture*   The histological picture in the cases of congenital X-linked agammaglobulinaemia, is characterized by the lack of plasma cells in the spleen, intestinal mucosa, bone marrow and lymph glands, and also after antigen stimulation. This disease depends on a deficient development of B lymphocytes from pre-B cells resulting in a lack of plasma cells and an underdevelopment of the thymus independent part of the peripheral lymphoid tissue with lack of primary and secondary follicles. The number of lymphocytes in the tissue is decreased even if the lymphocyte count is normal in the peripheral blood where T lymphocytes normally dominate. The hypoplasia of the lymphoid tissue in lymph glands and intestinal mucosa in these patients is striking in comparison with normal tissue (*Figure 13.2A–D*). Hyperplasia of reticular cells can result in enlargement of the lymph glands.

*Clinical picture*   Symptoms often appear during the second half of the first year of life in patients with sex-linked agammaglobulinaemia. Before that they are protected by the maternal transplacentally provided IgG antibodies. The clinical picture is dominated by an increased frequency of infections, especially bacterial purulent infections such as pyoderma, otitis media, sinusitis, pneumonia, life-threatening sepsis and meningitis. Gastroenteritis is common, as is recurrent pneumonia resulting in chronic lung damage, especially bronchiectases. The infections are often caused by Gram-positive cocci, or *Haemophilus influenzae*. Fatal echovirus infections have occurred, however, and oral vaccination with live polio vaccines has caused paralytic poliomyelitis, as has wild virus. The antibody deficiency does not result in an increased frequency of mycotic, or viral infections, Measles, rubella, influenza and upper respiratory tract infections run the same course as in normal children and also leave immunity.

Children with congenital agammaglobulinaemia have an increased frequency of arthritis which is similar to rheumatoid arthritis, but without rheumatoid factor (this auto-antibody against IgG appearing in rheumatoid arthritis is further described in chapter 21). It is striking that arthritis improves or normalizes when the patient is given substitution in the form of immunoglobulins. Other conditions regarded as immunological diseases, i.e. caused by immunological mechanisms (cf. chapters 16, 17, 19 and 21), have been seen in cases of congenital agammaglobulinaemia, for instance dermatomyositis, polymyositis, scleroderma and atopic allergies. Malignancies also

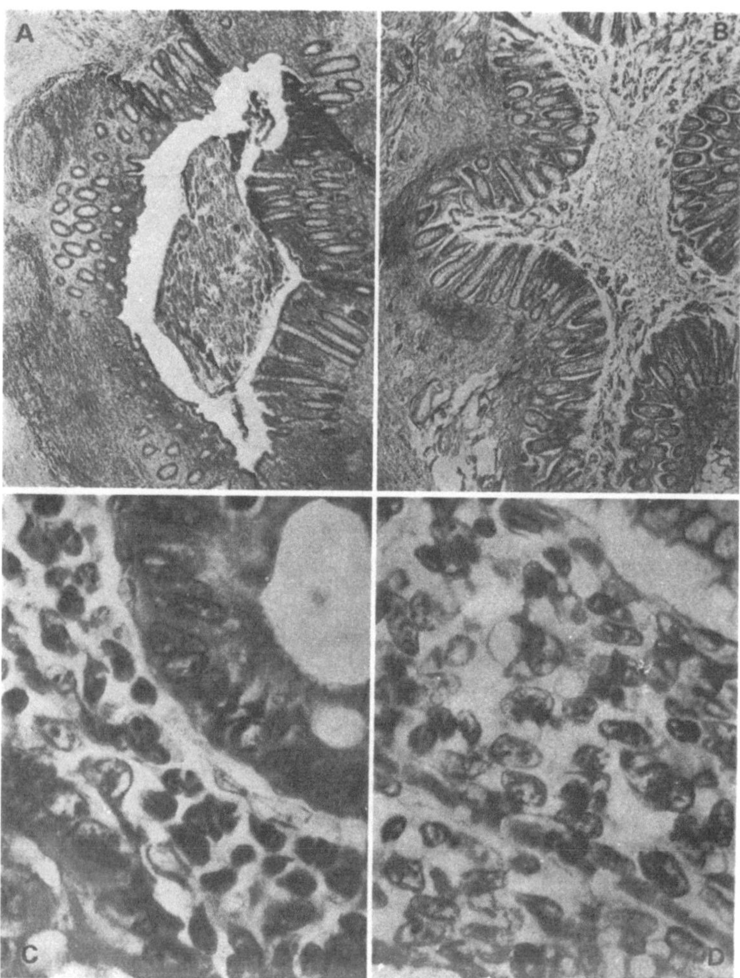

*Figure 13.2* Comparison between lymphoid tissue in appendix from an immunologically normal individual (A and C) and from one with Bruton's agammaglobulinaemia (B and D). A shows the many cells in the lymphoid tissue and appendix
from a normal individual. The follicles, diffuse lymphoid tissue and large numbers of
cells in the lamina propria are evident. B shows in contrast how a patient with
agammaglobulinaemia almost completely lacks lymphoid tissue in the appendix.
There are no follicles and lamina propria is deficient in lymphoid cells. C shows in
greater magnification the lamina propria from the appendix of a normal individual.
The many plasma cells are clearly seen. D finally shows lamina propria in the appendix
from the patient with agammaglobulinaemia. There are many reticular cells, but very
few lymphocytes and no plasma cells. (From R. A. Good *et al.* (1962), *Progress in
Allergy*, **6**, 187)

appear in an increased frequency in these patients. The tumours are usually
mesenchymal with lymphomas and leukaemias, but a few are also epithelial.

BCG vaccination can be given without complications and results, as do tuberculosis
and mycotic infections, in the development of delayed hypersensitivity reactions. This

demonstrates that cell-mediated immunity appears in patients with antibody deficiency syndromes. This is also illustrated by the fact that patients can reject allogenic transplants, even if rejection may be slower than in normal individuals. The patients' T lymphocytes respond normally on exposure to mitogens or antigens. They have normal inflammatory reactions and their phagocytosis is normal. During infections leucocytosis as well as leucopenia has been noted. Complement, interferon production and properdin are found at normal levels.

### Diagnosis

The diagnosis is reached by means of the typical appearance of repeated bacterial infections, decreased levels of serum immunoglobulins and a deficient antibody response after antigen stimulation. IgG is usually below 1.0, often below 0.15 g/l and IgM as well as IgA are usually below 0.02–0.03 g/l. Bacterial antibodies and alloagglutinins cannot be demonstrated at all or only in very small amounts in serum. With sensitive techniques antibodies can at times be found against some viruses. No, or only a few, B lymphocytes with immunoglobulin receptors are found in the blood, but pre-B cells can be seen in the bone marrow. In contrast the T lymphocytes are usually normal. The lack of plasma cells in a local lymph gland after antigenic stimulation is typical.

### Treatment

Treatment of patients with congenital agammaglobulinaemia includes the use of antibiotics to fight the acute infection. Furthermore the patients should be given immunoglobulins at regular intervals throughout their lives to improve their defence against infections. The intramuscular preparations sooner or later seem to give side effects, sometimes rather dramatically with back pain, dyspnoea, erythema and occasionally a drop in blood pressure in patients with antibody deficiency syndromes. Now preparations are available that can be given intravenously. Some of these preparations have shown very few side effects. The smallest dose given is 25 mg/kg per week. Some patients may require higher doses, around 100 mg/kg per week. Most patients do well on injections every third week but with intravenous preparations larger doses can be given such that every fourth to fifth week can be sufficient.

With adequate doses of immunoglobulin most patients remain in a good condition. Without the immunoglobulin prophylaxis or if it is given in inadequate doses retarded growth, subnormal weight and height may result. More serious, however, is the fact that they develop chronic lung damage which can so severely impair the lung function that they become chronically ill with a poor prognosis.

### Common variable immunodeficiency

Common variable immunodeficiency (I (4) in *Table 13.1*) is less well defined than the infantile sex-linked form. It is really a provisional term, probably including several forms of antibody deficiency syndromes. Some of these were previously designated sporadic, or primary 'acquired' hypogammaglobulinaemia. Most patients with antibody deficiency are given this diagnosis, both children and adults of either sex. The inheritance is not quite clear, but even in the closest family there are usually no other cases.

In many patients with variable immunodeficiency the decreased antibody production is probably due to a defect in the maturation of the B lymphocytes. In some cases the cell deficiency is due to a lack of T helper cells, in a few cases it may be due to an increased T suppressor activity. Autoantibodies against B or T lymphocytes have also been demonstrated as a cause of the abnormality. A disturbance in the development of B lymphocytes to plasma cells has been noted in patients with an autosomal recessive form of deficiency of transcobalamin II. This also results in megaloblastic anaemia and deficient granulocyte function.

On *histological* examination the patients with variable immunodeficiency usually lack plasma cells and secondary follicles in their lymphoid tissues similar to those with the congenital form of the antibody deficiency. The thymus-dependent system usually appears normal.

*Clinical picture*    The symptoms of variable immunodeficiency are dominated by bacterial infections, especially repeated sinusitis and pneumonia. Many of these patients develop bronchiectasis as well as emphysema and lung fibrosis. Symptoms from the intestine in the form of malabsorption, diarrhoea and steatorrhoea are relatively common. Prolonged intestinal infections with *Giardia lamblia*, *Campylobacter* and rotavirus are more common among these patients.

Various haematological abnormalities such as anaemia, leucopenia and pancytopenia have been noted, as well as lymph gland enlargement and hepatosplenomegaly. Thymoma has been reported in several cases. The cause of this remarkable combination of immunodeficiency and thymus tumour is unknown. There is an increased risk of tumours, mainly lymphomas and leukaemias, but also epithelial tumours primarily in the gastrointestinal tract.

In patients with variable immunodeficiency and also in relatives there is an increased frequency of autoimmune diseases such as rheumatoid arthritis and systemic lupus erythematosus. The reason for the combination of immunodeficiency and these immunological diseases is still unknown.

*Diagnosis*

The diagnosis is based on the same criteria as in the congenital form of hypogammaglobulinaemia. The symptoms are, however, often more varied and less striking and the level of IgG in the patient's serum is usually higher: 2–5 g/l. Small amounts of IgA and IgM can also usually be found in the serum. The patients have in their blood normal to increased numbers of B lymphocytes with immunoglobulin receptors on their surface. The cases with thymoma lack pre-B as well as B lymphocytes. In about half of the patients there are signs of a deficient T lymphocyte function such as decreased responsiveness to phytohaemagglutinin, or decreased capacity to react with delayed hypersensitivity reactions on skin testing.

There are no reliable figures for the frequency of hypogammaglobulinaemia. A recent survey in Sweden has shown a frequency of at least 2–3 per 100 000 with about half of the cases starting before the age of 15. The delay in diagnosis was about 12 years and undertreatment had resulted in unnecessary development of lung damage in a majority of cases. Active antibiotic treatment of acute infections and *adequate* immunoglobulin prophylaxis is vital and can keep the patients in a very satisfactory condition. Trimethoprim with or without sulphonamides seems to have a very good effect on the lung infections.

## Acquired hypogammaglobulinaemia

Hypogammaglobulinaemia can appear secondary to other conditions (I (5) in *Table 13.1*). It may be due to disturbed maturation of the lymphoid system caused by intrauterine rubella infection, or to increased loss of normally produced antibodies through the kidneys in patients with nephrosis, via the gut in protein-losing enteropathy or via large wounds such as burns.

Secondary hypogammaglobulinaemia can also be caused by a decreased production of immunoglobulins. This can be seen in extreme malnutrition and may occur in patients with multiple myeloma, lymphoma and chronic lymphatic leukaemia. In patients with myeloma mononuclear cells, which are not T lymphocytes, have been noticed, which can suppress B lymphocytes in their capacity to produce antibodies. It is possible that this explains the decreased levels of polyclonal immunoglobulins in these patients.

One explanation for the increased frequency of infections in patients treated with immunosuppressive drugs is that certain of the drugs may influence the antibody production, although other effects on the defence against infections may be more striking (cf. chapter 22).

## Selective immunoglobulin deficiency

Antibody deficiency syndrome where the deficiency is selective and only affects one or two of the three dominating immunoglobulin classes IgG, IgM and IgA used to be called dysgammaglobulinaemia. Depending on which immunoglobulins are lacking, these conditions have been divided into different forms.

Of these *isolated IgA deficiency* is especially common and occurs in approximately 1 per 600 in a normal population. IgA deficiency is combined with a number of conditions and the frequency among hospitalized patients may be about 1 per 200.

In some patients with IgA deficiency in blood and secretions an increased frequency of sinopulmonary infections occurs. Several of these patients also seem to have an IgG2 deficiency which possibly explains the increased frequency of infections. Furthermore gastrointestinal conditions such as coeliac disease, malabsorption and tumours, allergies and autoimmune diseases, including systemic lupus erythematosus are seen in combination with IgA deficiency. This may be due to the lack of mucosal protection via the secretory IgA antibodies, resulting in an increased contact with exogenous antigenic material enhancing the risk of these diseases.

Many individuals without IgA are healthy, probably because the immunodeficiency can be compensated by local production of IgM and also increased transfer of IgG antibodies through the mucous membranes in the presence of inflammation. Furthermore mucus-producing goblet cells are increased in the mucosa.

In the blood one can find B lymphocytes with IgA receptors in the same amount as in normal individuals, but the cells cannot release IgA antibodies. Several different pathogenic mechanisms such as disturbance of B cell maturation, increased T suppressor activity or lack of T helper cells may be causative. T lymphocytes are usually normal. Some cases of IgA deficiency have a genetic background, whereas others are caused by exogenous factors such as penicillamine and certain anticonvulsive drugs. In healthy IgA deficient individuals there is a strong association with HLA B8 and DR3. In those with recurrent respiratory tract infections there is only an increased frequency of HLA B40.

In IgA deficient patients antibodies against IgA are occasionally found. These cause severe side effects on blood transfusions, but also infrequently on injection with IgA containing immunoglobulins. Recently IgA–IgG2 deficient patients with IgA antibodies have been put on immunoglobulin prophylaxis without side effects, using a preparation very low in IgA.

Few cases of *selected IgM or IgG deficiency* are known. They seem to result in a similar clinical picture with a dominance of bacterial infections.

*Deficiencies of IgG subclasses*    These seem to be more frequent than common variable immunodeficiency. Isolated deficiency of IgG2 which contains most antibodies against bacterial carbohydrate capsules is followed by an increased occurrence of bacterial infections especially in the respiratory tract. These patients improve after immunoglobulin prophylaxis, but the diagnosis is easily missed, since it may not be apparent from quantification of total serum IgG. Often they are also deficient in IgG4. Cases of IgG1 and IgG3 deficiency are also commonly found. It is not yet clear whether or not they are always related to an increased frequency of infections and if they are improved by immunoglobulin prophylaxis.

The designation selective immunoglobulin deficiency has been used as well for a few cases with antibody deficiency syndromes where immunoglobulins are found at normal levels in serum. The defect in these patients is suggested to be limited to a deficiency in the production of antibodies against certain micro-organisms.

# Deficiencies in cell-mediated immunity

Primary defects in cell-mediated immunity have been observed in single cases with congenital immunodeficiency syndromes, but much more commonly in acquired forms as part of various diseases (II, in *Table 13.1*). These immunodeficiencies are schematically illustrated by B in *Figure 13.1*.

### Congenital deficiencies

*Thymus hypoplasia with hypoparathyroidism (Di George syndrome)*    Thymus as well as the parathyroid glands are formed from the third and fourth pharyngeal pouches. A defect in these pouches can lead to underdevelopment of both the thymus and parathyroid glands. In this syndrome the lymphoid tissues of the antibody-producing system are morphologically intact, but the thymus-dependent system is defective.

Thymus hypoplasia is characterized clinically by repeated severe infections with various bacteria, *Pneumocystis carinii* and fungi. Severe candidal infections are especially characteristic of defects in the thymus-dependent system. Virus infections also have a severe course in patients with such deficiencies. The hypothyroidism causes convulsions. In addition these patients often have heart malformations. With the complete syndrome the patients often die early.

As a consequence of the deficiency in the thymus-dependent system the patients cannot develop delayed hypersensitivity reactions. Nor do they reject incompatible skin transplants and their T lymphocytes show a deficient capacity to react to mitogens. The antibody response against a number of bacterial and viral antigens is also depressed in some of these infants. This may be due to the deficient T helper lymphocyte function.

In some cases of the Di George syndrome thymus transplantations have been successful and in some cases a spontaneous cure has occurred.

*Chronic mucocutaneous candidiasis*   This is seen in some individuals with a more or less selective defect in the capacity of T lymphocytes to react with candidal antigens. The relation between the mycotic infection and the T cell deficiency is unknown. Some patients have a mannase deficiency in their monocytes; mannans can inhibit cytotoxic lymphocytes. Several patients have been reported to improve on injections of transfer factor and thymosin (a thymus hormone), others by transfusion of compatible lymphocytes. In a few severe cases fetal thymus or bone marrow transplantations have been performed successfully. Most patients improve strikingly with the antimycotic drug ketoconazol.

## Acquired defects in AIDS, Hodgkin's disease, sarcoidosis, certain virus infections and malnutrition

AIDS (*acquired immunodeficiency syndrome*) has now appeared in more than 8000 persons, most of them in the USA but some also in Europe and Africa. Most patients are homosexuals, but some cases have occurred among drug addicts and in patients with haemophilia. The aetiology is due to a retrovirus HTLV III, or LAV (human T cell leukaemia virus III, or lymphadenopathy-associated virus), which infects T helper cells. The patients develop severe lymphopeniaand T cell deficiency, but the humoral immunity is intact. A decreased T helper/T suppressor cell ratio is common. They have fever, general lymph gland hyperplasia and lose weight. Opportunistic infections with bacteria, fungi and parasites occur, as well as tumours, especially Kaposi's sarcoma. The mortality rate may be close to 100%. There is no known cure at present, but vaccines are being developed.

In patients with active Hodgkin's disease it is difficult to induce delayed-type hypersensitivity reactions. Such an activity cannot be transferred passively to them. As a further sign of their deficiency of cell-mediated immunity these patients show a delayed rejection of skin transplants and their lymphocytes have a reduced responsiveness to phytohaemagglutinin. In contrast the immunoglobulin levels in serum are usually normal. They produce antibodies against most antigens. Patients with *Hodgkin's* disease have an abnormally increased sensitivity to infections, especially caused by fungi, viruses (including herpes zoster) and Gram-negative bacteria. Tuberculosis is said to be more common in these patients.

In patients with *sarcoidosis* (lymphogranulomatosis benigna) there is a deficiency in cell-mediated immunity similar to that occurring in *Hodgkin's* disease. During active disease a positive tuberculin reaction turns negative. When the patient is recovering from the sarcoidosis his capacity to develop delayed-type hypersensitivity reactions and to reject transplants normalizes.

During the course of some *virus infections* such as measles, influenza, varicellae, mumps and rubella it has also been observed that a positive tuberculin reaction can become weaker, or negative temporarily. This is due to effects of the virus on T cells as well as macrophages. Also in trypanosomiasis and onchocerciasis such a decreased lymphocyte reactivity has been noted. Various immunosuppressive agents can influence cell-mediated immunity (*see further* chapter 22).

In malnutrition and iron deficiency anaemia a decreased T lymphocyte reactivity has been noted. Deficiency of trace elements such as zinc, copper, selenium and magnesium as well as vitamins, e.g. vitamin A, C, pyridoxine and folic acid impair the immune response. The increased frequency of infections in malnourished individuals may be related to the decreased cell-mediated immunity, deficient phagocytosis and low C3 levels. The secretory IgA, but not the serum antibody response is impaired, unless the malnutrition is extreme. Malnutrition primarily occurs in countries with poor hygiene and continual exposure to micro-organisms. The resulting frequent infections seem to be an important cause of malnutrition. The problems of malnutrition, secondary immunodeficiency and infections are obviously intertwined.

# Deficiencies in immunity mediated via humoral antibodies and cell-mediated immunity

## Severe combined immunodeficiency (SCID)

The first cases of the combined immunodeficiency including immunity mediated via humoral antibodies as well as cell-mediated immunity, were described in Switzerland. These patients have thymus alymphoplasia as well as hypogammaglobulinaemia (III (1) in *Table 13.1*) which, in some cases, is due to a stem-cell deficiency causing a deficient development of T and B lymphocytes (C in *Figure 13.1*). The sex-linked recessive form is often called 'Swiss type'; autosomal recessive inheritance, as well as sporadic cases are also seen. About 50% of the latter cases have a *deficiency of adenosine deaminase* (ADA). This enzyme deficiency results in damage on T and B lymphocytes via abnormalities in the purine metabolism. A few cases of *nucleoside phosphorylase deficiency* have shown a disturbed lymphocyte function, especially in T lymphocytes. The cause of the abnormal development in the lymphocytes in the other cases is still unknown. In some the abnormality occurs in prethymocytes, in others at the thymocyte level. In some cases added interleukin-2 seems to increase the activity in the T lymphocytes of the patient, suggesting that a deficient interleukin-2 production may be part of the pathogenesis in some patients with T cell deficiency.

*Histological pattern* The underdevelopment of both immune systems is very apparent. Few lymphoid cells are seen in the bone marrow. The thymus is often very small weighing less than 1 g. It lacks differentiation in cortex-marrow and consists only of epithelial cells with a few lymphocytes (*Figure 13.3*). There are no developed Peyer's patches or tonsils. The peripheral lymphoid tissue is lacking in lymphocytes and plasma cells. There are no follicles (cf. hypogammaglobulinaemia in *Figure 13.2*).

*Clinical picture* This immunodeficiency results in severe infections which may be lethal in the first or second year of life. Widespread candidiasis is common, as well as bacterial bronchopneumonias and therapy resistant diarrhoeas. Virus infections such as varicellae may also prove to be fatal.

Smallpox vaccination used to kill these infants because it resulted in a progressive vaccinia. BCG vaccination with live mycobacteria of low virulence can cause generalized progressive BCG infection in a very low frequency. This complication seems to occur primarily in patients with severe combined immunodeficiency. They obviously lack the capacity to stop the progressive infection because of their deficiency in cell-mediated immunity, which normally provides the protection against tuberculosis.

The patients have very small amounts of immunoglobulins in their serum. Antibody responses or manifestations of cell-mediated immunity cannot be induced. They usually have leucopenia with numbers below $1 \times 10^9$ per ml$^3$.

*Treatment*

Treatment of combined immunodeficiency with antibiotics and immunoglobulins is

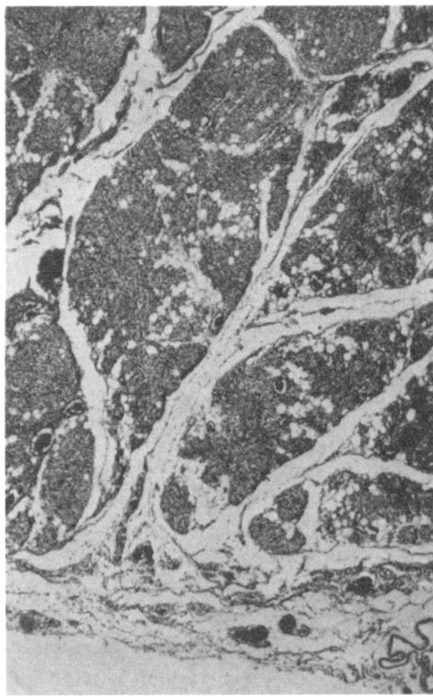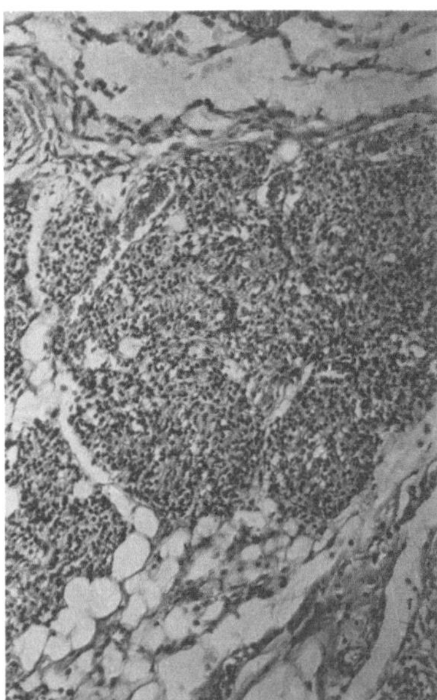

*Figure 13.3* Section through thymus from an infant with thymus alymphoplasia and hypogammaglobulinaemia. There is no differentiation between cortex and marrow. The tissue is dominated by reticular cells and contains only a few mature lymphocytes and no Hassal's corpuscles. It is grossly abnormal compared with a normal thymus (magnification × 50 left, × 200 right. Photo: S. Olling)

insufficient. Only transplantation of stem cells in the form of compatible bone marrow has compensated for the deficiency in B and T lymphocytes. Since these patients lack the capacity to reject transplants graft-versus-host reactions easily occur after the transplant, or if they are given transfusions of incompatible blood, which has not been irradiated to eliminate the lymphocytes. It is difficult to find compatible marrow for transplantation, and various techniques are now successfully being tried to eliminate the cells causing the graft-versus-host reaction. Transplantation of fetal liver and thymus epithelial cells have also been tried.

In patients with ADA deficiency the enzyme deficiency has been compensated by repeated transfusions of frozen irradiated normal red blood cells. The lymphocyte function and the patients have improved temporarily in some cases. Bone marrow transplantation is more efficient.

### Reticular cell dysgenesis and the bare lymphocyte syndrome

An even more severe immunodeficiency than SCID has been observed in a few cases. These patients have in addition to the T and B lymphocyte deficiency a granulocytopenia. They usually die within a few days of birth. It is probably a stem cell deficiency and has been called reticular cell dysgenesis (cf. *Figure 13.1*).

Bare lymphocytes, i.e. lymphocytes without HLA antigens, are found in connection with a rare form of severe combined immunodeficiency.

## Ataxia–telangiectasia (Louis–Barr syndrome)

In the syndrome ataxia–telangiectasia is included cerebellar ataxia, oculocutaneous telangiectasia, ovarial dysgenesis and occasionally an increased risk of infection. In these patients deficiencies in antibody-mediated, as well as cell-mediated immunity have been described but with great variability (III (4) in *Table 13.1*).

*Histological picture*   In autopsies of patients with ataxia–telangiectasia there is either a thymus aplasia, or hypoplasia with few lymphocytes and a lack of Hassal's corpuscles. The peripheral lymphoid tissue shows a reduced number of lymphocytes in the thymus-independent as well as the thymus-dependent areas.

*Clinical pattern*   The increased risk of infections mainly results in recurrent otitis, sinusitis and pneumonia. The patients usually have quantitive changes of serum immunoglobulins, often with lack of IgA. More important as an explanation for the infections may be that they usually have a decreased IgG2. The antibody response against various micro-organisms varies from normal to reduced, or non-existent. The deficiencies in the thymus-dependent immune system in patients with ataxia–telangiectasia is illustrated by prolonged survival of allogenic skin transplants, deficient capacity to develop cutaneous delayed-type hypersensitivity reactions and most importantly an inability to produce cytotoxic T lymphocytes against viral pathogens. They also have an increased frequency of autoantibodies as do individuals with hypogammaglobulinaemia and selective IgA deficiency. Good diagnostic support is provided by the fact that over 95% of the patients have an increased $\alpha$-fetoprotein in serum.

Tumours, mainly lymphomas and leukaemias but also epithelial tumours occur in about 10% of patients with ataxia–telangiectasia. Among patients with immuno-deficiency (cf. hypogammaglobulinaemia, Wiskott–Aldrich's syndrome and Chediak–Higashi's syndrome, *see below*) tumours are 10–200 times more common than in the normal population.

In ataxia–telangiectasia patients, as well as heterozygotic carriers, there is an increased sensitivity to ionizing irradiation with a deficient capacity to repair DNA. This defect together with the immunodeficiency may explain the increased risk of developing tumours and they should not be exposed to irradiation, including radiology. Carriers may be as common as 1% and might even explain 5% of all cases of cancer.

## Wiskott–Aldrich's syndrome

Wiskott–Aldrich's syndrome is characterized by repeated infections, eczema and thrombocytopenia. The patients show abnormalities in cell-mediated and antibody-mediated immunity (III (5) in *Table 13.1*).

*Histology*   Histological examination of the lymphoid tissue shows secondary follicles and plasma cells of normal appearance. During the course of the disease, a progressive reticular hyperplasia of the lymphoid tissue occurs and tumours appear in 10–20%. The thymus is normally developed in some patients with Wiskott–Aldrich's syndrome, while others have thymic hypoplasia or atrophy.

*Clinical picture*   Individuals with Wiskott–Aldrich's syndrome seem to have a deficient host defence against viruses, bacteria and fungi and many succumb early to infections. Others die because of bleeding due to the thrombocytopenia, or of tumours. Quantitative analyses of the serum immunoglobulins often show decreased values for IgM, while IgA and in particular IgE are often increased. The reason for these changes in the immunoglobulin levels is found in an increased synthesis, as well as increased catabolism. The decreased IgM levels are reflected by low or non-detectable alloagglutinin titres (anti-A, anti-B, cf. Appendix 1). Antibody production against various micro-organisms has been demonstrated in these patients, but decreased against polysaccharide antigens.

In all patients there are signs of deficiencies in the thymus-dependent immune system with lymphopenia and decreased lymphocyte reactivity *in vivo* and *in vitro*. Recently, it was found that the patients' lymphocytes lack a surface sialoglycoprotein found on normal lymphocytes. Morphological and functional defects have also been demonstrated in the monocytes as well as signs of abnormal metabolism in lymphocytes and platelets with a decreased hexokinase activity. Immunoglobulin prophylaxis seems useful. Bone marrow transplantation has been successful.


# Deficiencies in non-specific host defence

Deficiencies are also found in components of host defence other than the two effector mechanisms for specific immunity. Various forms of deficiencies in phagocytosis (D in *Figure 13.1*) and complement are known, as is lack of lactoferrin in granulocytes, probably explaining an increased frequency of infections. Another example is the recurrent respiratory tract infections in patients with non-functioning cilia as part of the congenital immotile cilia syndrome, also including immotile sperms and *situs inversus*. In some cases deficiencies can be secondary to other diseases, such as the decreased granulocyte chemotaxis in diabetes. Complement deficiencies are described in chapter 20.


### Granulocyte abnormalities

*Agranulocytosis and granulocytopenia*

Agranulocytosis and granulocytopenia can appear as inherited conditions or be acquired (IV (1) in *Table 13.1*). The acquired forms are usually caused by toxic effects (e.g. irradiation, cytostatic drugs), or allergic reactions to drugs (cf. chapter 18). Ulcerating stomatitis and gingivitis are characteristic of the clinical picture of agranulocytosis. In the severe forms bacterial invasion with sepsis may be lethal in spite of antibiotics and immunoglobulins being given. The infections may cause limited inflammatory reactions and suppuration, probably due to the role of granulocytes for the inflammatory response. The deficient defence against bacterial infections in agranulocytosis in spite of treatment illustrates the importance of the granulocytes in host defence. Granulocyte infusions can be successful.

Several other abnormalities are described concerning granulocyte function. Deficient motility and adherence especially of the neutrophilic granulocytes is noted in Chediak–Higashi's syndrome (*see below*), in Shwachman's disease in combination with abnormalities of the pancreas and skeleton, in abnormalities of the cell's actin and deficiency of a glycoprotein (GP110) in the cell wall. Lack of bacterial uptake and killing is seen in chronic granulomatosis (*see below*), myeloperoxidase deficiency and lack of another glycoprotein (GP150) in the cell wall. The hyper-IgE syndrome with eczema and repeated infections, especially *Staphylococcus* abscesses, may be due to an inefficient phagocytosis.

### Chronic granulomatous disease

Fatal granulomatosis is usually a sex-linked recessively inherited disease characterized by an increased tendency to attract infections and to develop granulomatous infiltrations in inner organs. Autosomally recessive inheritance has also been noted.

*Clinical picture*    The infections usually occur in the form of chronic suppurating lymphadenitis and infected eczematous dermatitis, but pneumonia and sepsis are not uncommon. The infections are caused by bacteria of relatively low virulence such as staphylococci, coli, *Klebsiella* and *Aerobacter* strains. The patients with this form of chronic granulomatosis often have hypergammaglobulinaemia and give a normal antibody response on antigen stimulation. They also have normal cell-mediated immunity and a normal inflammatory response.

*Pathogenesis*    The abnormality explaining the increased frequency of infections is localized in the granulocytes. They engulf bacteria, but the micro-organisms are not killed as in normal granulocytes. The phagocytes have a deficient $O_2$ metabolism and do not produce the free oxygen radicals which are so important for bactericidal activity. The mothers of the patients are carriers and their granulocytes have a capacity of bacterial killing which is intermediate to that of normal individuals and the children with the disease. The deficiency can easily be demonstrated with a specific test, the nitroblue–tetrazolium reduction test (NBT, *see* Appendix 2).

The appearance of severe infections with bacteria of low virulence in these patients again illustrates the importance of phagocytic granulocytes in the host defence against many micro-organisms. Viral infections do not have a more severe course in these patients. Trimethoprim–sulpha seems to efficiently get into the phagocytes of these patients and functions well therapeutically and prophylactically. Bone marrow transplantation has been successful in a few cases.

### Chediak–Higashi syndrome

The Chediak–Higashi syndrome is a rare autosomally recessive disease characterized by partial oculocutaneous hypopigmentation, severe recurrent infections and abnormal lysosomal granules.

The patients usually die before the age of ten, either of infections, or after development of malignant tumours in the lymphorecticular system. There is no deficiency in their immune response, but they have a much decreased function in their NK cells, which is not improved by interferon. Bone marrow transplantation seems to normalize this defect.

Their granulocytes have a decreased response to chemotaxis and they engulf bacteria slower than is normal. The increased risk of virus and bacterial infections is presumably related to the granulocyte abnormality. In the cytoplasm of these cells there are abnormal giant granules, which are of lysosomal nature and contain enzymes. Such abnormalities are also found in other cells including melanocytes which may explain the pigmentation abnormality.

# Bibliography

CHANDRA, R. K. (ed.) (1983). *Primary and Secondary Immunodeficiency Disorders.* Churchill Livingstone, London.
HAYWARD, A. R. (1977). Immunodeficiency. *Current Topics in Immunology Series* (Turk, J. ed.), **6**, 1.
HOROWITZ, S. D. and HONG, R. (1977). The pathogenesis and treatment of immunodeficiency. *Monographs in Allergy* (Kallos, P., Inderbitzin, T. M., Trunka, Z., de Weck, A. L. and Waksman, B. eds), **10**, 1.
IUIS/WHO Committee (1983). Appropriate uses of human immunoglobulin in clinical practice. *Clin. exp. Immunol.*, **52**, 417.
STIEHM, E. R. and FULGINITI, V. A. (eds) (1980). *Immunologic Disorders in Infants and Children*, 2nd edition. Saunders, Philadelphia.
WHO Committee (1983). Primary immunodeficiency diseases. *Clin. Immunol. Immunopath.*, **28**, 450.

# Chapter 14

# Clinical transplantation immunology

Erna Möller

Immunology has become very important in clinical transplantation. The problem with transplantations are not only surgical but rather, or even primarily, immunological. The recipient of an incompatible transplant reacts immunologically and the transplant is rejected whether it consists of an organ or single cells. This is called the HvG (host versus graft) reaction. The reason why immunological reactivity against a foreign transplant is so strong and difficult to surmount has been discussed in chapter 9. T cells find transplanted tissue foreign in the same way they would if their own tissue was changed. for example by a virus infection, and the number of T lymphocytes participating in a single alloreaction is very large. Furthermore the polymorphism between the MHC (Major Histocompatibility Complex) antigens of different individuals is so extensive that there is only a very slight chance that two unrelated individuals would have the same class I and class II molecules. As previously mentioned it is primarily the incompatibility of class I antigens which initiates an immune reaction, but the specificity of, for instance cytotoxic T cells, is mainly directed against class I target antigens.

In many countries renal transplantation of patients with terminal renal insufficiency has become routine. The survival of transplanted kidneys, which at the beginning of the 1960s was quite low, is now, with the techniques used for immunosuppression and the new immunological methods of selecting proper donors, about 80% after one year and around 60% after three years. As a rule kidneys from related donors have a better survival rate than transplants from deceased donors (necrotransplants). Since each individual has a unique constellation of strong, as well as weak, transplantation antigens it is impossible to avoid incompatibilities (antigen differences) for most transplantations. Therefore all transplant patients must be treated with drugs which suppress the immunological reactivity and hamper the rejection.

During the last few years bone marrow transplantations have also become important. The indications for bone marrow transplantation are severe combined immunodeficiency, Wiskott-Aldrich's syndrome, therapy resistant aplastic anaemia, certain forms of acute and chronic leukaemia and some congenital metabolic disorders. In patients with immunodeficiency and aplastic anaemia a non-functioning or damaged organ is replaced by normal tissue. In metabolic disorders the patient can be given cells synthesizing the lacking enzyme.

In leukaemia it is possible to kill all the leukaemia cells by drastic cytotoxic treatment and whole body irradiation. This results in an irreversible damage to all cells in the bone marrow including the normal ones. The patients must be given normal stem cells to redevelop all blood cells. Transplantation of pancreatic tissue to patients with severe diabetes is being tried and transplantation of heart, as well as heart plus lungs, and liver are being done.

## Kidney transplantation

The advantage of renal transplantation in patients with chronic renal insufficiency is that a successful transplant will return the patient to a normal life, whereas the alternative therapy, dialysis, is only life-sustaining and often does not reconstitute the patient fully. The disadvantage with transplantation is that all patients must be continuously treated with immunosuppressive drugs to prevent rejection.

As mentioned in chapter 9, the HLA antigens are the strong transplantation antigens in man. But not even HLA compatibility between donor and recipient is sufficient since there are weak, not yet well characterized transplantation antigen systems, which may induce a rejection. The immunosuppressive treatment given today is non-specific, i.e. a general suppression of immunoreactivity is induced, resulting in a severe sensitivity to infections in the transplanted patients. It is a delicate task to find the dose of the immunosuppressive drug for each patient which reduces the risk of rejection, without causing severe infections.

Blood group compatibility is also essential in renal transplantations. The A and B antigens are present on nucleated cells and 'natural' antibodies against A and B blood group antigens may cause hyperacute rejection of a transplanted ABO-incompatible organ. Such a rejection is probably mediated via the antibody-dependent cell-mediated cytolysis reaction (ADCC, *see* chapter 16).

Polymorphism of the genes of the HLA system makes it very unlikely that two unrelated individuals are HLA compatible. In contrast 25% of all siblings are HLA-identical since all HLA antigens are determined by coupled genes. This means that from the immunological point of view the best donors for a renal transplant are found among siblings. The great importance of genes of the HLA region and their products for the survival of transplanted kidneys is demonstrated by the almost 100% survival rate during five years of HLA identical transplants from siblings. Unsuccessful immunosuppression, or rejection of an HLA-identical sibling transplant due to the incompatibility of weak transplantation antigens is rare. Since many patients with chronic renal insufficiency do not have organs available from live related donors, necrokidneys from unrelated persons must be used.

### Necrotransplantation

Most renal transplants in Scandinavia are performed with kidneys from a deceased person, so-called necrokidneys. These kidneys, which are taken from individuals who have died recently, are refrigerated and perfused in a special solution within 15 minutes after death. The kidneys can be kept in the cold, or special perfusion machines for up to 40 hours. In the meantime the HLA antigens of the necrodonor can be determined and the immunologically best suited recipient can be selected from the patients on the waiting list for transplantation.

A large problem in necrokidney transplantation is that of finding an HLA compatible donor for each patient. The most common HLA phenotype (in Sweden HLA-A1,3 B7,8 Cw7 DR2,3 DQw1,3 DPw1,4) is found in a frequency of approximately 0.1%. This means that for a patient with this HLA phenotype, every 1 per 1000 necrodonors is suitable. Other HLA phenotypes are found in a much lower frequency and it is much more difficult to find a suitable donor for them. These problems are to some extent surmounted by international cooperation. For instance in Scandinavia all countries cooperate within the Scandiatransplant Organization, which also collaborates with the Eurotransplant Organization. All data concerning patients waiting for renal transplantation are computerized and on each occasion the donor's ABO and HLA phenotypes are checked in the computer providing information about the best suited recipient. The laboratory then arranges for the kidneys to be transported immediately to the recipient.

In spite of this extensive activity to provide as suitable transplants as possible, the transplant survival rate has not improved as drastically as expected. Furthermore it has been found that some transplants survive very well in spite of poor compatibility. Certain transplantation centres have not even taken into account HLA compatibility between donor and recipient and can still obtain transplant survivals of 60–70% after several years. There are many explanations for this. Patients with terminal renal insufficiency—uraemia—have a basic disease which *per se* results in a pronounced immunodeficiency, which may as a consequence make the patient unable to react against an incompatible transplant. Furthermore it was found that compatibility for the class I molecules, HLA-A, B and C antigens was of minor importance in renal transplantation. Evaluation of the transplantation results was performed at a time when the knowledge about the class II antigens, only discovered in 1975, was very limited. The situation was as if the results of ABO blood group compatibility in blood transfusions were evaluated knowing only about blood groups A and O, but not B.

Now it has been found that class II antigens are of major importance for the induction of T cell-mediated immune reactions. If there is class II antigen compatibility no immune reaction can be induced against the transplant and since cytotoxic T lymphocytes which react against class I antigens need T cell help for their differentiation, there is no rejection. In accordance with this theoretical background a number of studies have now demonstrated that identity between the donor and recipient concerning HLA-DR antigens give a very good survival rate in spite of incompatibility in the HLA-A, B and C antigens.

Each patient in need of a renal transplant is tissue typed to determine class I, as well as class II antigens. However, it is important to note that we do not yet know in detail all the HLA genes of importance for the induction of the rejection reaction. The recently discovered loci DQ and DP which together with the DR locus direct the synthesis of class II molecules have not been evaluated clinically yet as they cannot be determined adequately with serological techniques. It is possible that direct molecular genetic determinations will give us better and quicker information about the genes which are the most important, not only in transplantation, but also concerning the risk of developing HLA associated diseases (*see below*).

**Transplantation of organs from live donors**

Before transplantation of an organ from a live related donor, tissue typing is performed on all family members. Those siblings who are HLA and ABO compatible with the recipient are ideal donors. But since it is possible that a sibling through recombination in the HLA chromosome is identical with the recipient regarding HLA-A, -B and -C, but incompatible regarding HLA-D, MLC tests are also performed on all the family members. In 99% of all cases HLA-A, -B and -C identical siblings are also HLA-D identical, since the recombination frequency between B and D locus reflecting the chromosomal distance between these loci only is 1 cM (centiMorgan − 1 cM meaning a recombination frequency of 1 per 100).

As previously mentioned, survival of kidneys from HLA identical siblings is very good. But also kidneys from parents have a better survival rate than unselected kidneys from unrelated donors. This is because parents and children are always identical as to one haplotype. Kidneys from parents have a survival rate of 70–80%.

**Occurrence of antibodies before transplantation**

Certain individuals have in their serum antibodies reacting with allogenic HLA antigens. HLA antibodies do not occur naturally but are induced by immunization. Such immunization may occur after blood transfusion, pregnancy or previous transplantation. Patients waiting for renal transplants who have uraemia, often have anaemia too, and at times require blood transfusions. This creates a risk of immunization that later can limit the possibility of the patient to be successfully transplanted with a partly incompatible kidney. An immunological cross-match is therefore always performed before the transplantation to prevent cytotoxic antibodies against the HLA antigens of the transplant from causing hyperacute rejection of the kidney as can occur in ABO incompatibility. Serum from the recipient is mixed with the donor's lymphocytes in the presence of complement. A positive reaction is a contraindication against transplantation from that donor.

**Treatment of patients following transplantation**

Rejection occurs in many patients who have been transplanted with an allogenic kidney. Decreased urine production is often an early sign of a threatening rejection.

All patients with a renal transplant are treated with various immunosuppressive drugs. Specific immunosuppression is not yet available.

Standard treatment for the transplanted patients includes prednisone (a cortisone preparation) and another non-specific immunosuppressive agent, azathioprine (Imuran). Immediately after the transplantation high doses of prednisone are given which are later brought down to a low maintenance dose. Azathioprine is given in the same dose during the entire post-transplantation period. If a rejection appears high doses of prednisone are given. This usually results in a good restitution of the kidney function, but if that does not happen and the rejection crisis cannot be stopped the transplant is removed. The patient can be transplanted again and the result of the retransplantation is often as good as with first transplantations. Some patients have been transplanted more than three times.

During the 1980s a new immunosuppressive drug has been introduced, cyclosporine A. This drug is presently used for patients receiving kidney, liver, heart or pancreas grafts. The use of cyclosporine A has clearly improved graft survival. Unlike azathioprine, it does not seem to be myelotoxic. It is a cyclic oligopeptide isolated from a fungus. It seems to be quite selectively immunosuppressive on the T lymphocyte population, making it suitable in transplantations. The results are promising.

The problems with immunosuppression are manifold. Non-specific immuno-suppression always brings a risk of infection, but cyclosporine A also has severe side effects on the kidneys and liver, making it important that the physician responsible has experience with the drug.

In addition to chemical immunosuppression biological methods are used, e.g. treatment with antibodies directed specifically against T lymphocytes, socalled antithymocyte globulin, often prepared against human T lymphocytes in rabbit or horse and demonstrating a good immunosuppressive effect. Drainage of T lymphocytes from the thoracic duct over three to six weeks can eliminate up to 10% of the total lymphocyte pool and has demonstrated its clinical value (chapter 22).

## Bone marrow transplantation

The immunological problems in renal transplantation are still, in principle, unsolved even if there has been great progress during the last two years. The problems with bone marrow transplantations are even greater.

Bone marrow transplantation is performed in patients with severe immunodeficiency, or in those who after treatment with certain drugs have acquired persistent severe bone marrow damage resulting in aplastic anaemia.

Bone marrow transplantation is performed as an intravenous injection of bone marrow from an immunologically suitable donor. Bone marrow cells are aspirated from the pelvic bone of the donor. About $3 \times 10^8$ cells/kg should be given, which requires one litre of marrow or more. The marrow is filtered to eliminate any bone fragments or lumps of cells and is poured into ordinary transfusion bags. Transfused bone marrow cells home into the bone marrow of the recipient.

One prerequisite for a successful bone marrow transplantation is that the recipient cannot reject the foreign marrow and that the transferred marrow, which contains some immunocompetent lymphocytes, does not react against the antigens of the recipient in a graft-versus-host reaction (GvH). To prevent rejection of the transplanted marrow the recipient is treated with very high doses of cytostatic drugs before the operation. These patients also receive high doses of immunosuppressive drugs after the operation to prevent a GvH reaction.

Possible donors of bone marrow transplants are HLA-identical siblings, or in rare cases monozygotic twins. More recently, donors who have not been completely HLA-identical have been used. A prerequisite in these transplantations to avoid a lethal GvH-disease is to remove most of the immunocompetent cells in the bone marrow by passage on lectin-columns or by monoclonal antibodies directed against mature T lymphocytes. ABO incompatibility is not a contraindication for bone marrow transplantation in contrast to renal transplantation. A successful bone marrow transplantation leads to a replacement of the whole blood producing organ with donor tissue. ABO incompatible transplantation results in a change of the patient's blood group to that of the donor. Exchange transfusions (plasmaphaeresis) must be performed before the transplantation so that the recipient's natural ABO haemagglutinins do not lyse the given erythrocytes. In addition red cells can be removed from the recovered bone marrow cells by selective centrifugation.

The patients who are transplanted with bone marrow usually have a very small, or no chance of surviving without treatment. The survival rate of patients with aplastic anaemia who have been transplanted with marrow from HLA-identical siblings is about 80%. The mortality rate is partly due to GvH disease occurring also in HLA compatibility, causing damage to the recipient's intestinal epithelium, liver, etc., which eventually can lead to death. Infections are a cause of death. Pretreatment results in severe disturbances of the host defence of the recipient. This immunodeficiency remains after transplantation until the transferred bone marrow has developed new immuno-competent cells, which repopulate the secondary lymphoid organs. The high risk of infections in these patients is prevented by strict isolation during the first two to three weeks after transplantation, until there is a 'take' of the new marrow.

## Treatment of leukaemia

For several years bone marrow transplantation has been the treatment of choice for patients with certain forms of acute leukaemia. This includes primarily ANL (Acute Non-lymphocytic Leukaemia) and certain forms of ALL (Acute Lymphatic Leukaemia). ALL is one of the most common causes of death in children. About half of all children who contract ALL have a stable remission with the cytostatic treatment usually employed. The other half have a relapse of their leukaemia after varying periods of time. A second remission can often be induced with the cytostatic drugs, but in those children who have a relapse the risk of further relapses is very great. An alternative is to give the child very intense treatment with high doses of cytostatics and also whole body irradiation, usually 10 Gy, which is a lethal dose. This treatment kills the leukaemia cells, but also damages other vital organs such as the stem cells in the bone marrow. Death would follow within a short period of time if fresh bone marrow could not be provided. A child with an HLA-identical sibling can be given a bone marrow transplant.

In addition to the risk of GvH disease and infections, which may occur in all bone marrow transplant patients, these children can also have a relapse of their leukaemia. The survival rate varies for different forms of ALL, but seems to be around 50%. Immunosuppressive treatment to prevent GvH disease is given for a while after the transplantation, but in contrast to the kidney transplant patients those transplanted with bone marrow can stop immunosuppressive treatment after about a year. Successful transplantation brings the patient back to full health.

ANL is a form of leukaemia which often gives a relapse after a first remission has been induced with cytostatic drugs. These patients are therefore all potential bone marrow transplantation candidates. The risk of relapse after transplantation in these patients is less than for the ALL patients and the results of the transplantations are very good with about 70–80% becoming completely healthy.

One of the major problems is that the results are really only good if the patient has an HLA identical sibling as a donor. In the future methods must be found making it possible to also transplant those patients who do not have a sibling as a donor, as this is more than half of the patients. In certain cases comparatively good results have been attained using other relatives, or even unrelated donors. One possibility could be to use unrelated, but relatively HLA compatible donors. The ethical problems concerning these possibilities have not been solved.

## Autotransplantation of bone marrow

Autotransplantation means that the patient's own bone marrow is transplanted. This is being tried in leukaemia patients who do not have an HLA identical donor of marrow available. The bone marrow is instead collected from a patient with leukaemia who has been successfully treated with cytostatics inducing a complete remission leaving no malignant cells in the blood or bone marrow. The patient's bone marrow is frozen in liquid nitrogen keeping the cells alive. In a later relapse of leukaemia the patient can be treated with very high doses of cytostatics and possibly with whole body irradiation followed by reconstitution of the bone marrow with the autologous cells collected earlier.

Trials with this treatment have been performed in many institutes, but most of the transplanted patients have had a new relapse of their leukaemia and died. There have probably been a few leukaemic cells remaining in the marrow during the remission causing the relapse. The collected bone marrow has therefore been treated with various forms of antibodies against the leukaemia cells, sometimes in combination with toxins or radioactive isotopes coupled to antibodies to kill the remaining leukaemia cells in the marrow before it is transfused back into the patient. The results of such treatment are still very preliminary.

Autotransplantation has also been tried in patients with tumours which are difficult to operate upon, or tumours which metastasize early, but rarely leave metastases in the bone marrow. Ovarian cancer is such a tumour. Efficient chemotherapy, possibly combined with irradiation can damage all malignant cells. This damage caused by the treatment in the marrow can be compensated by transplantation with the patient's own previously collected marrow.

## Transplantation of an organ to an immunologically privileged site

Transplantation of allogenic cornea has been performed for many years with good results. The cells in the cornea contain alloantigens and should initiate an immune reaction in the recipient resulting in a rejection. Usually there is no rejection, but it can occur if the cornea becomes vascularized. The survival of the transplant is believed to be due to the fact that the transplanted cornea does not come into contact with the immune system of the host and therefore no immunization follows. The anterior chamber of the eye is regarded as a 'privileged site' for foreign transplants. In the cases where vascularization appears circulating immunocompetent cells can initiate a reaction resulting in destruction of the cornea. HLA compatible transplants survive after vascularization which destroys HLA incompatible transplants. Other areas in the body where immunologically privileged sites can occur are, e.g. uterus, muscles and other areas with inefficient lymph drainage, such as skin flaps or scarred tissue.

## The fetus as a transplant

The relation between mother and fetus in mammals seems to contradict fundamental principles of transplantation immunology, since the implanted fetus is a histo-incompatible transplant, which is exposed to, but tolerated by the potentially aggressive immune system of the mother. It has previously even been suggested that parturition is the result of an immunological rejection of the fetus, but this is disproved by the fact that the length of pregnancy is the same for mice with incompatible and compatible fetuses.

The part of the fetus which comes into contact with the mother's tissues is the trophoblast cell layer in the placenta.

Transplantation antigens are developed early during fetal life and the trophoblasts should contain alloantigenic structures and be immunogenic. A possible reason why immunization of the mother would fail to appear during pregnancy could be that the trophoblast cell layer does not expose its cell surface antigens, or that they are blocked, e.g. by a lipoprotein layer. This may not be the explanation either, since pregnant females have a depressed immunological reactivity indicating that humoral factors with immunosuppressive activity are produced during pregnancy. Such factors can be hormones, e.g. chorionic gonadotrophin (HCG), chorionic somatotrophin (HCS), or other factors appearing in high concentrations during pregnancy such as $\beta_2$-microglobulin or $\alpha$-fetoprotein. Yet another possibility is that the mother develops specific T lymphocytes which suppress development of cell-mediated, as well as humoral immunity during pregnancy, or that she develops antibodies which can inhibit cell-mediated immune reactions. It is clear, however, that the length of pregnancy is not influenced by previous immunization against any of the antigens. The explanation of this privileged situation of the fetus in relation to the mother's immune system is unknown, but interesting findings suggest that the mother's serum contains blocking IgG antibodies, and that, e.g. $\alpha$-fetoprotein has a selectively inhibiting effect on the activation on such T cells, that function as helper cells, for the development of the rejection reaction. The fetal T lymphocytes with strong suppressive activity on maternal T lymphocytes could also be important.

## Association between clinical disease and HLA antigens

In the 1960s it was demonstrated that leukaemia virus causes diseases in certain mice but not in others. The difference in resistance to this virus infection depended on genes linked to the H-2 region of the mouse. The discovery that immunological reactivity was genetically determined and to a certain extent (through IR and IS genes) was coupled to the H-2 region, resulted in an intense search for connections between human disease and certain HLA genes.

Leukaemia and malignant lymphoma were the first diseases in man to be investigated for an HLA association. No association was found. The activity in this area of research increased at the beginning of the 1970s when several laboratories demonstrated independently that psoriasis vulgaris (a chronic and relatively common eczematous disease), as well as ankylosing spondylitis, pelvospondylitis ossificans—a chronic arthritis including primarily the vertebrae—were strongly associated with certain HLA antigens. Later research has demonstrated that a large number of chronic autoimmune diseases have a clear relation to genes in the HLA system.

In Stockholm over 300 patients with ankylosing spondylitis have been investigated without finding a single patient lacking the antigen B27. The frequency in controls in Sweden is 9%, which means that only these run the risk of attracting the disease, B27 negative individuals cannot get it. Large studies have shown that objective signs of arthritis occur in about 30% of 'healthy' first degree relatives of sick individuals and that about 25% of healthy B27 positive blood donors have radiologically detectable changes usually without any subjective symptoms. A number of other inflammatory joint diseases, e.g. post-infectious arthritis, are associated with the B27 antigen, but not with the same high relative risk. This also includes arthritis as a complication to intestinal infections with *Salmonella*, *Shigella* and *Yersinia* bacteria and arthritis after certain urogenital infections as well.

Association with diseases follows the normal frequency of these extremely polymorphic antigen systems in different populations. As for the ABO blood groups the frequency of various alleles is specific for different racial groups. The antigen B27 which is relatively common in northern Europe and the USA, almost does not exist in Japan. In spite of this a few Japanese patients with ankylosing spondylitis have B27. All of them have Caucasian blood, showing that the risk of attracting the disease is genetically 'imported'.

**TABLE 14.1. Association between HLA antigens and certain diseases**

| Disease | HLA | Frequency in | |
|---|---|---|---|
| | | Patients (%) | Controls (%) |
| Ankylosing spondylitis | B27 | 100 | 9 |
| Post-infectious arthritis | B27 | 90 | 9 |
| Reiter's disease | B27 | 79 | 9 |
| Acute uveitis | B27 | 52 | 9 |
| Rheumatoid arthritis | DR4 | 70 | 20 |
| Pemphigus (Jews) | DR4 | 87 | 32 |
| Juvenile rheumatoid arthritis | DR8 | 23 | 8 |
| Psoriasis vulgaris | Cw6 | 87 | 33 |
| | DR7 | 50 | 23 |
| IDDM | DR3 | 56 | 28 |
| (insulin dependent | DR4 | 75 | 32 |
| diabetes mellitus, type I) | DR2 | 10 | 31 |
| Thyrotoxicosis | DR3 | 56 | 26 |
| Coeliac disease | DR3 | 79 | 26 |
| Addison's disease | DR3 | 69 | 26 |
| SLE | DR3 | 70 | 28 |
| Myasthenia gravis (females) | B8 | 80 | 25 |
| IgA deficiency (healthy blood donors) | DR3 | 81 | 25 |

The control frequency varies somewhat with where the investigation was performed. The figures are in certain cases means (%) between several different studies. (The material is taken partly from Svejgaard, A. and coworkers—HLA and disease 1982—a Survey. *Immunol. Rev.*, **70**, 1983)

A compilation of some of the most common associations between disease and HLA antigens is shown in *Table 14.1*. The diseases, which are associated with a single A or B allele, often show a heredity which is autosomally dominant but with limited penetrance, i.e. the inheritance is not X-linked (the HLA genes are found in the autosomal chromosome pair number 6). Furthermore, not all members of a family having the HLA haplotype combined with an increased risk of disease show signs of the disease. The penetrance varies from very high, e.g. for psoriasis vulgaris, to very low, e.g. for multiple sclerosis (MS).

A large group of autoimmune diseases are associated with the socalled 'super-haplotype' A1, Cw7, B8, DR3, one of the most common haplotypes where the separate genes within the A-DR loci show strong positive linkage disequilibrium (*see* chapter 9). This is true for insulin dependent diabetes in children (type I diabetes), thyrotoxicosis (goitre), Sjögren's syndrome, SLE, Addison's disease, coeliac disease (gluten intolerance) and myasthenia gravis. All these diseases are statistically significant, but not 100% associated with B8 and DR3.

It was previously thought that the HLA region contained many more genes than those that could be determined immunologically. With hybrid DNA techniques it has been found that the number of genes within the HLA region determining either class I or class II antigens is limited. This means that the actual genes B8 and DR3 probably have importance *per se* for an increased risk of developing autoimmune diseases. That the association is not 100% may indicate that what is today called a clinically homogeneous disease entity in reality is a combination of two or more diseases of different aetiology, where one disease is HLA associated and another one is not. An example of such heterogeneity is found in patients with Addison's disease. Seventy per cent of the patients have B8 and/or DR3, but 70% of patients with the disease have autoantibodies against the adrenal cortex, while 30% lack them. The 70% who have antibodies are those who have the antigens B8 and DR3

Psoriasis is associated with two different HLA genes, Cw6 and DR7. These are present in a certain linkage disequilibrium, but not to a sufficient extent to explain the increased frequency of both Cw6 and DR7 in patients with psoriasis. This probably means that psoriasis is the result of a cooperation of two genes within one haplotype or between genes in two different haplotypes that predispose to the disease, one being identical with or closely coupled to Cw6 and another one which is present together with DR7. If both of these genes are found on one haplotype the inheritance seems to be autosomally dominant with limited penetrance. If they are present on two different haplotypes the inheritance seems to be recessive.

Cw6 is present in about 70% of patients with psoriasis. The frequency in the control material is about 30%. The question is how many healthy Cw6 positive individuals have signs of the disease. One study showed that about half of all investigated healthy Cw6 positive persons had either one parent, a sibling or a child with psoriasis. Some of them had psoriasis themselves without knowing. Psoriasis can appear as a transient disease with few symptoms (e.g. increased scaling from the scalp), but it can also be a chronically debilitating disease with symptoms from both skin and joints. The presence of Cw6 does not give any hint about the severity or prognosis of psoriasis.

A disease which clearly shows an HLA-linked recessive inheritance is diabetes type I. The disease is associated with DR3 and 4. This means that a child with juvenile diabetes has inherited a gene DR3, or a tightly coupled gene) from one parent and another gene from another parent predisposing to the disease. Both parents are then carriers of a gene which increases the risk of developing the disease, but they are healthy. Only the HLA-identical siblings (25% of all) will have a clearly increased risk of attracting diabetes. The concordance for the disease in monozygotic twins is about 30%. Almost as high a concordance is found in HLA-identical siblings of the patient, which means that all the genes that give an increased risk of diabetes are HLA-linked. Within a family where one child has diabetes it is possible to predict the risk for the other siblings of getting the same disease. Unfortunately there is at the moment no possibility of preventing the development of diabetes and therefore this knowledge is of little or no clinical value, but of great theoretical interest. In patients with diabetes type I it is also clear that DR2 is found in a significantly decreased frequenty. This decrease is not secondary to the elevated frequency of the alleles 3 and 4. It means that the DR2 gene induces an increased resistance against the development of the disease. The mechanism of this phenomenon is not known.

HLA determination is used more and more for diagnostic purposes. Several diseases, some very rare, have a strong HLA association but have not been mentioned here. The mechanism behind these associations is not known. It is generally thought that HLA associated diseases are multifactorial, e.g. they depend on several factors. One such factor is the genetic predisposition (presence of special HLA genes), and another one may be environmental factors, for instance a special infection. It is still not known which—if any—infectious agents may be related to the onset of, e.g. diabetes or psoriasis, but the ensuing autoimmune reactivity could possibly be influenced at an early stage of immunosuppression.

Diseases with an immunological pathogenesis show HLA associations, since the immunological repertoire of the individual and his specific immunological reactivity is directed by MHC class I and II genes. Also certain complement factors are encoded by MHC genes and may be of importance for the appearance of disease. Some autoimmune diseases are much more common in individuals with deficiencies in the complement system. The association between DR3 and IgA deficiency in healthy blood donors that has been recently found is quite interesting. It probably means that the IgA deficiency is secondary to a deficient T cell function, since the MHC genes primarily regulate T cell mediated reactivity.

Not all the diseases with HLA association have an immunological pathogenesis. 21-Hydroxylase deficiency (adrenogenital syndrome) and idiopathic haemochromatosis (pathological deposition of iron in tissues) are examples of this. These enzyme deficiencies are clearly HLA-linked in family studies and therefore the HLA regions or closely linked genes code for the normal enzymes. Both of these diseases are recessive and the conclusion has been drawn that all patients with idiopathic haemochromatosis, which is quite common for instance in northern Sweden and parts of France, have common HLA haplotypes which contain defective genes. This may have arisen through a single point mutation. It can be estimated that all the people with this disease may have a common ancestor and an identical genetic defect resulting in the disease in homozygous carriers of this haplotype. The deficiency in idiopathic haemochromatosis patients can be calculated to have occurred in an individual about the year 1000. These findings clearly show how well the HLA system suits anthropological investigations.


## Bibliography

MÖLLER, G. (ed.) (1982). Structure and Function of HLA-DR. *Immunological Reviews*, **66**.
MÖLLER, G. (ed.) (1983). HLA and Disease Susceptibility. *Immunological Reviews*, **70**.
MÖLLER, G. (ed.) (1983). Allogenic Bone Marrow Transplantation. *Immunological Reviews*, **71**.

# Chapter 15

# Clinical tumour immunology

Hans Olov Sjögren

Clinical tumour immunology may come to encompass three main areas: prophylaxis, diagnostics and therapy. Of these it is currently only the diagnostic aspect that has any practical, clinical usefulness. It is quite probable that immunotherapy will also be of clinical importance in the future, whereas the prospects for immunological prophylaxis still seem limited.

It is important to differentiate clearly between *tumour associated antigens* (TAA), which are immunogenic in the patient, and *tumour associated molecules* (TAM), which can be demonstrated and quantified by means of polyclonal or monoclonal antibodies, but which are not immunogenic in the patient. Those types of molecules have diagnostic as well as therapeutic potential. The basic mechanisms in tumour immunology have been presented previously in chapter 10. The diagnostic methods based on various types of testing of the immunoreactivity in a patient against his own tumour requires the presence of TAA. Similarly TAA are a prerequisite for certain types of immunotherapeutic measures, such as immunization of a patient with tumour antigens, elimination of antigen-specific suppressor cells or suppressor products and transfer of *in vitro*-activated lymphocytes or lymphocyte products. Experience from animal experiments suggests that certain tumours have detectable TAA. The strongest rejection reactions can be expected to occur against unique individual antigens, against virus induced antigens, and against certain oncofetal antigens. The heterogeneity of the antigen expression in tumours may make the rejection reaction inefficient, however, by allowing quick selection of cells, which lack the critical antigen(s).

Against this background it seems that action should be directed towards isolating a battery of antigens from the tumour of each patient. The therapeutic potential of this approach is clearly shown by results with spontaneous leukaemia in the AKR-mouse strain. This tumour has been thought to be weakly antigenic since it is difficult to induce a rejection reaction against it. The reason is that these tumours contain antigenically different cell clones, of which one represents 98% of the whole population. Immunization with such a tumour results in good immunity against the dominating clone, but not against the others, which therefore will grow in an unrestrained manner. Immunization against the other two cell populations carrying two other antigens results in a strong rejection reaction. These three different antigens have been defined also with monoclonal antibodies. Treatment with an antibody against one of the antigens does not lead to any obvious therapeutic effect, whereas a pool of the three antibodies is quite efficient. These results illustrate a problem existing in most tumour systems, but they also indicate possible solutions.

## Demonstration that a patient reacts immunologically against his own tumour

*In vitro analysis*

Various *in vitro* techniques have to be used to demonstrate that a patient reacts immunologically against live tumour cells or various types of preparations from his own tumour. These techniques include antibody tests where serum antibodies can be shown to bind to tumour cells or tumour antigens. Such antibodies have been demonstrated in the serum from patients with certain tumours, e.g. melanoma. In these cases some antibodies are directed against the cell surface, others against cytoplasmic antigens. The antibodies also often react with melanoma cells from other patients. One of the safest ways of studying the specificity of these reactions is to do adsorption experiments with different cells and tissues.

Sensitization against TAA has also been demonstrated by tests for cell-mediated immunity based on lymphocyte cytotoxicity, leucocyte migration inhibition, leucocyte adherence inhibition and lymphocyte stimulation. These techniques show a relatively large proportion of patients with tumours such as melanoma to be sensitized against their tumours and also against antigens common to the same type of tumours from other patients. Unfortunately it is not known whether this type of reaction reflects a reactivity that may lead to tumour cell elimination *in vivo*.

*Direct analysis of tumour tissue*

It is well known that lymphocyte–macrophage infiltration of tumour tissue varies between different types of tumours and different patient. It is natural to see this infiltration as an indication of the sensitization to TAA, although it may sometimes be a reaction to tissue damaged by non-immune mechanisms.

The type of the infiltrating cells can be determined with reagents against markers on the cell surface. Their function can be analysed by *in vitro* tests after separation from other cells. So far it has been found that NK cell activity is often low and that cytolytic effector cells, as well as suppressor cells can be present.

## TAM and TAA defined with polyclonal and monoclonal antibodies

Molecules associated with a large number of different forms of tumours have been defined by means of antisera produced in various animal species. Particularly important has been a number of monoclonal mouse antibodies directed against glycoproteins and glycolipids with a varying degree of specificity for different tumours. Usually it has been possible to demonstrate low concentrations of these molecules on normal cells from healthy donors. It is more a question of quantitative rather than qualitative association with cancer.

Some examples illustrate the multiplicity of different forms of molecules. *α-Fetoprotein* (AFP) is a normal glycoprotein (molecular weight 70 000 dalton) similar to albumin and found in the fetuses of various mammals. In normal adults there are only very low concentrations in serum. In patients with certain tumours such as hepatoma and teratocarcinoma, AFP is found in high concentrations. In agreement with this, production of AFP can be demonstrated early during chemical hepatocarcinogenesis in experimental animals. Increased concentrations can also be seen, however, in toxic liver damage, hepatitis and cirrhosis which is important to take into consideration when using AFP diagnostically.

*Carcinoembryogenic antigen* (CEA) is a glycoprotein with a molecular weight of 175 000, containing 50–60% carbohydrate. It is found on the surface of normal colon in fetuses and in adults, on colon cancer cells and a number of other cancers, e.g. pancreas cancer, breast cancer and lung cancer. In most cases there is an increased concentration in the circulation of these cancer patients but this can also be seen in various types of inflammatory conditions. Several molecules have been identified in normal tissues cross-reacting with CEA.

*Fetal sulphoglycoprotein antigen* (FSA) has been demonstrated in gastric cancer cells and in cells from the mucous membrane of the fetal stomach as well as in the gastric juice from patients with gastric cancer. *Oncofetal pancreas antigen* (POA) is a cytoplasmic protein with a molecular weight of 40 000 that can be isolated from pancreatic cancer. It is excreted and present in the circulation in individuals with pancreas cancer as a high molecular weight complex (molecular weight 900 000).

With monoclonal antibodies several different glycoproteins and glycolipids have been identified as associated with melanoma. Many different monoclonal antibodies are directed against different parts of a glycoprotein with a molecular weight of 97 000 found in increased concentration on the surface of more than half of all melanoma tumours. This molecule is very similar to transferrin and also binds iron. The corresponding gene has been localized in chromosome 3 as has the transferrin gene. With gene cloning technology this molecule is now being analysed in detail.

A 350 000 glycoprotein is another TAM in melanoma and seems to be present independently of the 97 000 molecule. Monoclonal antibodies which recognize the carbohydrate moiety of the ganglioside GD3, whose structure is known, bind to the surface of viable cells from 80–90% of all investigated melanoma and also to sections of melanoma tissue. All melanomas so far investigated have had an increased concentration of one or several of these three molecules. A certain heterogeneity with regard to the expression of these molecules has been demonstrated within the same tumour and in metastases from that patient. It has not yet been excluded that small subpopulations of melanoma cells may exist, lacking all three different structures.

Two further glycolipids called OFA-I-1 and OFA-I-2 have been demonstrated in increased concentration in melanoma cells and in fetal brain tissue. They have been identified as gangliosides GM2 and GD2, respectively. They are of special interest in two ways. They are immunogenic in patients with the spontaneous appearance of antibodies demonstrable in melanoma patients. 'Immunization' with allogenic melanoma cells increases the titre. Assay of these antibodies has been reported to be of prognostic use in that patients with high titres have a better prognosis compared to other melanoma patients. Besides in melanoma OFA-I-2 is detected in tumours of neuroectodermal origin, while OFA-I-1 is present in a variety of neoplasms. Similarly about half of all healthy adults have low antibody titres against at least one of them. The reason for this sensitization is unknown.

Two lymphocyte clones from melanoma patients have been isolated after transformation with Epstein–Barr virus (EBV). They produce monoclonal antibodies, one against OFA-I-1 and the other against OFA-I-2. The latter appears to have a good specificity for melanomas.

A number of other monoclonal antibodies against TAM in cancer from various organs including colon, pancreas, kidney, lung, urinary bladder, brain and breast have been described. Their clinical usefulness is presently being assessed.

A large number of monoclonal antibodies are available which react with human leukaemia/lymphoma cell surface antigens. One type of antibody reacts with subpopulations of both normal and malignant B cells and therefore appears to detect differentiation antigens. None has been convincingly demonstrated to be directed against molecules exclusively present on neoplastic cells. However, it is clearly demonstrated by these antibodies that the B leukaemia/lymphoma subtypes defined by conventional histopathology and cytology are quite heterogeneous. Of practical significance is the demonstration that some of the monoclonal reagents, e.g. the antibody detecting the transferrin receptor, recognize neoplastic cells of a group of patients with poorer prognosis. Other monoclonal antibodies detect differentiation antigens of T cell malignancies and show a similar great heterogeneity with morphologically defined subtypes. Analogous reagents against differentiation antigens of myeloid, monocytic and erythroid cells are also available.

## Diagnostic potential

A large number of polyclonal and monoclonal reagents against TAM are available which in tissue sections can show a relatively high degree of specificity in binding to various tumour cells. Simultaneous usage of several reagents produces good sensitivity. As an example a combination of three different monoclonal reagents against melanoma gives full sensitivity, i.e. all tumours were discovered in a series of some 100 melanomas. The specificity in relation to various normal tissues seems to be good.

Of even greater potential is the use of such antibodies to demonstrate TAM or TAA in the circulation, or for instance in urine. Only a few antibody reagents have yet been extensively tested and some, as those against CEA and AFP, have been shown to be of practical use in the follow-up of initially positive patients receiving therapy. An increase in the concentration of CEA is an early sign of recurrence of, for instance, colon cancer. In contrast it has not been possible to attain sufficient sensitivity and specificity to use CEA for screening purposes.

In China a large investigation has been carried out on AFP in 344 000 persons. Out of 149 with increased serum AFP levels, the diagnosis of primary liver cancer was confirmed in 129 (88%). Unfortunately surgical resection was possible only in a few of these patients.

Another diagnostic principle is the demonstration of TAA common to a group of tumours. This could be achieved by analysis of serum antibodies but also through demonstration of reactivity in, for instance, leucocyte migration inhibition tests, leucocyte adherence inhibition tests or lymphocyte stimulation tests, in which the *in vitro* responsiveness of patient lymphocytes to specific antigen exposure is determined. None of these tests have so far become clinically useful, mainly due to insufficient sensitivity and specificity, which may be because of the TAA used. The further development of this assay technology is very important to make it possible to monitor immunotherapeutic effects.

On the basis of the development of a number of monoclonal antibodies against TAM, the tumour localization *in vivo* is being tested. Intravenous injection of isotope-labelled antibodies, intact or preferably as Fab fragments, is followed by repeated testing of the radioactivity over various parts of the body with a gamma camera. Fab fragments are advantageous because there is less non-specific uptake and delayed development of antibodies against the mouse antibodies. This area is rapidly developing and a much improved localization of small metastases can be expected through the combination of monoclonal antibodies directed against several different TAM.

# Therapeutic potential

Experience from animal experiments clearly indicates that it is possible to induce immunity in healthy individuals, resulting in efficient elimination of a transplanted isograft. It is also clear that it is much more difficult and often impossible to eliminate an already established tumour mass with the same procedures. The animal experiments point to three different principles which all function for certain types of tumours with demonstrable TAA. The first principle is the enhancement of immunity through improved immunization procedures including combinations of tumour material and immunological stimulators, for instance BCG. In certain animal models such treatment results in the elimination of already established small metastases. Analogous procedures have been tested in patients with various tumours with variable and doubtful effects. Evidence of increased tumour growth has also been reported. The conclusion is that mechanisms for this form of therapy must be further clarified and more efficient immunological techniques must be established to analyse the effects before these techniques can be adequately evaluated in humans.

Another therapeutic possibility is to utilize the patient's spontaneous reactivity against TAA. Elimination or decrease of T cell suppressor function has been tried in the mouse using antibodies against I-J antigens which are selectively found on suppressor T cells. This has had therapeutic effects. Similar therapeutic trials in man must await production of antibodies specific for T suppressor cells in the human. The recent progress concerning *in vitro* cultures of lymphocytes provides the possibility to select lymphocytes from patients with reactivity against TAA, to clone these lymphocytes and activate them *in vitro* and test them for possible therapeutic activity.

A third possibility is based on the transfer of antibodies against TAA or TAM. Therapeutic effects have been reported in certain systems with such antibodies. One type of antibodies was produced in mice through immunization with cells that were hybrids between a mouse myeloma and a human B cell lymphoma. The lymphoma surface immunoglobulin was present on the cell surface of the hybridoma. The mouse antibodies were found to bind to viable lymphoma cells and to the immunoglobulin produced by them and were thus anti-idiotype antibodies. Inoculation of the antibodies has resulted in a very good therapeutic effect in some lymphoma patients with complete regression of all lymphoma manifestations.

Antibodies against TAM are of major immunotherapeutic interest. The cytolytic effect of such antibodies can be used. Alternatively the antibodies can be employed as carriers of radioactive isotopes, a cytolytic agent, toxins such as ricin, cyctostatic drugs, or of boron atoms which on subsequent irradiation with slow neutrons emit $\alpha$-irradiation. Treatment with certain antibodies against TAM has resulted in clearly beneficial effects against transplants of human tumours in T cell deficient animals.

Monoclonal antibodies against differentiation antigens on blood cells have in certain cases given temporary therapeutic effects. The potential of such antibodies is still difficult to evaluate.

As mentioned above, a relatively good tumour localization has been attained with monoclonal antibodies in animals and man. This also suggests that a therapeutic use may become possible. A rapid development should be expected for this form of therapy and it is possible that specially tailored combinations of different monoclonal anti-TAM antibodies will be employed. The optimal combination will be possible to determine on the basis of binding tests on sections of tumour biopsies or against viable tumour cells.

## Conclusion

Clinical tumour immunology is still at a research level and only a few practical clinical applications have been established. Testing for the presence of AFP and CEA for prognostic purposes and follow-up of patients is already in use. At the research level there is a rapid development of monoclonal antibodies against TAM which may make it possible to

(1)   diagnose at least some tumour types by the use of sensitive radioimmuno-techniques and to support the histopathological diagnosis in other cases,
(2)   localize tumours *in vivo*, and
(3)   hopefully become a component in future cancer therapy because of the capacity of being enriched in tumours.

Due to the heterogeneity of most tumour cell populations, it will become necessary to use batteries of monoclonal reagents both diagnostically and therapeutically. Monoclonal human antibodies are being established which will become especially important when the antibodies can be injected into patients.

## Bibliography

ROSENBERG, S. A. (ed.) (1980). *Serologic Analysis of Human Cancer Antigens.* Academic Press, New York.
SELL, S. (ed.) (1980). *Cancer Markers. Diagnostic and Developmental Significance.* Humana Press, Clifton.
SELL, S. and WAHREN, B. (eds.) (1982). *Human Cancer Markers.* Humana Press, Clifton.

# Chapter 16

# Immunological diseases: immunological reactivity, inflammation and tissue damage

Lars Å. Hanson

The capacity of the lymphoid system to recognize and react with foreign material, such as micro-organisms, is of great importance for survival. This system must function for man to live a normal life. The defence reactions against exogenous material initiated via specific T and B lymphocytes are enhanced through several systems including soluble substances and cells. Antibodies, complement components, lymphokines and macrophages, granulocytes, mast cells react together and cooperate to fight and eliminate the 'non-self' material which has released the activity via the recognizing lymphocytes. This total reaction, which appears as *inflammation*, involves the host's own tissues to an extent which is dependent on the magnitude of the inflammatory reaction and which cells and humoral factors predominate.

In the presentation of the host defence in chapter 11, it was emphasized that the inflammatory reaction in many ways has positive effects, but also may be dangerous to the host and result in more or less pronounced tissue damage. This is true for inflammation released by and directed against exogenous material such as bacteria or viruses, which can induce immunological reactions directly hitting host tissues, as exemplified by T lymphocytes destroying the host's virus infected cells, or by disturbances in the control of the antibody response resulting in autoantibody production.

As a consequence of immunologically mediated tissue damage various diseases may appear. Such conditions are designated *immunological diseases* and include primarily allergies, immune complex diseases and autoimmune diseases. They will be described in the following chapters.

As a basis for the presentation a description is given of the various types of mechanisms that may be part of the pathogenesis of the immunological diseases. The first type reactions, nos. 1–4, originate from a classical description of Coombs and Gell. Later, further type reactions have been added, but they have not been given any generally accepted numbers and are presented separately after types 1–4.

**The immediate hypersensitivity reaction—type 1**

IgE antibodies bind to specific Fc receptors on mast cells and basophilic granulocytes and are found on the surface of such cells. These antibodies binding their antigen (allergen) induce a reaction mediated via various active components—histamine, leukotrienes—released from these cells (*Figure 16.1*). These mediators cause an *inflammation* which appears rapidly within 10–20 minutes, with swelling, redness and later eosinophilia. This reaction can cause hay fever, asthma, urticaria, etc., all

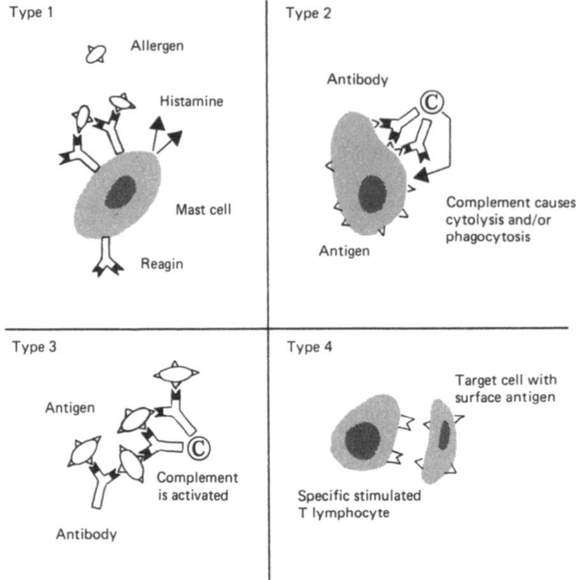


*Figure 16.1* Schematic representation of immunological mechanisms divided into four type reactions according to Coombs and Gell. *Type 1* is the immediate hypersensitivity reaction where binding of the antigen (allergen) to the reagin on the mast cell surface causes release of the symptom-inducing biologically active substances. *Type 2* is the cytolytic or cytotoxic reaction caused by complement activated by the reaction between antibodies and cell-bound antigen. *Type 3* is the immune complex reaction due to antibodies binding soluble antigen activating the complement system, inducing tissue damage. *Type 4* is the delayed hypersensitivity reaction caused by stimulated T lymphocytes. They produce lymphokines which are chemotactic for macrophages

manifestations of socalled *atopic allergy*. Such diseases are described in the next chapter.

## The cytotoxic or cytolytic reaction—type 2

Complement-activating antibodies reacting with an antigen on the surface of a cell can destroy this cell by complement-mediated lysis (*Figure 16.1*). Complement activation also enhances the neutrophilic granulocytes which can engulf and destroy the cell. The phagocytosis results in inflammation as described in chapter 11. This reaction type can cause tissue damage in a number of situations. A fetal blood group antigen which is lacking in the mother, can make the mother produce antibodies which are transferred to the fetus, destroying its red blood cells (cf. Rh immunization, chapter 9). Antibodies against erroneously transfused incompatible blood can have the same effect (chapter 9 and Appendix 1), as well as antibodies against drugs which have attached to the surface of red blood cells (*see* drug allergies, chapter 18). Genuine autoantibodies against thrombocytes, erythrocytes, or leucocytes can also mediate type 2 reactions as part of an autoimmune disease (chapter 21).

## The immune complex reaction—type 3

This reaction, as well as type 2, is mediated via complement-activating IgG antibodies, but with soluble, not cell-bound antigen (*Figure 16.1*). Antigen–antibody complexes are formed to eliminate the antigen, but complexes produced under certain conditions (i.e. in antigen surplus, tissue-bound antigen, *see further* chapter 19) may instead deposit in certain tissues. The complement activation causes aggregation of neutrophilic granulocytes, and their granular content together with the free radicals produced are toxic to tissues and induce a characteristic *inflammation* at the site. It appears after about 4–8 hours, much later than the type 1 reaction. Depending on where the reaction occurs, the individual will have various symptoms, possibly severe disease. In the kidneys there may be glomerulonephritis, in blood vessels vasculitis, in joints arthritis, etc. Immune complex diseases are presented in chapter 19.

## The delayed hypersensitivity reaction—type 4

While the three previously described reaction types are mediated via humoral antibodies, the fourth is dependent on T lymphocytes. Cell-mediated immunity can, in the same way as antibody-mediated immunity, protect as well as cause damage.

Antigen-activated T lymphocytes (*Figure 16.1*), which develop into lymphoblasts, appear as cytotoxic T cells and produce lymphokines with a number of activities, including chemotaxis for macrophages and macrophage activation. The aggregated macrophages induce an *inflammation* dominated by mononuclear cells. The reaction appears even later than type 1 and type 3 and is maximal only after 48–72 hours. It can cause disease in the form of contact dermatitis if it is directed against a material which via contact with skin and mucous membranes stimulates T lymphocyte-mediated immune reactivity (*see further* chapter 17). In connection with certain virus infections T lymphocytes are thought to cause exanthema, as well as post-infectious encephalitis. The granulomatous changes, for instance in tuberculosis, leprosy and schistosomiasis may have a similar pathogenesis. T lymphocytes can also play a role in certain autoimmune diseases (chapter 21), as they do in transplant rejection (chapter 14).

According to this description of the type reactions 1–4, the IgE antibodies, the complement activating IgG antibodies and activated T lymphocytes all cause inflammatory reactions of somewhat different characteristics (*Figure 16.2*). In the host all the reactions may occur more or less mixed. Neutrophil chemotaxis is induced both via the complement system and via leukotriene B4 from mast cells. Chemotaxis for eosinophilic granulocytes may come from mast cells, but probably also via T lymphocytes and the complement system, which in addition via C3b (fragment of activated C3) seems to be able to activate macrophages. Since macrophages produce C3 this connection can be important in several situations. There is much interest in the macrophages, not only because of their role in antigen presentation initiating rhe immune response and as effector cells for T lymphocyte mediated immune reactions, but also since they can play a central role in various mechanisms resulting in tissue damage. Apart from the toxic superoxide and hydroxyl radicals and the enzymes produced by the macrophages (collagenase, proteases, etc.), they can stimulate fibroblasts. This could be part of the pathogenesis behind certain forms of lung fibrosis. Macrophages can also activate osteoclasts, which results in degradation of bone tissue. This is seen in severe periodontitis due to a destructive inflammation in the supportive tissue of the teeth released by the active host defence against the bacterial deposits, plaques, on teeth.

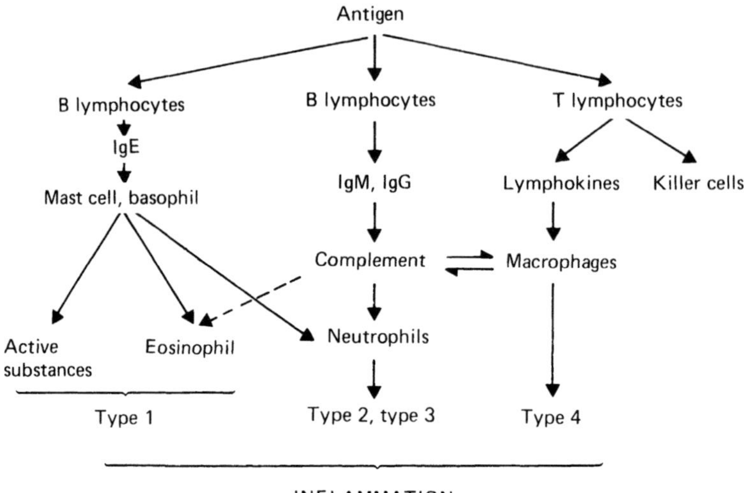


*Figure 16.2* The reaction of IgE antibodies with the allergen results in an inflammation, the immediate hypersensitivity reaction, dominated by eosinophilic granulocytes. Complement-activating antibodies binding to their antigens cause inflammation dominated by neutrophilic granulocytes. Antigen-stimulated T lymphocytes induce an inflammation with macrophages as the important effector cells

## Other type reactions

In addition to the four type reactions in *Figure 16.1*, there are also other immunological mechanisms that can be part of the pathogenesis of various diseases.

(1)   Antibodies directed against active molecules such as enzymes and hormones may cause symptoms of deficient enzyme or hormone activity (*Figure 16.3A*). This has been seen for antibodies against coagulation factors, against insulin and its cell receptor. Blocking autoantibodies against the acetylcholine receptor is an important part of the pathogenesis of myasthenia gravis. Autoantibodies against 'intrinsic factor' can prevent the uptake of vitamin $B_{12}$. This type reaction depends on the appearance of *blocking or inactivating antibodies*.

(2)   Disease can also be caused by *stimulating antibodies* (*Figure 16.3B*). Antibodies against the receptor for the thyroid-stimulating hormone are thought to induce thyroid hyperfunction with toxic goitre as a consequence (chapter 21).

(3)   Finally there is a reaction type called *antibody dependent cell-mediated cytolysis* (ADCC, chapter 7). Various mononuclear cells, such as certain lymphocytes and macrophages, as well as granulocytes, bound by their Fc receptors to IgG antibodies on a target cell become cytotoxic against the cell (*Figure 16.3C*). This reaction is probably part of the defence against certain virus infections and may also cause haemolytic anaemia. The fact that Rh antibodies mostly belong to the efficiently complement activating IgG subclass 3, may explain at least part of the Rh immunization as an ADCC-mediated destruction of the Rh-positive fetal red cells.

Most probably all immunological mechanisms in one form or another are part of the host defence against infections. This is clearly true for neutralizing and complement activating antibodies as well as cell-mediated immunity. IgE antibodies, together with

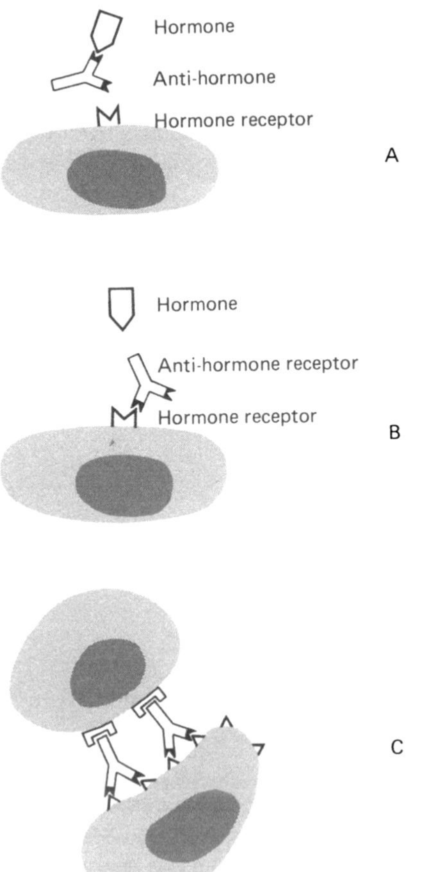


*Figure 16.3*A Autoantibodies against a hormone can block its activity and the patient will have symptoms of a hormone deficiency. B. Autoantibodies against a hormone receptor can block the hormone effect and cause the same symptoms of deficient activity as under A, or induce the same effect as the hormone by stimulating the receptor. C. Antibody-dependent cell-mediated cytolysis (ADCC). A cytotoxic cells uses its Fc receptors to attach to the target cell via IgG antibodies

eosinophilic granulocytes can be part of the defence against certain helminths (chapter 11). These defence mechanisms are necessary for survival. At the same time they are dangerous, if not carefully directed and balanced. The increased frequency of immunological diseases, both atopic allergy and autoimmune diseases in patients with certain immunodeficiencies, illustrate this (chapter 13). Better knowledge of the various controlling and regulating mechanisms in the host defence may aid in understanding the pathogenesis of several common diseases such as atopic allergy, rheumatoid arthritis and glomerulonephritis. This should provide a basis for improved diagnostic techniques and possibilities for more efficient therapy and prophylaxis via immunological measures.

*The immunological diseases* are described as follows:

| | |
|---|---|
| *Mechanisms* | |
| Allergies | chapters 17, 18 |
| Immune complexes | chapters 19, 20 |
| Autoimmunity | chapter 21 |
| *Diagnostic methods* | Appendix 2 |
| *Anaphylactic shock* | chapter 17 |

# Bibliography

LACHMAN, P. J. and PETERS, D. K. (eds) (1982). *Clinical Aspects of Immunology*. Vol. I–II, 4 edn. Blackwell, Oxford.
SELL, S. (1978). Immunopathology, *Am. J. Pathol.*, **90**, 211.

# Atopic allergies and contact allergies

**Lars Å. Hanson**

The concept of *allergy* was introduced by von Pirquet in 1906 to designate the *changed capacity to react*, developed after contact with an antigen. On renewed contact with the same antigen, there is a different reactivity due to the immune response against that antigen. Some authors, especially in the UK, use allergy in this original wide sense since it permits a clear definition of the concept. Allergy then includes all manifestations of immunological mechanisms, both their positive functions providing host defence against infections and their untoward effects causing tissue damage and disease.

In other literature, especially American, allergy is used in a more limited, less defined sense only including atopic allergy, contact allergies and drug allergies. This may be the most common use of the word allergy and it is applied thus in this book. Allergy then comprises effects of hypersensitivity reactions, e.g. conditions with an abnormally increased reactivity via the immune response. These diseases mainly include those caused via reaction type 1: immediate type of hypersensitivity (*Figure 16.1*, p. 192). In connection with such reactions, the concept of *anaphylaxis* is occasionally used. It was introduced by Richet in 1902 to describe the lethal hypersensitivity reaction that he observed in dogs. Now the term is mostly used in connection with the generalized hypersensitivity reaction of immediate type i.e. anaphylactic shock.

Usually the immediate hypersensitivity reactions show their manifestations *locally* causing allergic rhinitis, conjunctivitis, urticaria, angio-oedema, atopic eczema, and asthma (*Table 17.1*).

Reaction type 4, the *delayed type of hypersensitivity* (*Figure 16.1*, p. 192), causes contact dermatitis as an allergic manifestation (*Table 17.1*).

Common to these allergic reactions, as to all immunological reactions, is that they appear only after the individual has been exposed to the antigen and become sensitized, developing a changed capacity to react. On challenge by new exposure to the antigen, the immunological reaction is released and the allergic symptoms appear.

## Immediate hypersensitivity reactions

A patient with allergic rhinitis who comes into contact with the material to which he is sensitive, has a hypersensitivity reaction localized to the mucous membranes of the nose with increased secretion, swelling and obstruction of the nose as a consequence. These symptoms are examples of an allergic reaction released via the mechanism of immediate hypersensitivity (reaction type 1 in *Figure 16.1*, p. 192). Conditions which appear as a result of this mechanism are designated *atopic allergy*.

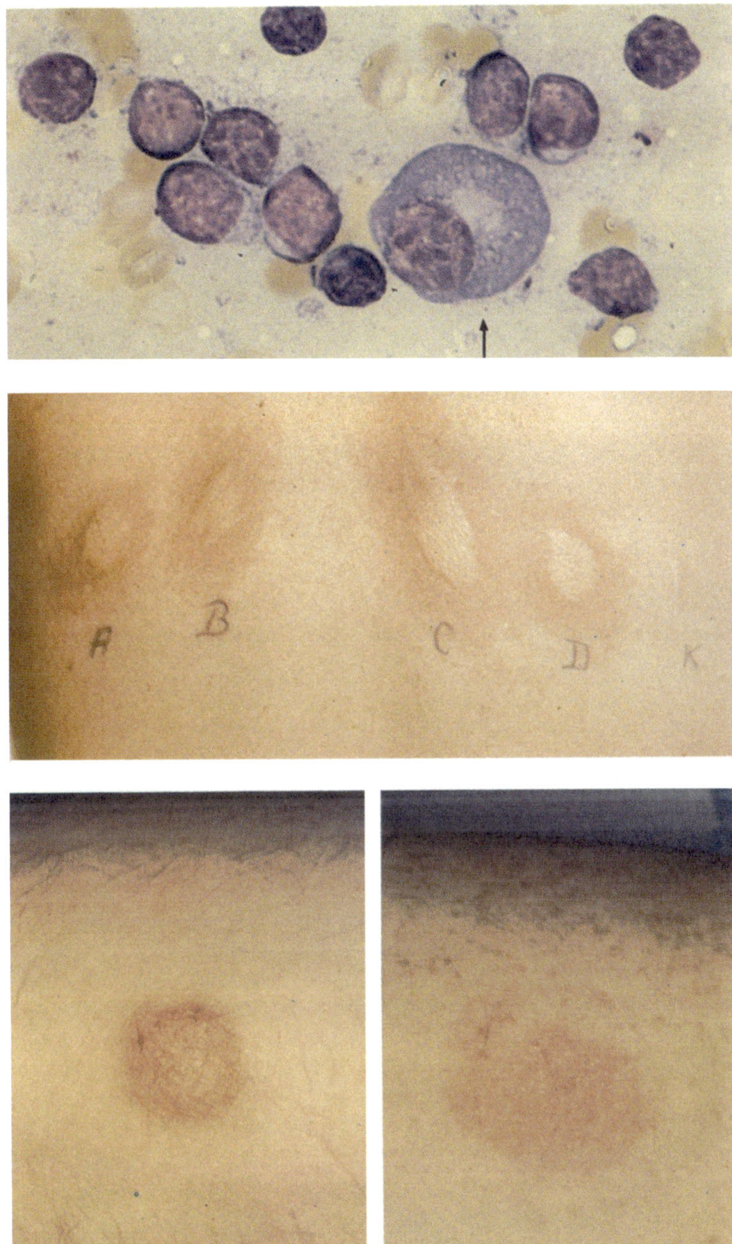

*Plate 1* A. Plasma cell (indicated by arrow) surrounded by small lymphocytes and red blood cells (the latter faintly red). (Photo: S. Persson, Göteborg). B. The typical weal and flare reaction induced by injection of an allergen into the skin of a person hypersensitive to this allergen (reaction type 1, immediate type hypersensitivity). The letters A, B, C and D indicate various allergens, the K stands for negative control. (Photo: H. Arnoldsson, Göteborg). C. Delayed-type hypersensitivity reaction (reaction type-4), to the left, after injection of tuberculin, redness, induration and papules. To the right a typical contact dermatitis with redness, scaling and small papules induced after sensitization with dinitrochlorobenzene (DNCB)

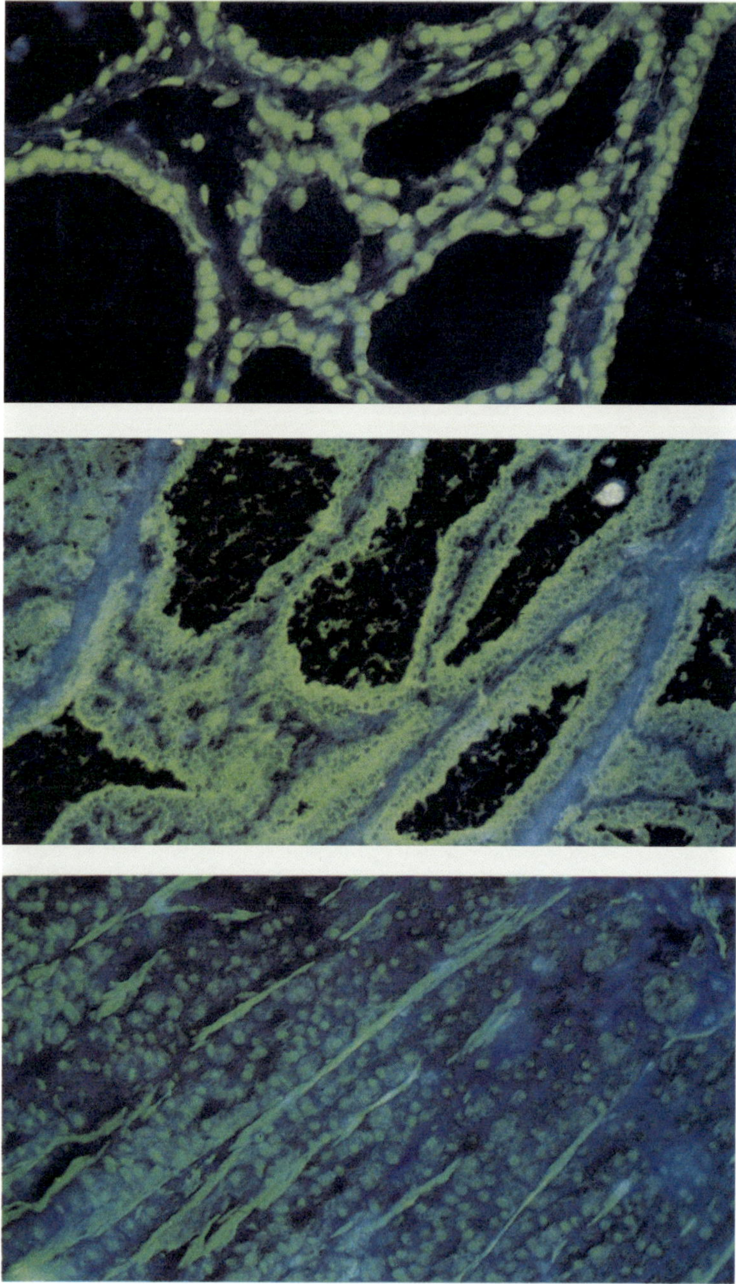

*Plate 2* Autoantibodies demonstrated by indirect immunofluorescence technique. Frozen sections of human thyroid. A. Antibodies against cell nuclei which are clearly stained, while the cytoplasma is unchanged. B. Antibodies against cytoplasmic antigens of thyroid cells. The nuclei are not stained and appear darker than the cytoplasm. The antibodies against thyroglobulin give a reticular fluorescence in the acini. C. Frozen section of gastric mucosa from rat. Antibodies against smooth muscle and against nuclear antigen. The muscle cells appear as illuminated streaks in the mucosa. Furthermore there is fluorescence of the cell nuclei

**TABLE 17.1. Allergic diseases**

---

**A.** *Immediate type hypersensitivity reactions* (reaction type 1)

*Released* by the binding of IgE antibodies, *reagins*, attached to mast cells, and their *allergin*, resulting in liberation of the *biologically active substances* which give the allergic symptoms, arising within 10–20 minutes after the challenge.
Can be passively transferred via serum.

*Causes* the atopic allergic diseases hay fever, asthma, urticaria, angio-oedema, atopic eczema, anaphylactic shock and some drug allergies (the latter can in certain cases also be induced via the reaction types 2, 3, and 4, *see* chapter 18).

**B.** *Delayed type hypersensitivity reactions* (reaction type 4)

*Released* via T lymphocytes.
The reaction develops 12–48 hours after the challenge.
Cannot be transfrred via serum, but with T lymphocytes.

*Causes* contact dermatitis.

---

The sensitizing material, the *allergen*, e.g. pollen, reacts with special antibodies, the *reagins*, which are produced by the atopic individual after sensitization and belong to the IgE class and bind to mast cells and basophilic granulocytes. The allergen–reagin reaction on the surface of a mast cell causes release from the cell of a number of *biologically active substances* (histamine, leukotrienes, etc, *see below*), which cause the allergic symptoms. Injecting the allergen into the skin of the hypersensitive individual, produces a typical swelling and redness (weal and flare reaction) which appears in a few minutes as a sign of the immediate hypersensitivity reaction when the allergen meets the mast cell-fixed reagins in the skin (*see* colour plate 1B, opposite p. 198). This inflammatory reaction mainly results from tissue oedema as a consequence of an increased blood flow in capillaries with increased permeability as described in detail below. Also typical for this allergic reaction is a local and general *eosinophilia*. The aggregation of these cells is due to a specific chemotactic factor released from the mast cells after the reaction of the IgE antibodies with the allergen.

## Heredity and pathogenesis

Various allergic diseases such as asthma, hay fever and urticaria can appear in one individual. There is a hereditary disposition for these allergic diseases, which were summarized under the designation *atopy* by Coca in 1922.

It is clear that atopic diseases are more common in individuals who have relatives with allergic symptoms of atopic type, than in those who do not. Children with one allergic parent run a risk of about 50% of attracting atopic allergy. If both parents are atopic the risk increases to about 60%. The mode of inheritance is not yet known.

The atopic individual produces IgE antibodies in large amounts against antigens, e.g. in pollen or household dust, which normal individuals do not. The explanation for this is not clear, but it is most probably due to a deficient control of the IgE production. Atopic individuals have a decreased number of T lymphocytes in the blood and presumably also an insufficient antigen-specific and/or non-specific T suppressor cell control of IgE production. It has recently been shown that T lymphocytes release IgE binding factors, which may participate in regulation of the IgE production.

Possibly one locus controls the general synthesis of IgE, whereas one or several specifically regulate the level of response against various allergens. It is not known how the IgE mediated reactivity against parasites mentioned in chapter 11 functions in atopic individuals.

Mechanisms other than IgE mediated ones can possibly be part of the pathogenesis in atopic diseases. Antibodies against $\beta_2$-receptors have recently been found in atopic patients. Such antibodies could block the receptors and support previous theories (Szentivanyi) about a $\beta$-adrenergic hyporeactivity in atopy, but there is currently no evidence that the receptor antibodies are of any biological significance. The permeability of mucous membranes to allergens may also differentiate atopic from non-atopic individuals. Again there are no conclusive data as to the importance of such factors in atopic diseases.


**Reagins–IgE antibodies**

In contrast to IgG or IgM antibodies, which are easily demonstrated and studied with precipitation and agglutination reactions (chapter 4), reagins can only be measured with more elaborate technology since they do not precipitate, agglutinate, or bind complement and are only found in concentrations of about $30\,\mu g/l$ in serum.

IgE antibodies are characterized by their specific capacity to attach to receptors on mast cells in the skin (skin-sensitizing antibodies) and mucous membranes, as well as basophilic granulocytes.

The IgE antibodies and their role as reagins were discovered in the 1960s. This finding formed a basis for an improved understanding of atopic diseases and resulted in the development of new diagnostic methods.

IgE has a molecular weight of 190 000 dalton and has, like IgM, five domains in its heavy chain (chapter 2). In contrast to most other antibodies the reagins are inactivated at a temperature of 56 °C for one hour. Like IgM and IgA antibodies, they do not pass through the placenta. They do not bind complement, but have on their heavy chain a structure which makes them attach to receptors on the surface of mast cells and basophilic granulocytes. Only 0.1–0.001 $\mu g/ml$ of specific IgE antibodies are required to cause a positive skin reaction after passive transfer of the antibodies (the Prausnitz–Küstner test, *see below*).

The IgE receptor on mast cells and basophilic granulocytes has been characterized. It is a glycoprotein of approximately 60 000 dalton. There are more than 100 000 receptors per cell. Each receptor can bind one IgE molecule. The higher the IgE concentration in serum, the larger the number of IgE molecules bound per cell. The binding is reversible. It is possible that the atopic allergic reaction in some cases can be released in other ways than via IgE antibodies. For instance there are controversial data that IgG4 antibodies can mediate immediate hypersensitivity reactions.


**Methods to demonstrate reagins**

In some cases of atopic allergy the history is so clear that further diagnostic work is not really necessary. Allergy to grandmother's cat can be quite obvious, but often further diagnostic support is required. Various ways of demonstrating the presence of reaginic IgE antibodies against the suspected allergens are then used.


*In vivo methods*

*Skin testing*    As already mentioned, an immediate type hypersensitivity reaction can be induced in the allergic individual giving the typical weal and flare reaction by introduction of the allergen in to the skin (colour plate 1B, opposite p. 198). These symptoms are caused by the active substances which are released when the allergen reacts with the specific reagins fixed to the mast cells in the skin. The prick test is usually used. Although the intracutaneous test is 10–100 times as sensitive, it is more painful and more often causes non-specific reactions, as well as severe allergic symptoms.

The patient is tested with the allergens suspected of causing the patient's symptoms on the basis of a detailed and careful history. A positive skin test demonstrates that the patient has reaginic antibodies in the skin against the allergen used, but it does not necessarily mean that the patient also has clinical symptoms caused by this allergen. As many as 30–40% of bakers finally develop positive skin tests against flour, but only a small number of them have a clinically manifest allergy to flour. As a screening test to implicate possible symptom-causing allergens the skin test is of great value in the work-up of an allergic patient. Its importance varies with the type of allergy. In pollen allergy skin testing gives useful information, while it is usually of little help in food allergy.

*Provocation test*   A careful history together with skin testing can bring out a number of allergens that can be suspected to be of aetiological importance in an individual with allergic symptoms. Often the positive tests can confirm the history making further tests unnecessary. In some instances however, further confirmation may be required. To prove that the suspected allergens really cause clinical problems a provocation test may be useful. The patient can inhale an aerosol containing the suspected allergen. If allergic symptoms in the form of coughing and dyspnoea of asthmatic type are induced, this can be seen as evidence that this allergen really can cause allergic symptoms of clinical relevance. In hay fever the suspected pollen can be applied directly onto the mucous membrane of the nose to verify the diagnosis.

It is important to realize that severe allergic symptoms, even life-threatening anaphylactic shock, can be released by provocation tests, as well as by skin testing, unless prick tests are used (*see further* Appendix 2).

*Passive transfer test in man—the Prausnitz–Küstner test*   In 1919 it was noted that reagins could be transferred from one individual to another through blood transfusion. The non-allergic patient who had had a blood transfusion from an individual allergic to horses had an asthma attack on his way home in a horsedrawn carriage. A few years later Prausnitz demonstrated on himself that he could obtain an immediate type hypersensitivity reaction in the skin on intradermal injection of a fish extract if he first injected at the same site serum from Küstner who was allergic to fish. This passive transfer test which was later called the Prausnitz–Küstner (PK) test has been of great use in allergy research.

### In vitro methods

*Quantification of IgE in blood*   Using a radioimmunosorbent technique (RIST or PRIST, *see Figure A2.1A* in Appendix 2) the level of circulating IgE is determined. Increased levels are found in about 60% of atopic individuals. The method is mainly of use in doubtful cases.

*Determination of reagins against certain allergens*   With the radioallergosorbent technique (RAST, *see Figure A2.1B* in Appendix 2), the level of IgE reagin against a certain allergen can be determined in serum. The method can be used for a number of well-characterized allergens. RAST gives, together with a careful history and clinical evaluation as good information as a correctly performed prick test, but is more expensive. In unselected materials RAST shows an agreement with the skin testing, provocation and history of approximately 75%, in certain groups over 90%.

**Allergens**

The allergens which sensitize atopic individuals are usually proteins of relatively low molecular weight, between 10 000–60 000 dalton, most are between 15 000–25 000 dalton. They are quite stable molecules, often relatively resistant to enzymic degradation. Their small size and stability may be of importance for their capacity to permeate mucosal membranes in immunogenic form.

Allergens are most commonly found in house dust, animal dander, food and pollen.

Pollen from ragweed, which is a very common plant in north America but not in Europe, is said to cause three-quarters of all cases of hay fever in the USA and half of all allergies there. What makes the constituents of these pollens so extremely potent as allergens is unknown. One reason may be the extensive spread of the plant and the large amount of pollen produced. Exposure to the ragweed pollen for three to five years is usually required before the allergy develops; for other allergens longer or shorter periods of time are necessary.

It is characteristic that the IgE response is released by very small amounts of allergen. During a pollen season it has been estimated that hay fever patients are exposed to only about 0.1 $\mu$g of the most common allergen from ragweed pollen.

Previously used allergen extracts from, for instance, house dust and various pollens contained a number of uncharacterized components. During the last few years many of the most important allergens have been identified and isolated. These purer allergen preparations of standardized strength and content have improved the diagnosis of allergic disease. The ten most common allergens cause about 95% of atopic allergies.


**Mechanism of the immediate hypersensitivity reaction**

In an individual allergic to a certain pollen as much as 30% of his IgE can be directed against the pollen allergen. Much of this IgE is found attached to the specific IgE receptors on the mast cells, which are found in the connective tissue around vessels, in the lung mainly in the submucosa, but also in the epithelium and in the lumen of the respiratory tract. The connective tissue mast cells differ morphologically and functionally from the mucosal mast cells, which are T cell dependent.

If two adjoining IgE antibodies bind to the same allergen molecule an enzyme is activated, serine esterase (*Figure 17.1A*). The enzyme causes production of phosphatidyl choline. Concomitantly there is an increase in the permeability of the cell membrane for calcium ions, which are required for the activation of phospholipase $A_2$. This enzyme hydrolyses phospholipids, such as phosphatidyl choline, to arachidonic acid and lysophosphatidyl choline. The calcium also activates enzymes which cause release of energy, aggregation of the microtubuli and contraction of contractile elements. As a result the granules of the mast cell, of which there can be 1000 per cell, move towards the cell membrane and fuse with it. The granules then release outside the cell their content of already produced substances: histamine, heparin, serotonin and a tetrapeptide with chemotactic effect on eosinophilic granulocytes (Eosinophil Chemotactic Factor, ECF-A), as well as a factor chemotactic for neutrophils (NCF-A). A thrombocyte activating component, PAF (Platelet Activating Factor) is produced (*Figure 17.1B*) and a number of enzymes are released including neutral proteases which stimulate the arachidonic acid cascade. Prostaglandins (PG) and thromboxane are then produced via cyclo-oxygenase and leukotrienes (LT) via lipoxygenase. The mast cells mainly make $PGD_2$, which stimulates the arachidonic acid cascade in macrophages. Prostaglandins $D_2$, $F_{2x}$ and thromboxane $A_2$ contract the smooth muscles of the bronchi, while $PGE_2$ has a weak dilating effect. $PGD_2$, $E_2$ and $I_2$ potentiate the increased vascular permeability caused by histamine. $PGD_2$ and $F_{2x}$ increase the secretion from exocrine submucosal glands and are chemokinetic for eosinophils and neutrophils. Alveoler macrophages also seem to be activated.

The production of leukotrienes adds even more strikingly to the immediate hypersensitivity reaction. The leukotriene $B_4$ is more strongly chemotactic for eosinophils and neutrophils than ECF-A and NCF-A. Furthermore $LTB_4$ stimulates the neutrophilic phagocytes to produce free oxygen radicals and enzyme liberation. The ensuing inflammation is enhanced by the eosinophils through their granular content of ECP and MBP (cf. chapter 11), which are cytotoxic and can damage the epithelium in the respiratory tract.

It has been discussed whether or not the eosinophilic cells can dampen or regulate the immediate hypersensitivity reaction. ECP can neutralize heparin, PGE can decrease further degranulation of mast cells, histaminase and arylsulphatase can possibly diminish the effects on histamine and the leukotrienes (*Figure 17.1C*). Histamine also has a feedback mechanism via $H_2$ receptors, which may inhibit further histamine release.

The leukotrienes $C_4$, $D_4$ and $E_4$, which are produced in parallel with $B_4$, contract smooth muscles in human bronchi 1000 times as efficiently as histamine. They also induce increased vascular permeability and mucus production. The discovery of the arachidonic acid cascade (Nobel prize 1982 to S. Bergström, B. Samuelsson and J. Vane) has added considerably to our understanding of the details of the immediate hypersensitivity reaction primarily through the description of leukotrienes. (The previously used designation SRS-A, Slow Reacting Substance of Anaphylaxis-A corresponds to the leukotrienes $LTC_4$, $D_4$ and $E_4$.)

Some authors claim that the platelet activating factor (PAF) is of great importance for the induction of the special inflammation of atopic allergy.


**Systems of atopic allergy**

*The local hypersensitivity reactions*   These are the most common manifestations of atopic allergy and are found in around 15% of the population.

The shock organ is the nose when the patient has *allergic rhinitis* and the eyes when the patient has allergic *conjunctivitis*. The symptoms from these mucous membranes are sneezing, running nose and eyes, swelling of the mucous membranes with obstruction of the nose and itching. Histamine is probably a major mediator of these symptoms. The allergens which commonly cause allergic rhinitis come from various pollens. The patients only have symptoms during the time of the year when the pollen causing their symptoms appears. Allergic rhinitis is very common, occurring in about 8–10%.

If the allergy is localized to the skin *urticaria*, or angio-oedema (Quincke oedema) may occur. The angio-oedema can also be localized in the larynx with risk of suffocation. *Eczema* can have an atopic pathogenesis, i.e. immediate hypersensitivity reaction in the skin.

In *asthma* the shock organ is the bronchi, at times appearing in combination with some of the other atopic conditions mentioned above. Asthma is also common occurring in about 1–4% of the population. In children causative allergens are found in 85–90%, among adults in only about 30%. These cases are called *exogenous asthma*. The allergens causing asthma are less often from pollen, which due to their size are mostly caught in the upper respiratory airways where they may induce hay fever. In contrast spores from moulds can get all the way down into the lungs and are together with allergens from house dust and animals the most common exogenous causes of asthma. The main allergen in house dust comes from mites, mainly *Dermatophagoides pteronyssinus* and *farinae*, but in house dust there are usually allergens from a number of animals such as horses, dogs, cats and cows.

During an asthma attack the bronchoconstriction dominates causing the typical wheezing breathing and the increased production of tenacious mucus which induces coughing. The leukotrienes have a central role, whereas histamine may be of minor importance compared to atopic reactions in skin and nasal mucosa. The immediate hypersensitivity reaction appears within some 20 minutes after the exposure to the allergen in the lung. The asthmatic symptoms have a later phase appearing after six to eight hours. Previously it was thought to be immune complex dependent (cf. chapters 16 and 19), but the late phase is due rather to the effects of leukotrienes, prostaglandins,

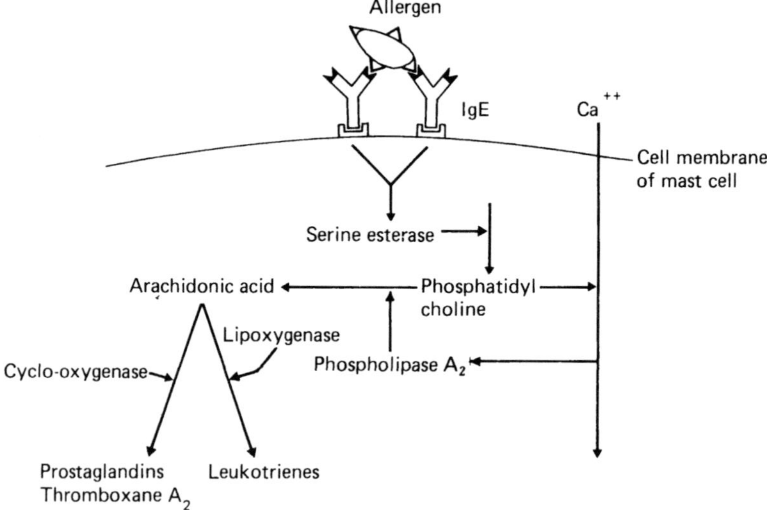


*Figure 17.1* A. Schematic and simplified picture showing two IgE antibodies bound to IgE receptors on a mast cell. When the IgE antibodies bind the allergen they recognize serine esterase is activated, resulting in formation of phosphatidyl choline. That increases the permeability of the cell membrane to Ca$^{++}$. The influx of Ca$^{++}$ activates phospholipase A$_2$, which is followed by production of arachidonic acid, and the synthesis of prostaglandins, thromboxane and leukotrienes.

B. The initial stage depicted in *Figure 17.1A* is followed by Ca$^{++}$ activating enzymes making the mast cell granules move towards the cell membrane. They fuse with the cell membrane and empty their content of active substances outside the cell. Drugs like *adrenaline* increase cyclic AMP via stimulation of $\beta$ receptors. *Theophyllamine* also increase cAMP, but through blocking of phosphodiesterase which normally degrades cAMP. Increased cAMP inhibits the movement of the granules to the cell membrane and the succeeding degranulation. *Sodium cromoglycate* inhibits the degranulation by prevention of the passage of Ca$^{++}$ into the cell, and *cortisone* inhibits phospholipase A$_2$ and thereby the production of prostaglandins and leukotrienes. *Antihistamine* competes with histamine for the H$_1$-receptors on the target organ.

C. The reagin–allergen reaction on the mast cell surface results in release of histamine, leukotrienes, etc. which, by their effects on the target organ, cause the allergic symptoms. The eosinophil chemotactic factor (ECF-A) and LTB$_4$ from the mast cell induce aggregation of eosinophilic granulocytes, which via PCE, ECP, aryl sulphatase and histaminase probably add to and/or regulate the atopic allergic inflammation

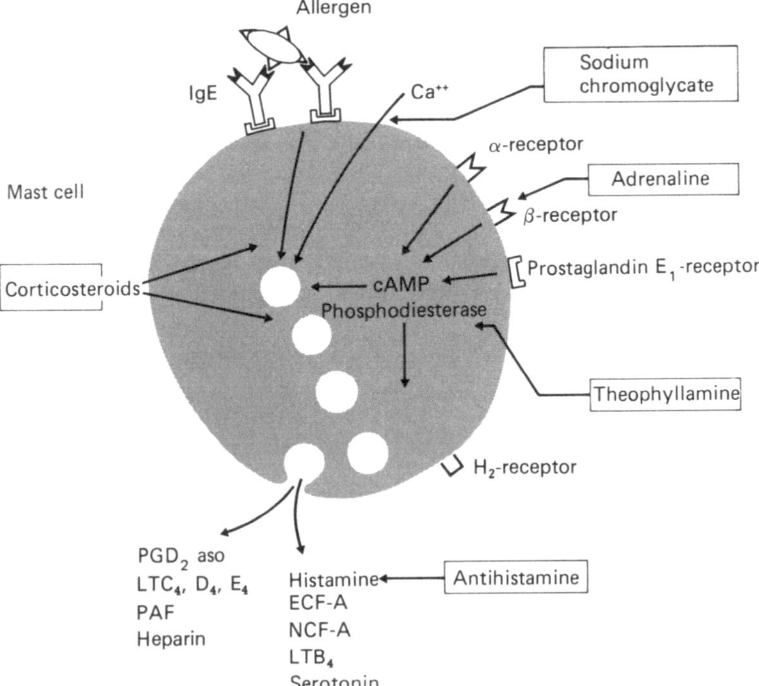



*Figure 17.1* B

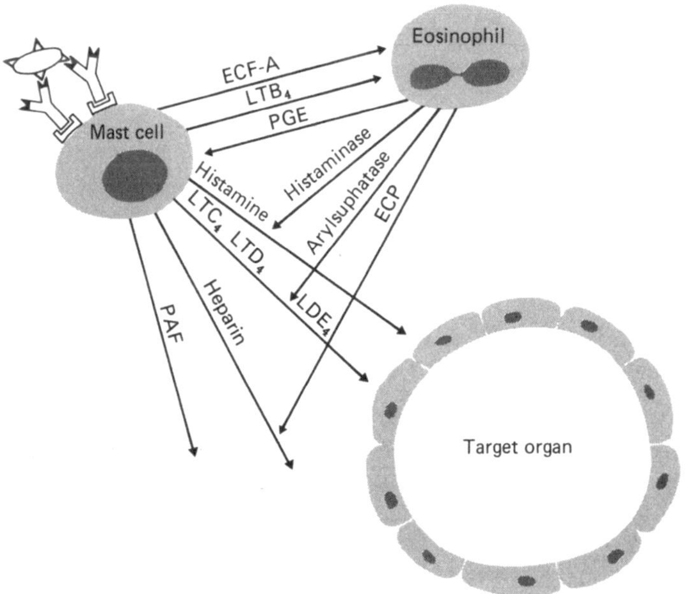



*Figure 17.1* C

thromboxane $A_2$ and possibly PAF. They may cause a long-standing bronchoconstriction, oedema in the submucosa and increased mucus production. The aggregation of neutrophilic granulocytes probably depends on the NCF-A from the mast cells.

In chronic, not therapeutically controlled asthma, tissue damage appears, which is probably due to the infiltrating eosinophils, neutrophils and monocytes. These cells presumably occur in response to the mediators $LTB_4$ and ECF-A.

*Endogenous asthma*, without demonstrable exogenous factors, is especially seen in adults. These patients have a hyperactivity in the bronchi for unknown reasons and a number of factors such as cold air, physical exercise and various irritating substances release bronchoconstriction with typical breathing problems. In small infants wheezing often occurs in connection with respiratory tract infections. This is at times called asthmatoid bronchitis, but does not necessarily develop into asthma. The reason may be a swelling of the mucosa in the respiratory tract caused by the infection. IgE antibodies have been demonstrated against, e.g. parainfluenzavirus, *H. influenza* and *S. pneumoniae* and it is possible that they are of pathogenetic significance, explaining bronchoconstriction in infections with these pathogens.

Adverse reactions of an allergic type to acetylsalicylic acid has been described in up to 20% of chronic asthmatic and urticaria patients. There is a preponderance in certain families. The mechanism of the reaction is not known. The reactivity is not dependent on IgE antibodies. Abberations in prostaglandin and leukotriene synthesis have been suggested, but are presumably not involved.

*Allergies to food* can cause urticaria and eczema, but also stomach pain, vomiting and diarrhoea. In infants such reactions caused by cows' milk proteins occur in about 0.5%. They usually vanish before the age of two.

Skin testing and demonstration of IgE antibodies does not give a good basis for the diagnoses of food allergies. It is usually necessary to prove the diagnosis by repeated trials with elimination of the suspected food from the diet and then challenge. There is reason to believe that food allergies are not only released, or even most often released via the immediate type hypersensitive reaction. An increase of prostaglandins $E_2$ and $E_{2\gamma}$ was recently found in the blood of individuals with egg allergy and intestinal symptoms.

In *coeliac disease* the symptoms from the intestine in the form of diarrhoea, malabsorption and villus atropy are caused by gliadin from wheat, rye and barley. Antibodies and T lymphocyte reactivity against components of gliadin develop and an immunological, possibly atopic allergic pathogenesis has been suspected, but is still unproven.

In *Crohn's disease* with inflammatory intestinal changes a deficient, or erroneously reacting host defence has been suspected. It has been assumed that micro-organisms in the intestinal mucosa could release tissue damaging allergic or other inflammatory reactions. The pathogenesis is still unknown.

*Anaphylactic shock*   This generalized hypersensitivity reaction is a rare life-threatening condition. In man the dominating symptoms are usually severe dyspnoea due to bronchospasm and a more or less pronounced circulation collapse with decreasing blood pressure. In addition there is often generalized urticaria, itching and sometimes vomiting and diarrhoea if the intestinal tract is also included as a shock organ. A severe reaction can be lethal.

It is not quite clear if this reaction is only released by the same mechanism as the local immediate hypersensitivity reactions. Even if the atopic reagins can be aetiologically important, it is possible that also other types of antibodies, e.g. IgG, can play a role for instance by activation of the complement system. In some cases of anaphylactic shock the complement level has been low, but it is not known if the activated complement system adds to the symptoms. In a number of cases with anaphylactic shock caused by penicillin all had reaginic antibodies. The severity of the anaphylactic reaction related to the level of the circulating IgE antibodies against penicillin.

The anaphylactic shock usually appears within one, or a few minutes after exposure to an allergen in an already sensitized individual. This provoking allergen has often been given parenterally, e.g. through injection of penicillin, intravenous injection of serum from a different species, skin testing or bee sting. The reaction can also be induced by a perorally given allergen.

For a period of time after an anaphylactic reaction, another one cannot be released with the same allergen. The patient is *refractory.*

## Treatment of atopic disease—hyposensitization

The treatment will only be discussed here in relation to the previously presented mechanisms.

*Allergen avoidance*   If the allergen which causes the atopic symptoms can be determined, avoidance of contact with this allergen will of course prevent the chain reaction of allergen–reagin-release of biologically active substances. Several allergens such as pollen, or house dust are difficult to avoid or eliminate from the milieux and therefore other strategies must be used.

*Immunotherapy—hyposensitization*   It was discovered many years ago that repeated injections of the allergen in very small doses, causing insignificant or no allergic reaction, decreases the sensitivity of that individual. This is called hypo- or desensitization. In pollen allergy the effect of this treatment is quite good, according to some authors an improvement is seen in up to 80% of the cases. Such results can be attained providing that the proper allergens have been defined and that well-standardized and characterized allergen preparations are employed.

The mechanism of the positive effect of hyposensitization is not quite clear, but may partly depend on the appearance of 'blocking' IgG antibodies, which are produced in response to the allergen injections. These antibodies, which on their own do not induce any hypersensitivity reaction, react with the homologous antigen/allergen and so block the allergen–reagin reaction. The blocking antibodies can inhibit a Prausnitz–Küstner test. Furthermore the synthesis of IgE antibodies against the injected allergen is decreased by hypersensitization, possibly through stimulation of T suppressor cells and/or production of inhibiting humoral factors. The hyposensitization treatment can decrease the hyperreactivity of the bronchi which is often seen in asthmatic patients. The mechanism which causes this is unknown.

A temporary desensitization can be carried through by means of repeated injections of the allergen over the course of a few hours. The available reaginic antibodies may be consumed by the large amount of allergen given. The refractory stage after anaphylactic shock may have a similar explanation.

In many cases of atopic diseases available methods do not permit demonstration of any causative allergen. In these patients the allergen cannot be eliminated or avoided and desensitization cannot be used. Various drugs are employed instead to try to eliminate or decrease the effects of the various mediators.

*Anti-allergic drugs    Antihistamines* compete with already released histamine for the $H_1$ receptors in smooth muscle and other tissues, while *catecholamines* function through the stimulation of $\beta$ receptors which increase the level of cAMP (*Figure 17.1B*). This prevents the degranulation through inhibition of the movement of the granules to the cell membrane. *Theophylline* which blocks the degradation of cyclic AMP by inhibiting the enzyme phosphodiesterase, has the same effect.

*Sodium cromoglycate* (Intal) may inhibit the release of mediators by blocking the passage of calcium through the cell membranes. Other data suggest that phosphorylation of a mast cell protein via cGMP turns off the release. Its effect on asthma does not primarily depend on the prevented release of histamine, but of other mediators such as leukotrienes (*Figure 17.1B*). The connective tissue, but not the mucosal mast cells are responsive to cromoglycate and theophylline.

The striking effect of *corticosteroids* in atopic allergy is not fully understood but most probably their capacity to inhibit phospholipase $A_2$ is important. This occurs through the production of the proteins macrocortin and lipomodulin which prevent the production of both leukotrienes, prostaglandins and thromboxanes. *Salicylates* are said to inhibit certain food-induced diarrhoeas, possibly through an inhibition of the production of prostaglandins and thromboxane from arachidonic acid.

# Delayed hypersensitivity reactions

Delayed hypersensitivity reactions (reaction type 4) which are a manifestation of cell-mediated immunity are induced by a number of bacterial, viral and fungal infections. Especially well known and studied is the delayed hypersensitivity reaction that can be demonstrated in tuberculosis which results in a positive tuberculin test (colour plate 1C, opposite p. 198). Furthermore cell-mediated immune reactions play an important role in transplantation rejection and tumour immunity (chapters 14 and 15). The delayed hypersensitivity reaction is also the mechanism causing *contact dermatitis*. The presentation here is limited to this allergic disease manifestation.

The theoretical background and the cellular reactivity behind the delayed type 4 hypersensitivity has already been described in chapter 7. It is caused by T lymphocytes without the participation of humoral antibodies. In contrast to immediate type hypersensitivity reaction, type 4 can not be passively transferred with serum from one individual to another. In addition the typical skin reactions which result from contact with the causative antigen or hapten, occur after 12–48 hours, whereas the immediate hypersensitivity reaction appears within some 20 minutes.

Contact dermatitis appears after repeated contact with a sensitizing substance on skin and mucous membranes. This may be a chemical, detergent, drug or plant material. After sensitization with certain substances such as extract of *Primula*, all individuals seem to develop a delayed hypersensitivity reaction, even though some require longer or repeated exposure. Application of penicillin on skin and mucous membranes induces contact allergy in as many as 10–15% of individuals. The difference in the tendency to become sensitized is probably genetically determined, but there is no relation between the heredity of atopic allergy and contact allergy. It seems that the atopic individuals have a rather smaller risk of developing contact dermatitis, possibly due to their decreased T lymphocyte reactivity.

It is remarkable that complete antigens rarely cause contact dermatitis. The offensive substances are usually simple compounds, such as dinitrochlorobenzene, formalin, picryl chloride or penicillin. How these compounds are taken up by the Langerhans cells in the skin is probably of central importance. These cells correspond to macrophages and form a network in the skin. They bind and present compounds taken up via the skin to T lymphocytes in local lymph glands and this may result in type 4 reactions.

Contact tests are used for the aetiologic diagnosis of contact dermatitis. Suspected substances are brought into contact with the skin for at least 24 hours. An allergic individual develops a typical delayed reaction with redness and papules, possibly vesicles and swelling (colour plate 1C, opposite page 198). The reactivity of T lymphocytes *in vitro* is not a useful test.

Cortisone is effective against contact dermatitis, which is probably the result of its anti-inflammatory activity.

### Shwartzman–Sanarelli's reaction

Endotoxin, which is a lipopolysaccharide complex from the cell wall of Gram-negative bacteria, has several biological effects. One of these is that an injection of endotoxin in the skin of rabbits, followed a few hours later by an intravenous injection of endotoxin results in a typical local skin reaction, called the *local Schwartzman reaction*. The skin becomes the site of a change which is reminiscent of an Arthus' reaction and vascular damage and invasion especially of leucocytes with necrosis, bleeding and intravascular coagulation occurs. It is remarkable that a number of substances other than endotoxin can be used for the second injection.

If both the first and the second injections are given intravenously a *generalized Schwartzman reaction* develops, and bilateral cortical necrosis of the kidneys and haemorrhagic necrosis in liver and spleen appears.

The mechanism of these reactions is unknown. It has been suggested that immunological mechanisms are involved, since immunization with endotoxin prevents the Schwartzman reaction in which complement is required for the reaction to appear. The fact that endotoxin activates complement via the alternative pathway may be of importance. Probably the activated complement system adds to the coagulation disturbances. Granulocytes also participate. On the other hand it has been suggested that it is a non-specific mechanism since the reaction can also be induced with a second releasing injection of agar, glycogen, or kaolin instead of endotoxin.

The generalized Shwartzman reaction has some similarities to certain diseases in man. A similar mechanism may be the cause of the disseminated intravascular coagulation, bilateral cortical necrosis of the kidneys and Waterhouse–Friedrichsen's syndrome (acute haemorrhagic necrosis of the adrenal glands in meningococcal sepsis).

# Bibliography

BUISSERET, P. D. (1982). Allergy. *Scientific American*, **247**, 82.
DUKOR, P., KALLOS, P., SCHLUMBERGER, H. D. and WEST, G. B. (eds.) (1982–1984). *PAR. Pseudo-Allergic Reactions. Involvement of Drugs and Chemicals*, Vols. 1–4. Karger, Basel.
ISHIZAKA, K. (ed.) (1982). Regulation of the IgE antibody response. *Progr. Allergy*, 32.
ISHIZAKA, K., YODOI, J., SUEMURA, M. and HIRASHIMA, M. (1983). Isotype-specific regulation of the IgE response by IgE-binding factors. *Immun. Today*, **4**, 7.
ISHIZAKA, K. (ed.) (1984). Mast cell activation and mediator release. *Progr. Allergy*, 34.
MÖLLER, G. (ed.) (1978). Immunoglobulin E. *Immunological Reviews*, 41.

# Chapter 18

# Immunological side effects of drugs

Göran Holm

Undesirable drug reactions are a major clinical problem. About 5% of all patients in internal medical departments are admitted with such reactions. Many of them have drug allergies. It is often difficult to differentiate between immunologically and non-immunologically mediated side effects of drugs. An immunological mechanism involves sensitization to the drug, or other related antigens and symptoms provoked by the drug. Even if immune reactivity against the drug can be demonstrated it is difficult to determine its relevance to the side effects. Untoward effects that are suspected to be allergic reactions can also appear without any immune reactivity being demonstrable. Toxic and other non-immunological side effects can occur in an immune individual. Therefore it is usually difficult and often impossible to substantiate an immunological cause of an adverse drug reaction. Drug allergy often remains a probable diagnosis based on clinical criteria including the appearance of urticaria, anaphylactic reactions, or serum sickness in persons with immune reactivity against the drug. Isolated damage of liver, lungs, blood cells and other organs occurring during the treatment with a drug can also have an immunological background.

Certain drugs can cause allergy-like symptoms in non-immune individuals through non-specific activation of inflammatory mechanisms (pseudo-allergic reactions). An example of this is acetyl salicylic acid, which in predisposed persons can cause type 1-like reactions possibly by release of mediators from mast cells and basophilic granulocytes. Polypeptide antibiotics and aminoglycosides can have similar effects. The rash, which often appears during ampicillin treatment of patients with various infections, also belongs to this group. Certain drugs like dextran can cause anaphylactoid reactions via type 3 reactions as well as non-immunological mechanisms, releasing mediators.

## Drugs as immunogens

The general requirements for a substance to induce an immune response are also valid for drugs. Most drugs are low molecular weight subtances (haptens) and are not immunogenic as such. A change of the molecule is required, which usually means that the drug is coupled with stable normally covalent bonds to amino, carboxyl or sulph-hydryl groups on a carrier protein (cf. chapter 3). It is well known from animal experiments that low molecular weight substances with a high chemical reactivity having the capacity to form covalent bonds at a physiological pH and to metabolize slowly, easily induce allergic reactions. Drugs usually do not have the same tendency as these substances to bind stably to micromolecules. It has therefore been assumed that reactive substances appearing during metabolization of the drug form immunogenic hapten–carrier conjugates. This hypothesis only seems to be partially correct. Even if reactive metabolites are produced during the catabolism of penicillin it is not clear to what extent they add to the immunization. Native penicillin can, after rearrangements, react directly with proteins producing penicilloyl, which is the main antigenic determinant of penicillin. Procainamide binds without metabolization and precipitates soluble nucleoprotein forming immunogenic conjugates. The concentration of the drugs should therefore be kept low so that few haptenic groups are bound to the autologous carrier macromolecules. Such conjugates are poor immunogens.

One cause of drug allergy is the presence of high molecular weight protein impurities present in penicillin and biological extracts such as non-synthetic polypeptide hormones. The frequency of allergic reactions has decreased with improved purity. Protein impurities in penicillin have large numbers of penicilloyl groups and are strongly immunogenic. Such penicillin-protein complexes probably play a major role for immunization against penicillin and for the appearance of penicillin allergy.

Low molecular weight drugs can also become immunogenic by polymerization. Ampicillin has a tendency to form polymers of varying size (*Table 18.1*). Larger polymers are immunogenic and can induce reactivity against the drug. Ampicillin polymers may be mitogenic as well, or have other non-specific effects on lymphocytes, explaining the ampicillin exanthema, which is a pseudo-allergic reaction. Drugs composed of high molecular weight heterologous proteins are strongly immunogenic. Antibodies against heterologous antilymphocyte globulin regularly appear after two to three weeks of treatment, when allergic reactions are common. Therefore the drug is of limited use for long-term treatment. Antibodies are produced during the treatment with heterologous enzymes such as streptokinase and L-asparaginase and can cause allergic side effects.

Autoimmunity is occasionally a consequence of treatment with certain drugs. One explanation may be that immunization against an autoantigen carrying the drug as a hapten breaks the tolerance against antigenic determinants of the carrier autoantigen

**TABLE 18.1. Immunity induced by drugs**

| *Drug* | *Immunogenic form* | *Immunity directed against* | *Examples* |
|---|---|---|---|
| Low molecular weight substance | (a) Conjugate between drug (hapten) and autologous carrier substance | Drug | Penicillin, procainamide |
| | | Carrier substance (autoimmunity) | Antinuclear antibodies under treatment with procainamide |
| | (b) Polymer of drug | Drug | Ampicillin |
| | (c) Conjugate between drug (hapten) and heterologous protein impurity | Drug | Penicillin |
| | | Carrier substance | |
| High molecular weight, heterologous substance | Drug | Drug | Antilymphocyte globulin, L-asparaginase |

(cf. chapter 8). This mechanism could explain the autoimmunization against nuclear antigens during the treatment with procainamide (*see below*). Another cause of autoimmunization may be changes of an autoantigen induced by a drug, making it appear as 'non-self' with immunization as a consequence. Autoimmune haemolytic anaemia occurring during the treatment with α-methyldopa may be an example of such a mechanism (*see below*).

## How is the allergic reaction induced?

Multiple antigenic determinants on the same molecule are required to induce an allergic reaction with antibodies, or sensitized lymphocytes. Univalent haptens in the form of a native drug or non-conjugated metabolite lack the capacity to induce allergic reactions and may compete with the conjugated drug for antibodies and sensitized T cells, possibly preventing the allergic reaction. The presence of blocking univalent antigen and allergy-inducing polyvalent antigens may be one of the factors determining whether or not an immunologic reaction will occur in an immune individual. Allergic reactions against dextran can be prevented by pretreatment with monovalent haptenic dextran.

## Predisposing factors

The risk for anaphylactic reactions is greater if the drug is injected rather than given perorally. This is one reason why parenteral treatment with penicillin is being used less. Drugs like neomycin, local anaesthetics and antihistamines can sensitize on local application. The dose of the drug is also important for the risk of developing immunological side effects. Coombs' positive haemolytic anaemia during treatment with penicillin or α-methyldopa, and antinuclear factors during the treatment with procainamide or hydralazine develop more often when high doses are given over long periods of time.

Genetic factors are probably of importance in the appearance of immune responses against drugs. IgE-mediated allergy is more common in individuals with a history of allergic reactions and an increased frequency of atopic allergic manifestation in the family. The metabolism and speed of the elimination of the drug is also genetically dependent and can influence the concentration of the drug and its metabolites, which is important for the development of immune reactivity. One example is the slow elimination of hydralazine in individuals with low acetyl-transferase activity in the liver, which enhances the risk of antinuclear factors appearing.

## Mechanisms for drug induced tissue damage

Tissue damage caused by drugs via immunological mechanisms does not differ from other immunologically mediated tissue damage, as shown in chapter 16.

### Type 1: Anaphylactic, immediate-type hypersensitivity

The best examples of reagin (IgE)-mediated allergy against low molecular weight drugs are anaphylaxis and urticaria caused by penicilling. The acting IgE antibodies are specific for penicilloyl, or other penicillin determinants. Anaphylactic penicillin reactions are rate. Since the late 1960s the risk of severe anaphylaxis is less than 50 in 100 000 injections according to WHO. Well documented anaphylactic or urticarial reactions have been described during treatment with heterologous serum, enzymes or polypeptide hormones. Impurities in hormones and enzyme preparations are important causes of sensitization and allergy. The risk of allergic side effects from injections of polypeptide hormones have decreased as a result of better purification procedures and the use of synthetic hormones.

### Type 2: Cytotoxic reaction

Antibodies against cell surface antigens damage cells with the help of complement and phagocytes. The antigen can be a cell surface bound drug, e.g. penicillin (*Figure 18.1*). Drugs can also induce autoimmunization against cell surface antigens (*Figure 18.4*).

### Type 3: Immune complex mediated damage

Soluble complexes between drugs and IgG antibodies can cause allergic side effects. Serum sickness was common when large doses of heterologous immune serum, usually from horses, was used to treat pneumococcal pneumonia and diphtheria. Recently serum sickness has been described during immunosuppressive treatment with heterologous antilymphocyte serum, but after purification of the antibodies and shortened courses of treatment it has become a rare complication. Serum sickness can also occur during treatment with other drugs, such as heterologous enzyme proteins.

Serum sickness can occasionally appear during treatment with low molecular weight drugs such as penicillin, sulphonamides and phenytoin. Isolated organ damage caused by drugs may at times also probably be caused via type 3 reactions, but are often difficult to distinguish from toxic effects of the drug. The nephrotic syndrome appearing during treatment with penicillamine, as well as certain drug-induced exanthemas and allergic vasculitis may be of this type. Immune complexes can also damage circulating blood cells and are discussed further below (*Figure 18.2*).

### Type 4: Cell-mediated tissue damage

Contact dermatitis caused by antibiotics, local anaesthetics and antihistamines exemplify this form. Cell-mediated immunity has been demonstrated, e.g. against proteins with penicillin as hapten and against procainamide–nucleoprotein complexes. It is not clear what role cell-mediated immunity plays in the allergic reactions against these drugs.

## Immunological reactions with blood cells under the influence of drugs

The original theories concerning drug-induced immunological damage of blood cells were based on studies of thrombocytopenia, but also seem to be relevant for haemolytic diseases and certain drug induced leucopenias. Drug-induced reactions against blood cells will be discussed here with the erythrocyte as a model. Four types of immunoreactions can be distinguished.

## Haemolysis of drug-coated erythrocytes (type 2 reaction) (*Figure 18.1*)

Investigations of thrombocytopenic purpura caused by the sleeping pill Sedormid (Apronal; Roche) showed that the thrombocytes were damaged by antibodies against the drug attached to the cell surface. Haemolysis during treatment with high doses of penicillin probably has a similar explanation. IgG, but rarely IgM antibodies, react

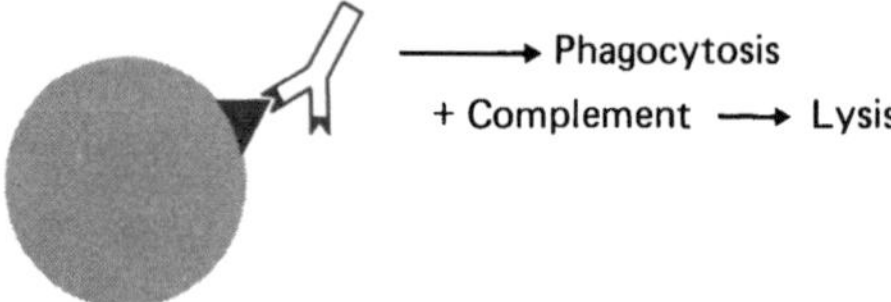


*Figure 18.1* Hapten mechanism. The drug (▲, e.g. penicillin) attached to blood cells reacts with antibodies (usually IgG), which lyse the cell (type 2). Coombs' reaction is positive with anti-IgG serum

with penicillin on the erythrocytes, which are destroyed by phagocytosis. Complement cooperates by enhancing the phagocytosis, but more rarely through haemolysis. The Coombs' direct reaction is positive with anti-IgG serum. Also cephalosporines are believed to give haemolysis of this type.

## Immune complex mediated haemolysis (*Figure 18.2*)

Thrombocytopenia appearing during treatment with quinidine bisulphate is considered to result from the loose attachment of immune complexes between antibodies and drug bound to cell membrane proteins. Complement is activated,

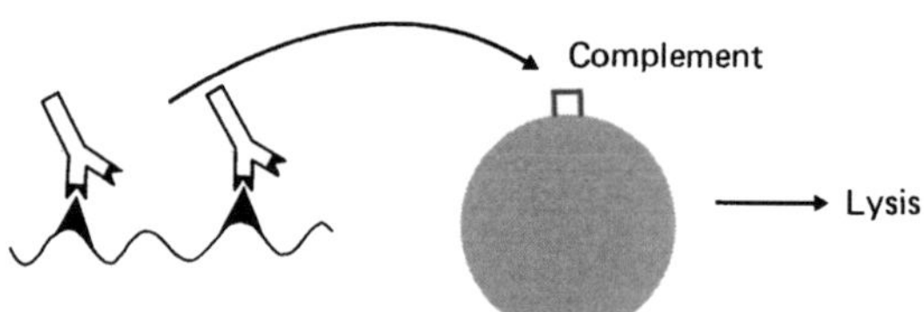


*Figure 18.2* Immune complex between drug (▲, e.g. stibophen, PAS, quinidine bisulphate) bound to a carrier protein and antibodies activating complement (☐) on the surface of blood cells, which are lysed (type 3, 'innocent bystander mechanism'). Coombs' reaction positive with anticomplement serum

destroying the cell. Drug-induced immune haemolysis is often of this type. Occasionally there is thrombocytopenia and haemolysis in the same patient. The Coombs' test is positive with anti-complement serum, but is negative with anti-immunoglobulin serum.

## Binding of IgG and other serum proteins (*Figure 18.3*)

Cephalothin and cephaloridine seem to change the erythrocyte membrane properties so that serum proteins attach to the cell surface. About 3% of patients treated with cephalothin have a positive direct Coombs' test, mainly due to absorbed IgG. Haemolytic anaemia has not been noted with this type of reaction.

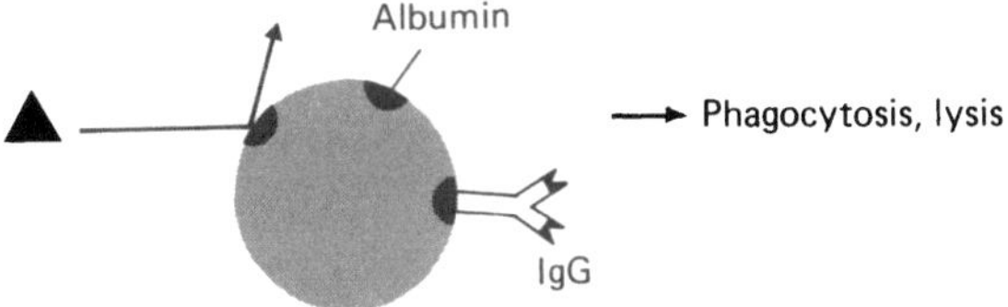



*Figure 18.3* Non-immunological binding. The drug (▲, e.g. cephalosporin) changes the erythrocyte membrane so that serum proteins, including IgG, are absorbed. Coombs' reaction positive with anti-IgG serum

## Auto-immune haemolytic anaemia caused by antibodies of warm type (*Figure 18.4*)

Drugs can also induce autoantibodies, usually of the warm type and occasionally with specificity for Rh antigen. The mechanism for the autoimmunization is not known. The tendency to form antibodies is connected with dosage of the drug and length of treatment; 20–35% of patients who have been given 2 g of α-methyldopa daily have a

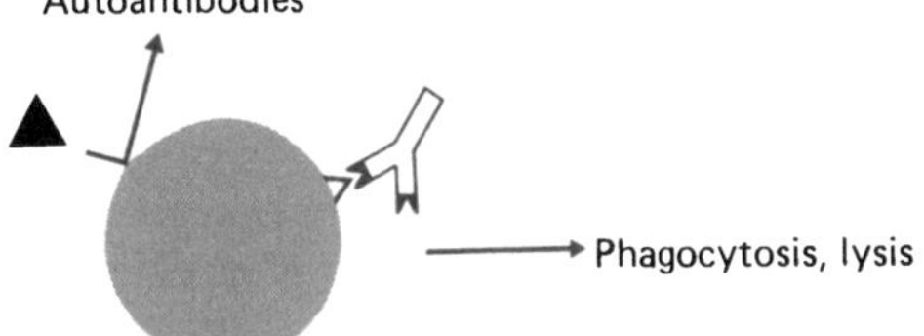



*Figure 18.4* Autoimmune haemolysis. The drug (▲, e.g. α-methyldopa) induces formation of autoantibodies (IgG) against red blood cell antigen (▷, e.g. Rh). Coombs' reaction positive with anti-IgG serum

positive direct Coombs' reaction with anti-IgG sera, while 1 g daily give Coombs' positivity in about 10%. Only a small number of patients get a clinically manifest haemolysis. The Coombs' reaction can remain positive for a year after termination of the treatment. This is the most common form of drug-induced haemolytic anaemia.

## Drug-induced systemic lupus erythematosus (SLE)

Drugs can cause several forms of autoimmunity and autoimmune disease. Best known is the appearance of antinuclear factors and the SLE syndrome during treatment with hydralazine, procainamide, isoniazide (*Table 18.2*). Several of these drugs can also induce autoantibodies against red blood cells. Patients with drug-mediated SLE have most of the symptoms of spontaneous SLE, although immune complex nephritis is

**TABLE 18.2. Drugs which can induce autoimmune disease**

| | |
|---|---|
| Hydralazine | Chlorpromazine |
| Procainamide | Trimethadione |
| Isoniazid | α-Methyldopa |
| Sulphonamides | Nitrofurantoin |
| Phenytoin | Penicillin |

**TABLE 18.3. Mechanisms for appearance of drug induced antinuclear factors**

Breakage of tolerance through immunization with (a) drug bound to nuclear antigen, (b) nuclear antigen changed by the effect of the drug

Antibodies against drug cross-react with nuclear antigen

Activation of latent SLE

Activation of latent virus infection

rare. Antibodies against native DNA which are typical of the spontaneous form are rare in the drug induced SLE. The symptoms usually vanish when the drug is stopped.

The mechanisms for autoimmunization against nuclear antigens are not clear. Several hypotheses have been presented with some experimental support (*Table 18.3*). Most likely is the suggestion that tolerance against nuclear protein is broken through coupling of the antigen to haptens, or some other change of the nuclear antigen under the influence of the drug. Treatment with a high dose over a long period of time increases the risk of SLE. Drug-induced SLE develops more easily in persons with a genetically determined low level of acetyltransferases, which participate in acetylation of drugs. SLE-like symptoms before treatment and such symptoms in relatives seem to predispose to the disease. Persons with the phenotype HLA Dw4 develop drug-induced SLE more easily.

# Allergy to penicillins

Allergy to a drug can occur with very different clinical pictures, either with an acute course or with slowly progressive symptoms. The side effects of penicillin illustrate this:

**TABLE 18.4. Allergic reactions induced by penicillin**

| Clinical patterns | Antigen | Antibody | Mechanism |
|---|---|---|---|
| Immediate type hypersensitivity reactions (2–30 minutes): Urticaria, shock, dyspnoea | Penicillin | IgE | Type 1 |
| Late urticarial reactions (3–72 h) | Penicillin | IgE | Probably type 1 |
| Late allergic reactions<br>(1)  Serium sickness: fever, joint pains, exanthema | Penicillin | IgG | Type 3 |
| (2)  Contact dermatitis | D-penicillamine | | Type 4 |
| (3)  Ampicillin exanthema | Ampicillin polymer | | Non-specific activation of lymphocytes? |
| (4)  Haemolytic anaemia | Penicillin | IgG<br>IgM | Type 2 |
| (5)  Nephrotic syndrome (membrane nephritis) | Penicillamine | IgG | Type 3? |
| (6)  Interstitial nephritis with tubular damage (mainly methicillin) | Penicillin?<br>Autoantigen from tubular basement membrane? | IgG | Type 3?<br>Type 4? |
| (7)  SLE syndrome | Penicillamine | ? | ? |

acute and life-threatening anaphylactic reactions via IgE antibodies can appear, as well as urticaria and other type 1 reactions (*Table 18.4*). The haemolytic anaemia is an example of a type 2 reaction, either in a mild form with extravascular haemolysis, or in an acute intense intravascular haemolysis. Penicillin can cause classical serum sickness and other manifestations of type 3 reactions as well.

Penicillamine nephrosis is another example of immune complex disease. Immune complexes may also be the cause of the interstitial nephritis that can appear during treatment with methicillin. Ampicillin and other penicillins can give skin reactions via cell-mediated immune reactions as well (type 4). Finally it seems that penicillin can induce autoimmunization against kidneys and an SLE syndrome.

## Bibliography

ACKROYD, J. G. (1975). Immunological mechanisms in drug hypersensitivity. *Clinical Aspects of Immunology*. Ed. by Gell, P. G. H., Coombs, R. R. A. and Lachmann, P. J. L., pp. 913–961. Blackwell Scientific Publications, Oxford.

DUKOR, P., KALLOS, P. and SCHLUMBERGER, H. D. (eds.) (1980–84). *PAR, Pseudo-allergic Reactions. Involvement of Drugs and Chemicals*, Vol. 1–4, Karger, Basel.

PARKER, C. W. (1975), Drug allergy, *N. Engl. J. Med.*, **292**, 511–514, 732–736, 967–960.

# Chapter 19

# Immune complex diseases

Renée Norberg

von Pirquet suggested around 1910 that simultaneous presence in the circulation of heterologous serum proteins and antibodies against them could give rise to 'toxic compounds', causing the symptoms of serum sickness. Serum treatment—usually serum from a horse immunized with diphtheria or tetanus toxin—was previously given in acute infections to quickly provide neutralizing antibodies. About a week after the serum infusion certain patients had symptoms in joints, heart, blood vessels and kidneys. However, direct support for the theory of von Pirquet was not provided until some 50 years later when it was demonstrated that antigen and corresponding antibodies could form soluble circulating complexes which deposit in small blood vessels. By the activation of complement and aggregation of granulocytes the immune complexes cause tissue damage, the socalled type 3 reaction, according to the classification of Coombs and Gell (cf. chapter 16).

The localization of the tissue damage depends primarily on where the antigen–antibody reaction takes place, while the severity is related to the amount of complexes produced. If the antigen is localized in a certain tissue the antibody will bind to it resulting in local damage. If the antigen–antibody complexes form in the circulation they have a tendency to localize in structures which function as physiological filters, e.g. the basement membranes of blood vessels and glomeruli.

A good example of immune complex induced tissue damage is the *Arthus' reaction*, which is a localized, acute, necrotizing vasculitis. One of the reactants, antigen or antibody, must be present in the circulation and the other one is injected locally. The produced antigen–antibody complexes are deposited in local vessels and react with complement. Granulocytes move in by chemotaxis. Phagocytosis and degradation of the immune complexes and release of toxic material from the granules of the phagocytes, together with free radicals from the cell membrane follow, resulting in inflammatory changes in the vessel walls.

Circulating soluble antigen–antibody complexes are most easily formed in the presence of an excess of multivalent antigens. The amount of antigen and the period of time the antigen is present in the circulation is of importance for the development of the tissue damage. It can be assumed that there are mainly three different quantitative relationships that may occur between antigen and antibody during immunization:

(1) The amount of antibodies produced is small in comparison with the amount of antigen. This results in the formation of few and small antigen–antibody complexes. These complexes may remain in the circulation for a long time—

usually their metabolic rate is similar to that of the antigen alone—but they do not elicit tissue damage as they are not complement activating. Due to their small size they also freely pass through the basement membranes of the blood vessels.

(2)    The antibody amount is large in comparison to the amount of antigen. Under these conditions the immune complexes formed can reach a considerable size. Such large complexes are rapidly eliminated from the circulation.

(3)    The antibody production is insufficient to completely neutralize all the antigen with antigen excess as a consequence. In this situation soluble immune complexes of medium size are formed. They have a tendency to get caught in physiological filters. It is usually in individuals with this type of antibody production that immune complex disease occurs.

The *classical serum sickness* can serve as a prototype for the disease that develops when an individual is exposed to an antigen during a limited period of time. Even if the complexes which induce serum sickness are formed, the tissue damage and the clinical symptoms are temporary. The cause of serum sickness has been followed in detail in experimental animals (*Figure 19.1*). The animal is given intravenously radioactively

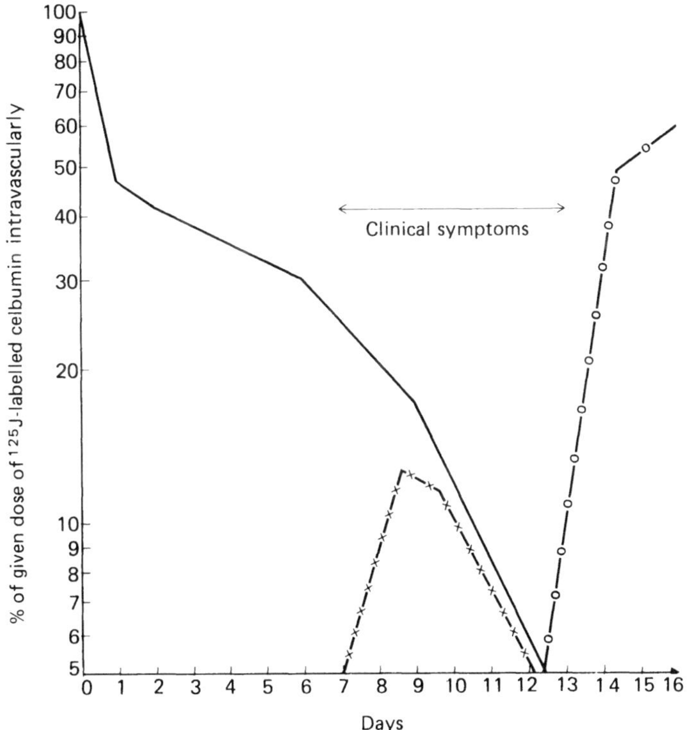


*Figure 19.1* Development of acute serum sickness in rabbit. On day 0, $^{125}\gamma$-labelled bovine albumin is injected intravenously. The level in the circulation is determined daily (———). During approximately one week the bovine albumin is catabolized as autologous albumin, then is rapidly eliminated from the circulation simultaneously with the appearance of albumin–antialbumin complexes (×). The complexes can be demonstrated during four to five days and are followed by the appearance of free antialbumin antibodies (○). Clinical symptoms appear together with the circulating immune complexes

labelled protein, e.g. bovine serum albumin. The first five to six days after the infusion the protein is catabolized in a normal manner. Then there is a phase of rapid elimination of the antigen before free circulating antibodies against the bovine albumin can be demonstrated. The antibodies produced first react with the antigen in a strong excess promoting formation of small immune complexes with a tendency to remain in the circulation. With increasing levels of antibodies the complexes increase in size, enhancing their elimination from the circulation. Simultaneously with the appearance of the antigen–antibody complexes in the circulation, the complement level decreases. Acute inflammatory lesions develop primarily in the kidneys, heart and joints where the antigen as well as the specific antibodies are demonstrable. The clinical symptoms are usually temporary and circulating immune complexes cannot be demonstrated after about a week.

There is another experimental model where daily intravenous antigen injections are given. This model may be more akin to the chronic conditions in man where circulating antigen–antibody complexes are thought to produce the diseases. In this model, some animals have symptoms from joints, heart and kidneys. These animals produce antibodies against the heterologous antigen, but not in such amounts that all given antigen can be neutralized. During the experiment there is a slight antigen excess in the circulation and circulating immune complexes are present. The symptoms as well as the histopathological changes persist long after completion of antigen administration. Reduced renal function can be detected for a year. On the other hand, progress of the disease can be prevented by changing the balance between antigen and antibody, either by decreasing or drastically increasing the antigen dose. In both situations the circulating immune complexes are eliminated. Animals lacking or with poor antibody response show no clinical symptoms, while the animals which produce many antibodies during the second week of the experiment, have temporary symptoms as in acute serum sickness. They change from antigen excess to antibody excess and in a few days circulating antigen–antibody complexes are present.

## Deposition of circulating immune complexes in tissues

Circulating antigen–antibody complexes are eliminated primarily through phagocytosis. Immune complexes are bound to phagocytic cells by Fc and/or C receptors mainly in the liver and spleen. Overloading or blocking of such receptors may contribute to the development of immune complex mediated diseases. Immune complexes produced in slight antigen excess are of limited size and may therefore more easily avoid the receptors of the phagocytic cells. It has been assumed that the immunological specificity of the complexes is without significance for their localization in tissues and that only their size determines where they deposit. Circulating complexes primarily localize in organs with a special vascular structure, such as the kidneys, skin, lungs, joints and arteries. The release of vasoactive amines, mainly from thrombocytes, induces the increased vascular permeability which is a prerequisite for the deposition of the circulating immune complexes in tissues. The release of amines can occur after direct interaction between thrombocytes and complexes, or after secretion of platelet activating factors, mainly from basophilic granulocytes (PAF, *see* chapter 17). The increased vascular permeability makes it possible for the immune complexes to pass through the vascular endothelium and to aggregate along the basement membrane of the vessel, where they induce the inflammatory changes which cause tissue damage. The vasoactive substances produced by complement activation, including C3a and C5a, contribute to a further increased vascular permeability.

It is clear that antigen–antibody complexes interact not only with platelets but also with all other cells equipped with Fc and C receptors, interfering with a number of biological activities and forming the basis for the development of symptoms.

At least in the case of immune complex-mediated renal damage it can be doubted that only the size of the complexes determines their localization. There is experimental as well as empirical support for free circulating antigens to have affinity for a certain tissue, due to their specific physical properties, e.g. their charge. Antibodies are bound to the antigen in the tissues and the locally produced antigen–antibody complexes induce the same reaction as the complexes deposited from the circulation. It has been shown recently that cationic IgG can bind to negatively charged components in the glomerular basement membrane and induce *in situ* immune complex formation accompanied by severe glomerulonephritis. This also means that the charge of the antibodies can be important for the local formation of immune complexes.

Exogenous as well as endogenous antigens can induce an immune response resulting in immune complex mediated tissue damage. During the last 10–15 years there has been great interest in these conditions and it has been thought that antigen–antibody complexes are of pathogenic importance in a large number of conditions, from acute infections to chronic neurological diseases (*Table 19.1*). In a number of conditions the immune complex aetiology can be proved; antigen as well as specific antibodies and complement factors have been identified in damaged tissues. In other instances the evidence for immune complex mediated tissue damage is more indirect. With various methods, circulating immune complexes have been demonstrated and this has been taken as evidence for the relationship between the complexes and the tissue damage.

On the other hand, no complexes have been demonstrated in the sera from many patients with apparent immune complex disease as judged from clinical symptoms. These sometimes rather unexpected results may have several explanations. Of major importance is the fact that there is still no ideal method to demonstrate all types of complexes. The increased capacity of patient serum in comparison to control serum to bind complement factor C1q or isolated IgM rheumatoid factor, as well as the capacity to react with Fc and complement receptors on large lymphoid cells has been taken as indirect evidence for the presence of antigen–antibody complexes. Only in a few cases

**TABLE 19.1. Examples of diseases in which there is direct or indirect evidence of circulating or locally formed antigen–antibody complexes of pathogenic significance**

Auto-immune diseases (SLE, polyarteritis nodosa, pemphigus, pemphigoid, myasthenia gravis, active chronic hepatitis, etc.), rheumatoid arthritis, Felty's syndrome, reactive arthritis, arthritis in patients with intestinal shunt.

Drug reactions (chapter 18).

Glomerulonephritis, various forms.

Lung diseases (allergic alveolitis, etc.).

Vasculitis of various aetiology.

Tumours.

Infectious diseases caused by bacteria (e.g. streptococci, meningococci, gonococci, lepra, etc.), as well as viruses (e.g. dengue fever, cytomegalovirus, mononucleosis, hepatitis) and parasites (malaria, trypanosomiasis, schistosomiasis, toxoplasmosis).

Other diseases, for instance dermatitis herpetiformis, ulcerative colitis, Crohn's disease, heart infarction, sarcoidosis, interstitial pneumonia, multiple sclerosis, uveitis, eclampsia, etc.

has it been possible to directly demonstrate the circulating complexes and analyse the participating components.

Obviously the prerequisites for formation of circulating antigen–antibody complexes may be present during immunization. The unexpected finding of circulating immune complexes is in many instances explained by their normal presence. It is important to be critical of the claim that the presence of circulating immune complexes proves the presence of a type 3 reaction with ensuing clinical disease.

## Joint diseases

In *rheumatoid arthritis* (RA) immune complexes of various sizes are demonstrated in the granulation tissue as well as in the synovial fluid. Varying numbers of IgG molecules are part of the complexes. Many complexes also contain IgM rheumatoid factor (RF). Extensive studies, so far without results, have tried to demonstrate a specific antigen in the complexes. IgG in the complexes have RF activity, i.e. they have specificity for antigenic determinants on the Fc part of the IgG. The complexes are complement activating and their importance for the appearance of the rheumatic joint disease has been much discussed, but not settled.

Complexes containing two to four IgG molecules, the socalled intermediary complexes are present in sera. Also larger complexes, often containing IgM RF, are common. The intermediary IgG complexes do not seem to be complement binding. They remain in the circulation for a long period of time and are obviously metabolized at the same rate as normal IgG.

The presence of large, circulating immunoglobulin complexes is often connected with severe joint disease and signs of vasculitis. In the vascular changes of patients with severe RA immunofluorescence techniques can demonstrate immunoglobulin with RF activity, as well as complement factors.

Joint symptoms of varying severity—from slight temporary pain to advanced joint inflammation with exudation—are not unusual after acute infections, socalled *reactive* or *post-infectious arthritis*. In many of these cases circulating immune complexes have been found. In single cases specific antibody activity has also been demonstrated in the complexes. However, circulating immune complexes are found in about the same frequency in post-infectious patients without any complicating joint disease. Therefore it remains to be proven that the detected immune complexes are of pathogenic significance. It should be added that patients with post-infectious arthritis are HLA-B27-positive in 70–80%.

In the acute stage of *erythema nodosum* of different pathogenesis antigen–antibody complexes are found in the circulation. In biopsy from fresh skin lesions intravascular deposits of IgG and complement have been seen.

## Systemic lupus erythematosus (SLE)

Although its aetiology is unknown SLE is in many ways the prototype for an immune complex mediated disease (*see* chapter 21). This is especially true for the tissue damage occurring as glomerulonephritis, vasculitis and arthritis.

Deposits of DNA, immunoglobulins with specificity for DNA and other nuclear antigens as well as complement have been demonstrated in glomeruli. Practically all

SLE patients show deposits of immunoglobulin and complement in skin biopsies. Circulating immune complexes are demonstrable in high frequencies and the findings are to some extent related to disease activity, although these findings are of limited diagnostic value in single individuals. In contrast, it may at times be useful in the individual case to follow the immune complex level in the serum to try to monitor therapeutic trials. Anti-DNA and other nuclear antibodies have been demonstrated in the circulating immune complexes.

Deposits of circulating DNA–anti-DNA complexes have been thought to be of special significance for the appearance of vascular and renal damage in SLE. In newer and more critical experimental studies, however, this has been partly questioned. Subepithelial glomerular deposits of immune complexes could be induced by free circulating antigens, which had affinity for structures in the glomerular basement membrane. Circulating antibodies reacted locally with the deposited antigen initiating the tissue damage. Moreover, cationic antibodies, e.g. DNA antibodies, may interact with the negatively charged glomerular basement membrane forming local immune complexes with circulating antigens.

## Vasculitis

*Necrotizing vasculitis* can occur in all systemic immune complex diseases, but vasculitis can also occur without any other signs of generalized disease. The vascular changes are characterized by fibrinoid necrosis of the vessel wall. Granulomas are occasionally formed in connection with necrotic vascular changes and can then be felt as an induration with or without simultaneous purpura. Occasionally the necrosis can be so extensive that there are ulcerations of the skin. Immunoglobulin and complement can be demonstrated in the vascular changes in approximately 50% of the cases. The aetiology is mostly unknown, but in some cases bacterial antigens have been identified. Among other agents of aetiological importance for the appearance of vasculitis are various drugs and in some cases food constituents. Hepatitis B antigen has been discussed as a possible initiator of vascular changes especially in *polyarteritis nodosa*. In single cases not only immunoglobulin and complement have been found to be deposited in the arteritis, but also hepatitis B antigen. In many cases of polyarteritis nodosa the antigen or antibodies against the hepatitis B can be demonstrated in the circulation. The frequency, however, varies in different materials from various parts of the world.

## Glomerulonephritis

Two immunological mechanisms of pathogenic importance for the generation of glomerulonephritis can be distinguished experimentally. Either antibodies react with antigen in the glomerular basement membrane (GBM), or complexes of antibodies and non-glomerular antigens are localized within the glomeruli. The histopathological picture is the same in both types of nephritis, but in immunological analyses there is a clear difference with a continuous deposition of immunoglobulin along the basement membrane in GMB nephritis (*Figure 19.2a*). In other types of nephritis immune complexes are found as irregular lumpy deposits along the capillary walls and/or in the mesangium (*Figure 19.2b*). Complement factors can often be demonstrated, but rarely specific antigens.

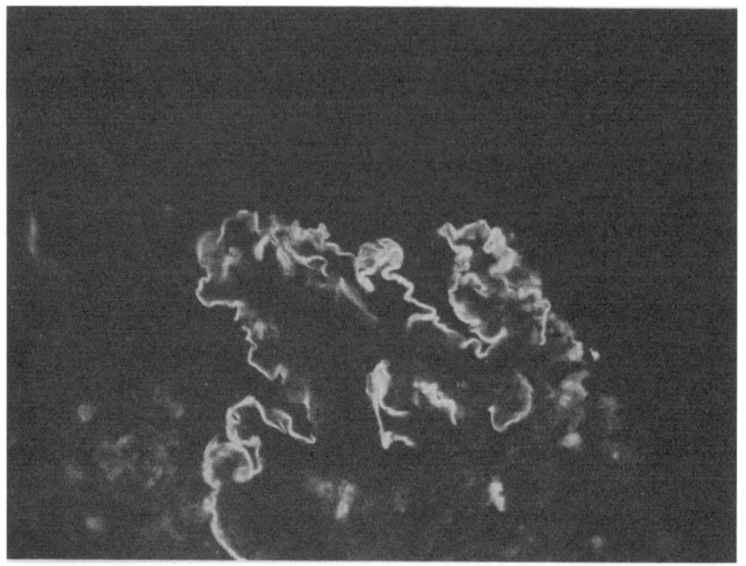

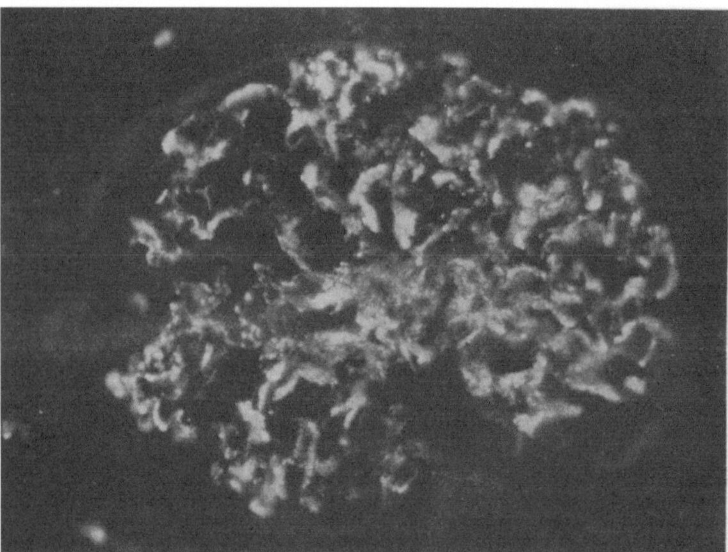

*Figure 19.2* Immunofluorescence analysis of renal biopsies (Photo: J. Wassermann, Stockholm) (a) Continuous linear deposits of IgG along the glomerular basement membrane in a case of GBM nephritis. (b) Diffuse lumpy deposits of IgG in the glomerulus of a patient with immune complex-mediated glomerulonephritis

## GBM nephritis

Antibodies against GBM are directly pathogenic. Transfusion of human GBM antibodies causes nephritis in the recipient. Patients who have been nephrectomized and transplanted because of GBM nephritis usually develop new nephritic changes in the transplant. This was prevented in some cases, where the nephrectomy was performed so long before the transplantation that the GBM antibodies were no longer present at the transplantation.

GBM nephritis is a relatively rare disease. About half of the cases also have severe, often fatal lung bleedings. This clinical pattern is usually called *Goodpasture's syndrome*. Obviously the lung symptoms are the result of damage induced by the GBM antibodies also reacting with the alveolar basement membrane.

The disease is rapidly progressive and it is important to make a correct diagnosis as soon as possible so that therapy can be instituted quickly. The prognosis has very much improved since the initiation of treatment with extensive plasma exchange and immunosuppression. Most patients respond to the therapy by lowering the amount of circulating antibodies against GBM and this reduction appears to be lasting. The diagnosis of GBM nephritis should be made immunologically. Circulating antibodies can be demonstrated in more than 80% with enzyme-linked immunosorbent assay (ELISA) or radioimmunoassay (RIA). The antibodies are species specific and human antigen must be used. On biopsy the glomerular immunohistological pattern with linear deposition of immunoglobulin along the basement membrane is typical (*Figure 19.2a*).

Single cases of GBM nephritis have been described after virus infections, in connection with drugs (penicillamine), or traumatic kidney damage, but usually the cause of the production of GBM antibodies is unknown.

## Glomerulonephritis induced by circulating immune complexes

The special circulation and filtration of blood in the kidneys, probably contributes to immune complexes being so commonly deposited in the glomeruli. It is rather surprising that the kidneys are not more often damaged by antigen–antibody complexes which surely are normally present in the circulation during for instance infections and after vaccination. This has been explained by the presence in the glomerular mesangium of cells with the capacity to engulf and eliminate macro-molecular complexes. Deposits of complexes in the mesangium usually do not cause any histologically or functionally demonstrable damage on the glomeruli. But with increased deposition of immune complexes surmounting the phagocytic capacity of the mesangium, complexes are deposited in the basement membrane with glomerulo-nephritis as a result. Support for these theories in man has been found from studies of the development of glomerulonephritis in patients with SLE.

Several different antigen–antibody systems have been considered in connection with glomerulonephritis in man. Only in single cases has the antigen in the complex been identified, including endogenous as well as exogenous antigens.

As previously mentioned it has been thought that the specificity of the antigen in immune complexes may be unimportant for the location of deposition. Any antigen–antibody complex can get caught in the glomeruli and cause an inflammatory reaction there (*Figure 19.2b*). But the deposition of circulating complexes can only explain some phenomena in glomerulonephritis. It is clear that glomerulonephritis is more common in connection with certain infections, such as those caused by haemolytic streptococci. The pathogenesis is obviously more complex than only deposition of complexes from the circulation. For instance streptococcal antigens may have an increased affinity to glomeruli where they bind antibody and complement. Local activation of complement via the alternative pathway may also occur under certain circumstances.

## Lung diseases

Inhaled organic material against which the individual has IgG antibodies (precipitins), can give rise to tissue damage resulting in coughing, fever, dyspnoea and cyanosis by an immune complex reaction locally in the bronchi and lungs. Radiological examination reveals typical micronodular changes which finally turn into lung fibrosis. A number of antigens, especially from moulds and dust of various origins, are important in this connection. Antigens often originate from micro-organisms such as *Micropolyspora* or *Thermoactinomyces* in individuals with farmers' lung or mushroom pickers' disease. Malt workers' lung is caused by *Aspergillus*, while people with wood trimmers' disease are exposed to moulds such as *Penicillium, Alternaria, Cladosporium, Botrytis* and *Micropolyspora*. In patients with bird fanciers' lung the antigens originate from doves, budgerigars, hens and parrots (*see also* Appendix 2).

It should be emphasized that the finding of precipitating antibodies against a certain inhaled antigen does not necessarily mean that the patient has an immune complex induced disease. Only some of the patients who produce antibodies against antigens, thought to be important in these conditions, really develop clinical symptoms and there may be several immunopathological reaction types involved in socalled *allergic alveolitis*.

In fact dust often contains Gram-negative bacteria and byssinosis for instance is most probably due to the inhalation of endotoxins. These endotoxins can activate complement via the alternative pathway and cause an immune complex-like reaction. It is possible that inhaled endotoxins are part of the pathogenesis in some cases of allergic alveolitis.

Interstitial pneumonia and occasionally granulomatous lung changes may occur in isolated cases, but usually the lung symptoms are seen together with other immune complex induced organ symptoms.


## Bibliography

COUSER, W. G. and SALANT, D. J. (1980). *In situ* immune complex formation and glomerular injury. *Kidney International*, **17**, 1–3.
NYDEGGER, U. E. (1985). A place for soluble immune complexes in clinical immunology. *Immunol. Today*, **6**, 80–82.
THEOFILOPOULOS, A. N. and DIXON, F. J. (1980). Immune complexes in human diseases. *Am. J. Pathol.*, **100**, 531–591.

# Chapter 20

# The complement system and disease

Anna-Brita Laurell

## Hereditary deficiency of factors in the complement system

Deficiencies inherited as autosomal recessive traits have been recognized for several of the proteins belonging to the complement system. Genetic deficiencies of the control proteins of the complement system are also well established.

*Selective C1q deficiency* has been described with, as well as without, inheritance. Individuals producing a deficient non-functioning C1q, with relatives being heterozygous for the abnormal component, have also been found. In selective C1q deficiency there is an increased risk of infections and immune complex diseases with skin and kidney manifestations.

Patients with agammaglobulinaemia or hypogammaglobulinaemia, or severe combined immunodeficiency (SCID) often have C1q deficiency. It is not clear if the C1q deficiency is in any way coupled to the immunodeficiency.

*C1r deficiency* has been reported in a few families. These patients have SLE-like symptoms and glomerulonephritis.

*C2 deficiency* is the most common inherited deficiency within the C system; the frequency is about 1 per 15 000 population. Around 50% of individuals with C2 deficiency have an SLE-like disease, most often with symptoms from the skin but no antinuclear antibodies.

*C4 deficiency* has so far only been found in nine cases from seven families. The blood group antigens Chido and Rodgers which consist of C4 bound to erythrocytes of normal individuals, are lacking in the C4 deficiency cases. In one patient the phagocytic capacity was decreased and abnormalities in the cell-mediated immunity were also present. Excessively high levels of IgM, especially 7S IgM was found in one of the patients. It is not yet clear if these immunological disturbances are related to the C4 deficiency. As in patients with C2 deficiency, SLE-like symptoms are a dominating feature.

*C3 deficiency* has been found in an inherited form in a few patients, who all had repeated severe bacterial infections. The important opsonization with C3b via the classical pathway was lacking and activation of the alternative pathway did not function at all.

*Deficiency in factors C5, C6, C7 or C8*   More than 40 individuals with one of these deficiencies have been described. In more than half of them there were repeated infections with meningococci or gonococci, in spite of high titres of specific antibodies and intact capacity of opsonization through C3b and C4b. Their infections are usually relatively mild.

*C9 deficiency* has also been demonstrated, but in contrast to the deficiencies of C5, C6, C7 or C8, the C9 deficiency has not been connected with any disease.

*Properdin deficiency* was recently found in a family where three members died in rapidly progressive meningococcal sepsis. Two healthy adult individuals with complete deficiency of P have been found in the family. There was an impaired function of the alternative pathway in these P deficient individuals. The inheritance seems to be sex-linked.


## Inherited deficiency of inhibitors within the complement system

*Inherited lack of C̄I inactivator, C̄I IA (C1 esterase inhibitor)* was early connected with hereditary angioedema (HANE). The inheritance is autosomal dominant and the patients are thus heterozygous. The disease is characterized by recurrent oedema in the skin, larynx or peritoneum.

Usually there is a deficient synthesis of the inhibitor, but there are also some families where a biologically inactive inhibitor is synthesized. With immunochemical methods levels of the inhibitor increased three to four times are found, but it lacks the capacity to bind activated C̄I. In crossed immunoelectrophoresis the inhibitor appears as two precipitation peaks, where the anodal peak is produced by a complex between the abnormal inhibitor and albumin.

Patients with HANE have low levels of C4 and C2, which is a direct consequence of the activation of C1 in the circulation. The C1 activation is probably caused by enzymes liberated in the tissues, for instance in infection or after trauma. Patients with HANE having constantly low levels of C2 and C4, also show an increased frequency of symptoms that are usually connected with immune complexes, for instance SLE, as do patients with C2 and C4 deficiency. It is possible that a long-standing decrease of the early C factors lowers the capacity to eliminate micro-organsisms, e.g. viruses or microbial antigens, which then can cause immune disease.

For some years danazol, an androgen derivative, has been used as prophylaxis in HANE. Most patients responded very well. The C̄I inactivator increases three to four times and reaches levels in the lower normal range. The low C4 and C2 levels, which are characteristic of the disease and a consequence of consumption by activated C̄I, increase during danazol treatment up to normal levels.

HANE patients can, in principle, synthesize half the normal amount of C1 inactivator, but usually the C̄I IA level is only 20–25% of the normal or even less. The effect of danazol is due to an increased C̄I IA synthesis in the liver, resulting in serum and tissue concentrations which keep the activation of C1 under control. This is reflected by a rapid increase of C2 and C4 in serum during treatment.

HANE patients can also be successfully treated with ε-aminocaproic acid. Two-thirds of the cases are relieved of symptoms or are clearly improved. ε-Aminocaproic acid is a known enzyme inhibitor, which inhibits for instance plasmin. It has no inhibiting effect on activated C̄I. Its therapeutic effect in HANE is probably due to inhibition of enzymes which are released in trauma, stress and which activate C1.

*Factor I deficiency (C3b inactivator, C3b IA deficiency)* results, as does C3 deficiency, in repeated severe bacterial infections. These patients have drastically decreased levels of C3, factor B and properdin. The reason for the repeated infections and the changed complement profile is that the C3b dependent feedback system of the alternative pathway is out of control. Due to the lack of factor I the C3b cleavage resulting in C3c and C3d cannot occur, which is followed by continuous intense activation and consumption of C3 and the subsequent factors. The principal opsonizing factor can therefore not be mobilized to meet the invading micro-organisms.

*Factor H deficiency* has been found in a few cases with strikingly increased sensitivity to infections. It is probable that the explanation is the same as in factor I deficiency, with inability to control the feedback system in the alternative pathway. The pattern in plasma of C3, factor B and properdin are about the same as described for factor I deficiency.

A patient with severe Quincke oedema has recently been found with a *lack of the anaphylatoxin inactivator*. It is not yet clear if it is an inherited deficiency.

It is obvious that deficiencies of the early components of the classical pathway predispose to diseases where circulating and tissue-bound immune complexes are of major importance. This is also true for patients with lack of C1 inactivator, resulting in chronic secondary consumption of C4 and C2. In all of these patients the alternative pathway is intact. Severe infections are not a major problem.

In contrast patients with deficiency of C3, factor I and factor H suffer from repeated fulminant bacterial infections. In these cases the important C3b opsonization of invading bacteria via the classical as well as the alternative pathway is lacking.

The reason for the recurrent *Neisseria* infections in individuals with deficiencies of the terminal factors C5, C6, C7, or C8 is not obvious. These patients have a normal immune response, the C system functions well through the C3 step via both activation pathways and the opsonization capacity is therefore normal. It has been suggested that the lytic function of the complement might protect against, or reduce the colonization of *Neisseria* on mucous membranes.


## Hyocomplementemia

### Activation and consumption of factors in the classical pathway

Immune complex diseases includes pathological processes where circulating or tissue deposited immune complexes seem to play a pathogenic role through activation of complement, mainly via the classical pathway. On binding of C to immune complexes deposited in the tissue there is a local release of chemotactic factors and anaphylatoxin, which add to and sustain the inflammatory reaction. To this group of diseases belong, e.g. immune haemolytic anaemia, systemic *lupus erythematosus* (SLE), cryoglobulinaemia, rheumatoid arthritis, certain manifestations of hepatitis B virus infections and haemorrhagic shock syndrome in dengue fever. In immune haemolytic anaemia there is often a decreased level of C3 and especially of C4 as a consequence of the binding of C to antibodies on the erythrocytes. The complement consumption is most extensive if the antibodies are of the IgM class.

SLE is characterized by depressed levels of C3 and C4 in plasma and C1q is often decreased. During clinical improvement the values normalize. C1q, C3 and C4 can be demonstrated together with immunoglobulins in skin lesions and in glomeruli of SLE patients with nephritis.

Normal or increased plasma levels of C3 and C4 are often found in rheumatoid arthritis when the disease is in an active phase. In synovial fluid the concentrations of C1q, C3 and C4 are low. This indicates a local complement consuming process in the joints, which is not reflected in plasma due to the increased synthesis of C3 and C4 during an acute phase reaction.

In immune complex diseases there may also be signs of engagement of the alternative pathway with decreased levels of properdin and factor B. This may be dependent on immune complexes or other substances activating the alternative pathway directly, or on activation of the feedback system of the alternative pathway via the C3 convertase of the classical pathway.

The acute poststreptococcal glomerulonephritis is characterized early in the course of low levels of C3, properdin and C5. The concentrations of C1q, C4 and C2 are at the onset of the disease roughly normal, but can later decrease to slightly subnormal levels. These findings demonstrate that both activation pathways are engaged and that the alternative pathway probably is activated before the classical pathway. The complement abnormalities are normalized within about ten weeks.

The haemorrhagic shock syndrome of dengue fever can appear in reinfected patients with remaining high antibody levels. Dramatically lowered levels of C1q, C3 and C4 are found. Factor B is decreased indicating activation of the alternative pathway. In the circulation there are active C5b6 complexes which by interaction with thrombocytes may add to the induction of intravascular coagulation. The massive activation of C3 and C5 with production of C3a and C5a probably surmounts the capacity of the anaphylatoxin inactivator, contributing to the development of the shock. Subnormal levels of the anaphylatoxin inactivator have been demonstrated.

### Activation and consumption of the factors of the alternative pathway

In severe Gram-negative infections such as *E. coli* sepsis and meningococcal sepsis, the properdin, factor B and C3 levels are low, whereas the C4 level is normal. These findings agree with the *in vitro* findings where the complement system is activated by endotoxin via the alternative pathway.

Anaphylactoid shock has been reported in some cases on dextran infusion. An acute activation of the alternative pathway takes place with consumption of properdin and C3, while C4 remains normal. The level of the anaphylatoxin inactivator may decrease to subnormal levels during shock.

In patients with membranoproliferative glomerulonephritis, the plasma C3 levels are decreased, whereas C1, C2 and C4 are normal. Serum often contains a factor—C3 nephritic factor, C3NeF—which contributes to the activation of the alternative pathway. C3NeF is an autoantibody of the IgG class, specific for C3bB and C3bBb complexes. On binding of C3NeF these complexes are stabilized and the feedback cycle of the alternative pathway is continuously activated.

The same chronic complement abnormality and presence of C3NeF are found in partial lipodystrophy. These patients often suffer from a membranoproliferative glomerulonephritis, but there are cases where the C change is fully developed without any renal disease. With this background it has been suggested that renal disease is not induced by activation of the alternative pathway, but is rather related to an acquired partial C3 deficiency.

In paroxysmal nocturnal haemoglobinuria there is an abnormality in the cell membrane of the erythrocytes, enabling activation of the alternative pathway on the cell surface leading to lysis of the erythrocytes.

## Aggregation of neutrophilic granulocytes

C5a which is split off from C5 through the C5 convertases can function not only as an anaphylatoxin and chemotactic factor, but can also aggregate neutrophilic granulocytes. The chemotactic and aggregating capacities remain after the anaphylatoxin inactivator has split off arginine from the C5a molecule forming $C5a_{desArg}$.

With C5a bound to the granulocytes they adhere to vascular endothelium, which results in sequestration and aggregation mainly in the lungs. These events have turned out to be an important component in the pathogenesis of 'shock lung', or adult respiratory distress syndrome (ARDS). After intensive C-activation granulocyte aggregates occlude the vessels in the lungs and tissue damaging free superoxide radicals leak out from the cells. This syndrome can appear in connection with Gram-negative bacteraemia, traumatic shock and acute pancreatitis—all conditions where there is an intense activation of the complement system. 'Sudden blindness' in connection with severe trauma has also been claimed to have this pathogenesis. High doses of corticosteroids is an efficient treatment, probably primarily due to inhibition of the production of free radicals in the granulocytes.

During haemodialysis the alternative pathway may be activated by the dialysis membranes. Repeated dialysis over long periods of time can be complicated by an increasing lung dysfunction with fibrosis of the lung parenchyma. A chronic ongoing destruction of lung tissue due to the same mechanism as in the acute symptoms in shock lung is assumed to be the cause of the damage. The same is valid for the lung dysfunction which can appear in connection with extracorporal circulation, 'cardiopulmonary bypass'.

## Disorders of the subcomponents of C1

Using crossed immunoelectrophoresis, it is possible to demonstrate in normal sera small amounts of complexes of $C\bar{1}r$, $C\bar{1}s$ and $C\bar{1}$ inactivator as an expression of a continuous, low-grade physiological activation of C1. In sera from patients with various immunological diseases, such as chronic urticaria, SLE, rheumatoid arthritis and glomerulonephritis, $C\bar{1}r$–$C\bar{1}s$–$C\bar{1}$ complexes appear in an increased concentration, indicating an intensified C1 activation by immune complexes, or C1 activators. In some patients one can also find complexes composed of C1r–C1s in the proenzyme form (*Figure 20.1*).

In recurrent pneumococcal otitis media in children, large amounts of the C1r–C1s complexes are present in serum and in most cases also complexes of $C\bar{1}r$–$C\bar{1}s$–$C\bar{1}$IA. The cause of the occurrence of the C1r–C1s complexes is not known. The findings point to a partial dysfunction of C1 which could imply a reduced capacity to eliminate the bacteria.

## Increased levels of the complement factors

In acute or chronic inflammatory processes, e.g. infectious diseases, tumours with tissue necrosis and rheumatoid arthritis several of the C factors in plasma are often increased. Both C1s, C3, C4 and factor B belong to the acute phase proteins. Normal or slightly increased values of C3 and C4 in plasma do not exclude a complement consuming process, for instance in rheumatoid arthritis. To interpret the C determinations, the results should be related to the levels of other acute phase proteins (C-reactive protein, orosomucoid, $\alpha_1$-antichymotrypsin, $\alpha_1$-antitrypsin.

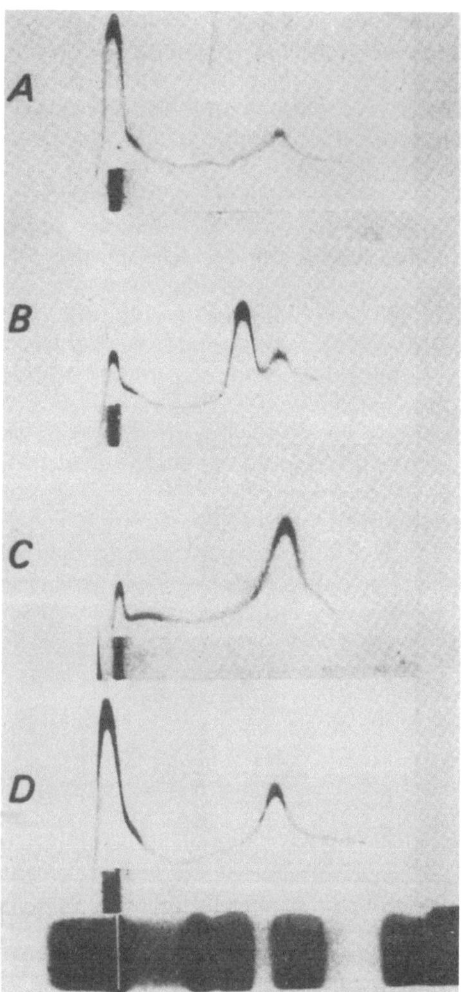

*Figure 20.1* Crossed immunoelectrophoresis with anti-Cls in agarose gel. A, Normal serum. B, C, D, Sera from patients with chronic urticaria. In normal serum there is a faint precipitate in the $\alpha_2$ region, which is more evident in the patients' sera (B, C, D). Also in the $\beta$ region there is a Cls containing precipitate originating from macromolecular Cl not moving into the gel

## Complement analyses in pathological conditions

The complement function can be examined by means of various types of haemolytic tests. By the CH50 test the function of the classical pathway can be analysed, but it does not permit evaluation of the feedback system of the alternative pathway. By means of simple haemolysis-in-gel tests, defects in both activation pathways can be analysed.

All factors within the C system, as well as the C$\bar{1}$ inactivator, factor I, factor H and the C4 binding protein, can be quantified by immunochemical tests such as the electroimmunoassay or the Mancini test. A combination of the haemolysis-in-gel tests and C3, C4 determinations can locate an abnormality within the system. Further immunochemical analyses of C1q, C1s, C2, factor B, C$\bar{1}$IA and properdin, will determine the disorder.

Activation of the classical pathway usually leads to reduced levels of C1q, C2, C4 and C3, while factor B remains normal. Activation of the alternative pathway causes decreased levels of C3, properdin and factor B, whereas C1q, C2 and C4 remain normal. However, analyses of the complement profile have their limitations. Thus a fast turnover of C factors, or C factor degradation may be compensated by an increased synthesis. In spite of these problems determination of complement factors can be used to detect disturbances in a number of diseases.

Immunochemical methods to directly determine and quantify cleavage products of C3, C4 and factor B are now available since antisera against the fragments have been produced. In rheumatoid arthritis, where the level of C3 and C4 in plasma often is normal or increased, it is now possible to detect and quantify C3d and C4d fragments by means of crossed immune electrophoresis or electroimmunoassay.

Radioimmunoassays have been developed to detect the small fragments of C3a and C5a. These methods are dependent on an initial separation of the fragments from the original molecules C3 and C5, since the antigenic determinants are the same on the fragments as on the original complete molecules. A commercial kit is now available. Also with this new procedure there are problems, since C3a, as well as C5a bind to different cells. This can result in a negative finding in spite of the fact that there has been a cleavage of C3 and C5 resulting in C3a and C5a.

On activation of C1r and C1s in the native C1qrs complex the C$\bar{1}$ inactivator is bound to these two activated components and the whole C$\bar{1}$r–C$\bar{1}$s–C$\bar{1}$ inactivator complex dissociates from C1q. Quantification of C$\bar{1}$r–C$\bar{1}$s–C$\bar{1}$IA by electroimmunoassay is a sensitive and safe method to demonstrate that C1 activation has occurred.

Other methods for quantitation of C1 activation have recently been described, in which C$\bar{1}$r–C$\bar{1}$s–C$\bar{1}$IA complexes were estimated by radioimmunoassay or an ELISA technique.

An ELISA technique for quantitation of activation of the alternative pathway has been reported. This method permits measurement of C3bBbP and C3bP complexes in serum and plasma.

## Bibliography

AGNELLO, V. (1978). Complement deficiency states. *Medicine (Baltimore)*, **57**, 1.

COOPER, N. R., NEMEROW, G. R. and JAYES, J. T. (1983). Methods to detect and quantitate complement activation. In *Springer Semin. Immunopathol.*, **6**, 195.

HACK, C. E., HANNEMA, A. J., EERENBERG–BEHMER, A. J., GUT, A. T. and AALBERSE, R. G. (1981). A C$\bar{1}$ inhibitor complex assay (INCA): A method to detect C1 activation *in vitro* and *in vivo*. *J. Immunol.*, **127**, 1450.

JACOB, H. S. (1981). The role of activated complement and granulocytes in shock states and myocardial infarction. *J. Lab. Clin. Med.*, **98**, 645.

LACHMANN, P. J. and PETERS, D. K. (eds) (1982). *Clinical Aspects of Immunology*. Fourth edition, **1**, 18. Blackwell Scientific Publications, Oxford.

OPFKERKUCH, W. and ROTHER, K. (1978). *Clinical Aspects of the Complement System*. Georg Thieme Publishers, Stuttgart.

# Chapter 21

# Autoimmune diseases

**Renée Norberg**

Autoimmunity is a condition where an immunological reaction is directed against 'self'. The famous immunologist Paul Ehrlich found at the turn of the century that experimental animals normally did not produce antibodies against their own tissue. Ehrlich thought that such autoimmune reactions would have led to severe tissue damage and he formulated the concept 'horror autotoxicus'. Still Ehrlich and other contemporary scientists realized that this tolerance against 'self' probably could be broken and that as a consequence various diseases might be explained. Not until 1957 did Witebsky convincingly demonstrate a connection between a thyroid disease and the simultaneous rise of autoantibodies against thyroid gland antigens.

We now know that autoimmune reactions can occur in a number of situations. These reactions do not necessarily cause disease and the immune system in fact utilizes certain autoimmune reactions in its normal activity (cf. chapter 8). The mechanisms behind the development of autoimmunity are multiple, and infectious agents, drugs as well as direct tissue damage, can be important. Cellular and humoral components of the immune system can be recruited for participation in autoimmune processes, but the prerequisite of the reaction varies with the underlying mechanisms of the disease in question. Furthermore there are important predisposing hereditary factors and certain autoimmune diseases show a strong linkage to one or several defined HLA antigens (cf. chapters 9 and 14). Measurable titres of autoantibodies are a relatively common finding even in healthy individuals, especially in middle-aged and older women. In several diseases, however, autoantibodies are linked to the disease process and their presence can be utilized diagnostically.

The autoimmune reaction can be directed against a special organ with symptoms originating from disturbances in the function of this organ (*Table 21.1*). An example of such an organ-specific disease is chronic thyroiditis with characteristic changes in the thyroid gland. Simultaneously there are antibodies in serum against thyroid tissue. The role of these antibodies in the aetiology is, as in several other organ-related autoimmune diseases, not clear. They may well be secondary to damage by non-immunological mechanisms. Other autoimmune diseases can engage several organ systems with multiple symptoms as a result (*Table 21.1*). Systemic lupus erythematosus (SLE) is an example of such a disease with a large number of different autoantibodies of varying specificity, some of which are neither organ nor species specific.

**TABLE 21.1. Autoimmune disease**

| Diseases | Autoimmunity demonstrated against |
| --- | --- |
| *Blood diseases* | |
| Haemolytic anaemia | Erythrocytes |
| Leucopenia | Granulocytes, lymphocytes |
| Thrombocytopenia | Thrombocytes |
| Pernicious anaemia | Intrinsic factor (IF) |
| *Endocrine diseases* | |
| Thyrotoxicosis | TSH receptor (stimulating antibodies) |
| Chronic thyroiditis | Thyroglobulin, thyroid epithelium |
| Primary myxoedema | THS receptor (blocking antibodies) |
| Gastritis | Parietal cells |
| Addison's disease | Adrenal glands |
| Polyglandular insufficiency | Endocrine organs (ovaries) |
| Male infertility | Sperms |
| Hypoparathyroidism | Parathyroid glands |
| Hypophyseal insufficiency | Hypophysis |
| Juvenile diabetes (type I) | Islets of Langerhans; insulin receptors |
| Insulin-resistant diabetes | Insulin receptors |
| *Skin diseases* | |
| Pemphigus | Intercellular substance of skin |
| Pemphigoid | Basement membrane of skin |
| Vitiligo | Melanocytes |
| *Muscle diseases* | |
| Myasthenia gravis | Acetylcholine receptors; (skeletal muscle) |
| *Kidney diseases* | |
| Glomerular basement membrane | Glomerular basement membrane |
| (GBM) nephritis (Goodpasture's syndrome) | |
| *Liver diseases* | |
| Primary biliary cirrhosis | Mitochondria |
| Active chronic hepatitis | Actin; cell nuclei |
| SLE | Cell nuclei, various other antigens |
| 'Mixed connective tissue disease' (MCTD) | Cell nuclei |
| Systemic sclerosis | Cell nuclei |
| Rheumatoid arthritis | IgG |

## Antigens

Autoantibodies have been demonstrated reacting with antigens present on cell membranes, in the cell cytoplasm or in the nucleus. Antibodies also appear against secretion products such as thyroglobulin, insulin and other hormones. Several human autoantibodies are specific for certain organ antigens. Some of these organ antigens are species specific. Antibodies against some thyroid antigens thus react only with cells from man or monkey. Other organ antigens show a close immunological relation between different species, even between species distantly related within the animal series. Classical examples of such antigens are found in the brain and the eye lens.

## Effector mechanisms

Autoimmune reactions cause tissue damage principally in the same way as other immunological reactions (*see* chapter 16). For tissue damage to appear the immunological reaction must include antigens available *in vivo*. Autoantibodies are rarely of pathogenic significance *per se*. Obvious exceptions are antibodies reacting with receptors of various kinds, e.g. those for hormones or transmitter substances (*Figure 16.3*, p. 195). Such antibodies have been demonstrated to be of importance for the development of symptoms in endocrinological diseases. Autoantibodies binding to a hormone receptor can induce the same activity as the corresponding hormone. In some cases the receptor antibodies can block the receptor preventing the reaction between the receptor and its hormone or transmitter substance, as in myasthenia gravis.

Tissue damage caused by the cooperation between autoantibodies and complement is primarily seen in haemolytic anaemia, but is also thought to be of importance in certain cases of leucopenia and thrombocytopenia. In patients with glomerular basement membrane (GBM) nephritis there are serum antibodies which react with the GBM and activate complement causing progressive nephritis. In some cases of male infertility there are complement binding autoantibodies against spermatozoa which can be of pathogenic significance.

Antibody-dependent cell-mediated cytolysis (ADCC) may be of importance for the development of chronic thyroiditis as has been demonstrated experimentally, and may well play a role in other conditions as well (cf. chapter 16).

Cooperation between autoantibodies of the IgG class and phagocytes with receptors for IgG can possibly be of pathogenic importance in certain haemolytic anaemias. Erythrocyte–antierythrocyte antibody complexes have been demonstrated experimentally to bind to macrophages in the spleen.

Cell-mediated immune mechanisms are of decisive importance for the appearance of experimental allergic encephalitis and allergic orchitis. Although in the latter condition there is evidence that autoantibodies against testicular tissue can also be of significance.

## Blood diseases

*Autoimmune haemolytic anaemia* can be primary or secondary to other diseases. Moreover, treatment with certain drugs can induce autoimmune haemolytic anaemia (*see* chapter 18).

According to the temperature sensitivity *in vitro* of the autoantibodies, the autoimmune haemolytic anaemia can be divided into two types. The 'warm' antibodies are optimally active at $37°C$, while the 'cold' antibodies have their reaction optimum at $2–10°C$. Primary autoimmune haemolytic anaemia with warm antibodies is a rarity. These antibodies are more often seen in connection with other diseases such as SLE, lymphatic leukaemia, or occasionally virus infections. The clinical symptoms which can be of short or long duration vary from insignificantly decreased numbers of red blood cells to severe haemolytic anaemia with icterus. Exacerbations are common, usually for unknown reasons. The warm antibodies are mainly of the IgG class and are demonstrable with Coombs' direct antiglobulin test. Free erythrocyte antibodies can occasionally be demonstrated, more often in the severe cases. Most warm erythrocyte antibodies react with antigens within the Rh system. The autoantibody specificity can be such that the patient's own erythrocytes have a shortened life-span, while transfused homologous erythrocytes with a very slightly different antigen set-up can survive normally. There are patients with IgG sensitized erythrocytes without any signs of haemolysis. This may be explained by a low antibody density on the surface of the erythrocytes, since a close contact is required between two IgG antibodies on the cell surface for complement activation and haemolysis to occur.

Antibodies agglutinating erythrocytes at low temperatures are often found in low titres in normal individuals. Cold-agglutininaemia with pathologically increased titres appear in one acute temporary and one chronic form. The acute form, appearing without any sex difference, is often seen in connection with infections caused by *Mycoplasma pneumoniae*. The patients rarely have signs of haemolysis but in those with very high levels of cold-agglutinins anaemia and icterus can appear.

Chronic cold-agglutininaemia may occur without any known cause, but it is generally secondary to a neoplastic disease. These cold-agglutinins are usually monoclonal and of the IgM class as in the acute form. They are often specific against I antigen. The symptoms are mostly moderate and can be directly explained by the presence of the cold agglutinins. When the temperature is decreased there is a local agglutination in superficial blood vessels causing stasis and pain, which vanish when the temperature is increased and the agglutination is reversed.

The most dramatic form of autoimmune haemolytic anaemia is the acute haemolysis seen in connection with cold exposure followed by haemoglobulinuria. The disease used to be related to congenital syphilis, but probably has a different pathogenesis in most cases.

*Autoimmune thrombocytopenia* can as haemolytic anaemia be primary or secondary. Secondary thrombocytopenia occasionally occurs in SLE and various lympho-proliferative diseases. It can also be induced by certain drugs. The primary thombocytopenia is seen in an acute form, usually in children after virus infections, but also in a chronic form. The symptoms, primarily petechia, ecchymoses and mucosal bleedings are the same in all forms. Free thrombocyte antibodies are rarely found, but IgG antibodies bound to the patients' own thrombocytes can occasionally be demonstrated.

Autoantibodies against *granulocytes* can be found in SLE and are thought to contribute to the granulocytopenia often seen in this disease. Free granulocyte antibodies are technically the most difficult to detect.

Antibodies reacting with membrane antigens of *lymphocytes* can be demonstrated in most SLE patients and often in different virus infections. Lymphocyte antibodies have been found in many relatives and also unrelated individuals living with SLE patients (*see below*).

Patients with *pernicious anaemia* have, in a high frequency, antibodies blocking the binding of vitamin $B_{12}$ to the intrinsic factor (IF). The pathogenic IF antibodies are of the IgA class and are found in the gastric and intestinal mucosa. IF antibodies in serum are of the IgG class and do not affect the uptake of the $IF-B_{12}$ complex from the intestine. Patients with pernicious anaemia have achlorhydria and there is pronounced atrophy of the gastric mucosa which is infiltrated by lymphocytes and plasma cells. Almost all patients also have antibodies which react with *parietal cells*. Recently parietal cell antibodies from patients with pernicious anaemia have been shown *in vitro* to block the gastrin receptors on the parietal cells, inhibiting the activity of gastrin.

## Endocrine diseases

Most patients with *Graves' disease* (diffuse toxic goitre) have antibodies (TSab) with thyroid-stimulating activity. TSab react with the receptor for the thyroid-stimulating hormone (TSH), imitating the stimulating effect on the thyroid metabolism of the TSH. The presence of TSab is considered to indicate active disease and determination of TSab can be of use for the follow-up of thyrotoxicosis. Remaining, or reappearing increased levels of antibodies show the need for continued therapy.

The *exophthalmus* often accompanying Graves' disease is also thought to be of autoimmune origin, even if the pathogenesis is unknown. There is no relation between the development of exophthalmus and the level of TSab. Recently patients with Graves' disease and exophthalmus were found to have in high frequency antibodies reacting with a soluble, not yet identified antigen from eye muscles.

Single cases of *primary myxoedema* occur with antibodies blocking the binding of TSH to its receptor. The transfer via placenta of such antibodies may explain why transient hypothyroidism may occur in infants of mothers treated for primary myxoedema.

*Chronic thyroiditis* or Hashimoto's goitre is characterized by enlargement of the thyroid with histologically demonstrable changes of the epithelial cells, lymphocyte infiltration and formation of lymphoid follicles with germinal centres. The tendency to develop fibrosis is pronounced in some cases. The thyroid gland is not always enlarged, but its firm texture is characteristic. The clinical symptoms are usually quite insignificant, but when they appear they are consistent with those of hypothyroidism. Thyroglobulin antibodies are demonstrable in high concentrations in almost all patients with chronic thyroiditis. High titres are rare in other diseases of the thyroid. Antibodies against thyroid microsomal antigens are found in about 80% of the patients but are also seen in lower titres in other diseases of the thyroid, as well as in patients with pernicious anaemia, SLE and rheumatoid arthritis. Low titres are often seen in apparently healthy elderly women. Antibodies reacting with the thyrotropin receptor but promoting thyroid growth have been demonstrated sporadically both in chronic thyroiditis and in Graves' disease.

In most patients with chronic thyroiditis there is cell-mediated immune reactivity against thyroglobulin and thyroid microsomal antigens. The significance of cytotoxic T cells for the appearance of the tissue damage is not fully known.

During the last few years evidence has accrued that *insulin-dependent diabetes* (*type I diabetes*) occurs in conjunction with autoimmune manifestations. There is a statistically significant relation between insulin-dependent diabetes and organ-specific autoimmune diseases, such as chronic thyroiditis, pernicious anaemia and Addison's disease. In type I diabetes antibodies appear, reacting with cells in the islets of Langerhans. The antibodies which are found in low titres, are transient and can usually be demonstrated only in recently discovered cases. In some patients, however, the antibodies persist long after the appearance of the symptoms of diabetes. These are the patients who often have other organ specific autoantibodies (in one study 67%). Antibodies against the islets of Langerhans are of the IgG class and react with all types of cells in the islets but not with hormones from the pancreas. Their aetiology has been discussed and it seems probable that they are secondary to cell damage.

In some cases of juvenile diabetes of recent onset there have been antibodies reacting with viable Langerhans cells. These antibodies are still incompletely characterized, but may be of pathogenic significance as they are likely to be involved in the cellular destruction because of their reaction with surface antigens. Antibodies to the insulin receptor competing with insulin for binding to the receptors have recently been demonstrated to occur in juvenile onset insulin-dependent diabetes. Receptor antibodies with insulin-like activity have also been demonstrated in a few cases of pronounced hypoglycaemia.

Autoantibodies against the adrenal glands can be shown in cases of idiopathic *Addison's disease* and against the hypoparathyroid glands in cases of *idiopathic hypoparathyroidism*, especially early in the course of the disease. The antibodies are organ specific, but their pathogenic significance is unknown.

Organ specific autoantibodies reacting with *ovaries* and various cells from the hypophysis have also been reported in single cases of polyendocrine disease.

## Skin diseases

Almost all patients with *pemphigus vulgaris* have circulating antibodies which react with an unknown antigen located intercellularly in the epidermis. In *bullous pemphigoid* there is a high frequency of antibodies which react with the basement membrane of the skin.

In both diseases skin biopsies, preferably taken at the rim of an intact new bulla, show deposits of IgG and complement demonstrable with immunological techniques. If circulating antibodies have been shown there is no need to take a biopsy.

Pemphigus antibodies are seen in 15–50% of individuals with burns, and also in single cases associated with the treatment of penicillin, penicillamine and phenyl-butazone. The aetiology of the autoantibody production in pemphigus as well as pemphigoid is unknown. In both conditions, however, these autoantibodies may be of pathogenic significance.

In *dermatitis herpetiformis* immunological analysis of biopsies from normal skin usually demonstrates granular deposits of IgA in the dermal papillae. The patients lack circulating antibodies against dermal antigens but for unknown reasons 15–20% of the cases have antibodies against reticulin (the collagen moiety of basement membranes).

Immunologic studies of skin biopsies can be of value to differentiate SLE from *discoid lupus erythematosus* (DLE). In both SLE and DLE there are granular deposits of immunoglobulin (IgG, often IgA and IgM as well) and complement along the dermal–epidermal junction of the affected skin. In SLE the same immunological findings can be made in biopsies from normal skin. It has been speculated whether or not these findings of immunoglobulin and complement are the result of deposition of circulating immune complexes in the skin. There are no definite data to clarify this point at present.

## Liver diseases

*Active chronic hepatitis* is a progressive disease where immunological mechanisms probably are significant for the development of the organ damage.

The disease appears in individuals of all ages, but mainly in women. The onset can be insidious or acute as in infectious hepatitis. In addition to signs of a disturbed liver function (icterus, increase of transaminases, etc.) there are often other symptoms such as arthralgias, pleuritis, thrombocytopenic purpura, nephritis and ulcerative colitis. There is a hepatocellular necrosis of the type called piecemeal necrosis with large vacuolated liver cells. Infiltration of plasma cells and lymphocytes with a tendency to form germinal centres is often striking, especially in the portal area. Early in the course of the disease there is nodular cirrhosis. Most patients have drastically increased levels of serum immunoglobulins particularly of IgG. Antibodies against nuclear antigens are demonstrable in high frequency.

The most useful serological reaction for the diagnosis of active chronic hepatitis is the demonstration of antibodies against the muscle protein actin. Actin is found not only in muscle cells but in all other mammalian cells. The antibodies are of the IgG class and not species specific. In untreated cases of active chronic hepatitis there are actin antibodies, usually in high titres, in more than 80% of the patients.

The actin antibodies are to some extent related to the course of the disease so that the titres decrease on remission and rise again on relapse. IgM antibodies against actin are common in acute infections with or without liver engagement. Actin antibodies do not react with live, intact cells and there is no evidence that they would cause tissue damage. Instead it has been discussed whether or not immunity against certain yet incompletely characterized liver specific antigens can be of pathogenic importance. There are autoantibodies, as well as T cell reactivity against these antigens in patients with chronic hepatitis and in experiments with rabbits liver damage occurs after immunization with such antigens.

*Primary biliary cirrhosis* usually has a gradual onset in middle-aged or older women. The most advanced cases have intrahepatic cholestasis, icterus, liver and spleen enlargement, steatorrhoea and itching. The earliest morphological changes with inflammatory, often granulomatous infiltrations are seen in the portal area. Antibodies against mitochondria, often in high titres, are found in more than 95% of the patients. The titres of these antibodies do not relate to the severity, or the stage of the primary biliary cirrhosis. Many patients with high titres of antibodies against mitochondria have no symptoms, but liver biopsy usually shows histological changes in agreement with the diagnosis of primary biliary cirrhosis.

It should be added that there are mitochondrial antibodies of different specificity (*see further* Appendix 2) and that only mitochondrial antibodies type M2 occur in connection with primary biliary cirrhosis.


## Muscle diseases

*Myasthenia gravis* is a neuromuscular disease with characteristic weakness in skeletal muscles. The basic defect in myasthenia gravis is a reduction of the number of available acetylcholine receptors. This is a rare disease, which occurs more frequently in females than in males. All skeletal muscles can be affected, but the first symptoms usually appear in the muscles of the eyes and eyelids. Symptoms from only one or a few groups of muscles can persist for a long period of time in some cases; in other cases there is a rapid progression of the disease resulting in general muscle weakness. It is characteristic that the activity of the disease fluctuates, often for unknown reasons.

Myasthenia gravis was quite early considered to be an autoimmune disease because of the frequent finding of histological changes in the thymus and the demonstration in many patients of antibodies reacting with skeletal muscles. About 10% of myasthenia patients have a usually benign thymoma and around 80% of the others have histological changes in the medulla of the thymus characterized by lymphoid follicles with germinal centres. Therapeutic thymectomy was already being performed at the beginning of this century and the improvement then noted has been confirmed retrospectively with 57% of the patients improving in one study and 86% in another following the operation. In some cases the improvement did not occur until several years later. More or less complete remission was found in 20 and 36% respectively.

Based on data from experimental models in animals, autoantibodies against the acetylcholine receptor were searched for and in 1974–75 they could be demonstrated in about 90% of all myasthenia gravis patients. The antibodies are pathogenic, as demonstrated by the development of muscle weakness in animals transfused with immunoglobulin from myasthenia gravis patients. Antibodies against the acetylcholine receptor can be transported across the placenta and transient myasthenia gravis symptoms can occasionally be seen in infants of diseased mothers.

The effect of the autoantibodies is due to blockage of the neuromuscular transmission via the receptor and by affecting the metabolism of the receptor cells. It seems logical to try to decrease the amount of circulating antibodies and good, but transient results have been reported with plasmaphaeresis.

Recent data demonstrate that in patients with *polymyositis* there are lymphocytes cytotoxic for fetal muscle cells in tissue culture. These studies probably provide the best example of the pathogenic significance of T cell-mediated immunity for the occurrence of tissue damage in an autoimmune disease. The specificity of the muscular antigen is unknown as is the clinical importance of the finding.

# Connective tissue diseases

### Systemic lupus erythematosus (SLE)

In systemic lupus erythematosus pathological changes can be seen in most organs. Symptoms from joints, skin, serous membranes, blood vessels and kidneys are especially common.

Up until 1950 the disease was thought to be rare and to have a very poor prognosis. With improved diagnostic methods it was found that the disease is much more common than previously realized and has a wide range of severity. With the use of corticosteroid therapy the prognosis has also been radically improved. The disease can start at any age in either sex, but it is most common in fertile females. It was originally described as a rapidly progressive, usually fatal systemic disease characterized by high fever, skin changes, polyarthritis, exudation in pleura and pericardium, as well as glomerulonephritis and symptoms from the central nervous system. Now patients are often seen with relatively vague symptoms, perhaps only with arthralgias, but symptoms of all degrees of severity can be compatible with the SLE diagnosis.

The spontaneous course is characterized by remissions and exacerbations, often without any obvious reason. The development of glomerulonephritis is prognostically unfavourable and often results in a progressive and finally fatal renal insufficiency. The tissue changes are fairly uncharacteristic, but IgG as well as complement factors can usually be demonstrated in the glomeruli, skin lesions and vessel walls. The complement level in serum is often decreased in active cases, as mentioned in the previous chapter.

The aetiology of the disease is unknown. The role of viruses has been much discussed, but there is no definite evidence for an aetiological role in SLE. The high frequency of lymphocytotoxic antibodies in SLE patients, as well as their relatives and unrelated household members has been seen as an indication of a virus infection relating to the onset of the disease. Drug-induced SLE was discussed in chapter 18.

Family studies have shown an increased frequency not only of SLE but also other immunological abnormalities in relatives of SLE patients. Studies of HLA antigens in patients with spontaneous SLE have hitherto only indicated an association to the DR3.

Autoimmune diseases similar to the human SLE syndrome which show haemolytic anaemia, production of nuclear antibodies and development of an immune complex induced nephritis, occur spontaneously in certain strains of mice. Genetic, as well as immunological and virological factors are of importance for the development of manifest disease in the mice. To what extent and in which way the various factors cooperate and influence each other is only partly known.

More than any other autoimmune disease, SLE is characterized by circulating antibodies, demonstrable *in vitro*, directed mainly against components of cell nuclei, but also against a number of other tissue antigens. Typically the nuclear antibodies lack organ or species specificity. Antibodies against several different nuclear antigens can often be demonstrated simultaneously. Nuclear antibodies are present in almost all cases of SLE with only rare instances of seronegative patients being described. In these instances nuclear antibodies can usually be demonstrated if repeated samples are investigated for the presence of less commonly occurring nuclear antibodies (*see further* Appendix 2). Antibodies against the Sm antigen and against native double-stranded DNA are seen almost exclusively in SLE. Changes in the titre of DNA antibodies— increases as well as decreases—can be a prognostically bad sign, indicating the likely exacerbation of the disease. On the other hand follow-up studies have demonstrated high DNA antibody titres remaining for long periods of time without appearance of symptoms of active disease.

Nuclear antibodies can also be demonstrated in more than 90% of patients with *systemic sclerosis*. In addition nuclear antibodies are found in a number of diseases, but with the exception of *Sjögren's syndrome* and some cases of rheumatoid arthritis, the titres are usually much lower than those seen in SLE.

Antibodies against nuclear antigens can also appear during treatment with certain drugs, especially procainamide and hydralazine (*see also* chapter 18). In a smaller number of these cases an SLE-like syndrome appears, which is clinically very similar to spontaneous SLE, although antibodies against double-stranded DNA are rarely seen. The autoantibodies as well as the clinical symptoms usually vanish after drug treatment has been discontinued.

There is little evidence that the nuclear antibodies can induce tissue damage. They are transported across the placenta, but leave no obvious signs of organ damage in the fetus. Neither do they damage cells in tissue cultures.

Antibodies reacting with membrane antigens on lymphocytes are demonstrable in about 80% of SLE patients. Whether or not the lymphocyte antibodies are pathogenic and add to the symptomatology of SLE is unclear. The correlation between lymphocytopenia and the presence of cytotoxic antibodies against lymphocytes is poor. In contrast, the presence of central nervous symptoms in SLE patients relates to the presence of lymphocyte antibodies. Several studies have in fact demonstrated that lymphocyte antibodies from patients with SLE of the CNS react with brain tissue *in vitro*, while antibodies from patients without any neurological symptoms lack this reactivity.

Circulating antibodies against coagulation factors that interfere with coagulation are seen occasionally in single patients with SLE. More common are the occurrence of antibodies reacting with phospholipids which act as 'lupus anticoagulants'. An increased bleeding tendency is rare in these patients, but they often have complications with thrombosis.

Other organ-specific antibodies are occasionally seen in SLE, but the frequency is relatively low.

About 30–40% of SLE patients have detectable rheumatoid factor. There is no difference in the clinical course between those with or without the rheumatoid factor.


**Rheumatoid arthritis**

It can be discussed whether or not rheumatoid arthritis (RA) should be included among autoimmune diseases. There are many similarities between RA and other autoimmune diseases, for instance concerning the production of autoantibodies. In 85% of RA patients there are increased titres of antigammaglobulins, rheumatoid factors (RF) or the IgM class and in most patients there are IgG RF in serum and/or synovial fluid.

The rheumatoid factors react with determinants within the constant portion of the IgG Fc; the binding is more efficient to immune complexes or aggregates of IgG than to native monomeric IgG. RF reacting with human IgG is often demonstrated in other chronic diseases such as active chronic hepatitis, liver cirrhosis, sarcoidosis and infections of long duration. The titre of RF correlates rather poorly with the activity of the disease, although the highest RF titres are seen in patients with advanced disease. A connection was recently found between the presence of HLA DR4 and seropositive RA.

Nuclear antibodies are found in 20–30% of RA patients without any correlation to the clinical symptoms. Nuclear antibodies are seen in about 40% of patient with juvenile RA. The presence of collagen antibodies is not sufficiently specific to be of diagnostic use, even if their appearance has been considered of importance for the development of arthritis.

## Bibliography

FELTKAMP, T. E. W. and SOMSENK, R. J. T. (eds.) (1985). Nuclear antigens and antinuclear antibodies. *Scand. J. Rheum.* suppl. 56.
LACHMANN, P. J. and PETERS, D. K. (eds.) (1982). *Clinical Aspects of Immunology.* Fourth edition. Blackwell Scientific Publications, Oxford.
SCHOENFELD, Y. and SCHWARTZ, R. S. (1984). Immunologic and genetic factors in autoimmune diseases. *New Engl. J. Med.*, **311**, 1019.

# Chapter 22

# Immunosuppressive therapy

**Göran Holm**

Immunological tissue damage is a common cause of acute and chronic disease in man. Immune reactions also hinder transplantation of bone marrow or solid organs between histoincompatible individuals. Since immunological disease and transplantation reactions often result in severe, occasionally life-threatening conditions, it is important to provide immunosuppressive therapy to prevent, or decrease the tissue damage. In spite of the fact that such treatment has been used for over 30 years, our knowledge about the mode of function of immunosuppressive drugs and the risks of long-term treatment is incomplete. Clear indications for immunosuppressive therapy are present only in transplant patients and in a few immunological diseases.

There are several reasons for the lack of information on how to use immunosuppressive therapy. We know too little about the immunological mechanisms behind diseases where an immunological pathogenesis is suspected. Only during the last few years have well-controlled clinical trials been performed permitting evaluation of some immunosuppressive drugs. Ionizing irradiation and immunosuppressive agents are limited in their applicability because of their non-specific effects on the immune system and other organs introducing the risk of severe side effects. In spite of its deficiencies *non-specific immunosuppression* is an important complement to other treatment and in many instances the only efficient therapy the patient can be offered.

The ideal immunosuppressive treatment is directed only against the immunological reaction causing the disease. Such immunologically *specific immunosuppression* has so far only been successful in Rh prophylaxis (*see* chapter 9). Induction of tolerance as another possibility has been discussed in chapter 8. The use of monoclonal antibodies may bring new possibilities for specific immunosuppression (chapter 6).

### Inhibition of immunological tissue damage

Immunological tissue damage is usually the result of a chain reaction in which immune and inflammatory cells and cell products participate. Since the reaction is inhibited if any of the links are eliminated or blocked, a number of different measures can inhibit immunologically induced tissue damage (*Table 22.1*). Immunosuppressive therapy usually influences several steps in the reaction.

Immunological tissue damage can obviously be inhibited by drugs preventing the inflammatory component, which is always part of the immunological tissue damage. The beneficial effect of anti-inflammatory agents does not permit judgement concerning the possible immunological aetiology of the disease. Also inflammatory diseases where the immune system does not participate can of course be influenced by anti-inflammatory drugs.

**TABLE 22.1. Mechanisms of non-specific immunosuppression (examples of immunosuppressive agents in parenthesis)**

*Mechanical elimination of lymphocytes*
Ductus thoracicus drainage
Splenectomy
Thymectomy

*Damage to, or changed distribution of, lymphocytes*
Lympholysis (ALG[a], ionizing irradiation, cyclophosphamide, glucocorticoids)
Opsonization, phagocytosis? (ALG?)
Changed distribution (glucocorticoids)
Decreased recirculation

*Functional inactivation of lymphocytes*
Receptor-blocking (azathioprine? Cyclosporine A?)
Inhibited proliferation (cell cycle specific cytostatic drugs)
Inhibited production of lymphocyte products, lymphokines, antibodies (glycocorticoids?)
Blocking of membrane interaction with other lymphocytes or with macrophages

*Inhibition of monocytes–macrophages*
Inhibition of phagocytosis (glucocorticoids)
Blocking of the effects of lymphokines on cells (glucocorticoids)
Decreased degradation of antigen (glucocorticoids)
Decreased production of cells (cytostatic drugs)
Decreased release of cells from bone marrow (azathioprine, glucocorticoids)

*Polymorphonuclear granulocytes*
Decreased production (cytostatic drugs)
Inhibited function (glucocorticoids)

*Inhibition of mast cells and basophilic cells*

*Inhibition of complement*

*Inhibition of coagulation*

[a] ALG = Antilymphocyte globulin


# Immunosuppressive measures

## Surgical immunosuppression

### Drainage of ductus thoracicus

Several litres of lymph containing as many as $10^9$ lymphocytes per litre can be drained over 24 hour periods via a catheter in the *thoracic duct*. Mainly circulating lymphocytes are eliminated (*see* chapter 1), resulting in lymphocytopenia with more loss of T than B lymphocytes. During the treatment delayed hypersensitivity and T cell-dependent lymphocyte functions in peripheral blood are decreased, while antibody production is well preserved. The method is not useful for long-term treatment and immunological functions normalize as a rule when the drainage is discontinued. The method has been used as part of the treatment of patients with severe SLE and transplant patients.


### Splenectomy

Splenectomy in young patients, especially before the age of two, increases the risk of sepsis dramatically. Earlier it was thought that splenectomy in adults did not decrease the immune defence. More recent studies have shown a persistent increase of the risk of attracting septicaemia after splenectomy in adults as well. In fact the risk in splenectomized adults has been estimated to be 500 times that of non-splenectomized. The risk increases if treatment with cytostatic drugs or ionizing irradiation is applied. The sepsis is usually caused by pneumococci and sometimes complicated by meningitis and acute adrenal insufficiency.

The immunodeficiency after splenectomy depends on the importance of the spleen for elimination of blood-borne encapsulated bacteria through phagocytosis and for the production of opsonic antibodies. The antibody production after immunization is decreased in splenectomized patients.

Because of the obvious long-term risks with splenectomy this procedure is used restrictively. The method has no practical application for immunosuppression.


*Thymectomy*

In certain animal species thymectomy during the neonatal period results in persistent T cell deficiency. Thymectomy in adults eventually results in an immunodeficiency. Adult patients who are thymectomized probably become immunodeficient after more than ten years.


## Ionizing irradiation

Ionizing irradiation inhibits antibody production in animals. The primary antibody response is more sensitive than the secondary. B lymphocytes seem to be more sensitive to ionization than T lymphocytes. The number of circulating B and T lymphocytes decrease during therapeutic irradiation of patients. The B lymphocyte level normalizes within a few months, whereas the T lymphocytopenia is slowly restored and can remain for several years. Helper T cells seem to be more sensitive to irradiation than suppressor T cells. Irradiation causes lymphocytopenia through damage to stem cells and lysis of mature lymphocytes (*Table 22.1*). Irradiation for immunosuppressive purposes has a limited use in man. Total body irradiation has been tried to prepare recipients of bone marrow transplants. It has also been tried to prolong the survival of transplanted organs by local irradiation and by pretreatment of the transplant with irradiation. Extracorporal irradiation of circulating lymphocytes has been tried to decrease immune reactivity without success.

Irradiation of lymph glands of the neck, axillae, mediastinum, abdomen and loins (total nodal irradiation) has been used during the last 20 years for treatment of malignant lymphoma. There is a small risk of severe side effects. Leukaemia and other secondary tumours do not show any noticeable increase after the treatment. The incidence of other severe complications such as virus and bacterial infections, is less than 1%. Immediately after treatment with 30–40 Gy the blood T lymphocyte level decreases dramatically, while the granulocytes remain unchanged. The lymphocyte numbers then increase successively, but lymphocytopenia can remain for ten years. Since helper/inducer T cells are selectively eliminated, T cell functions and T cell-dependent antibody production is inhibited. Induction of tolerance is facilitated. Total lymph nodal irradiation results in long-term remission of experimental autoimmune diseases, such as SLE in NZB/NZW mice and adjuvant arthritis in rats. Promising results have also been described in kidney transplant patients and in cases of severe rheumatoid arthritis.

**Antilymphocyte globulin (ALG)**

ALG consists of the globulin fraction of antilymphocyte serum prepared by heterologous immunization. ALG is a potent inhibitor of cell-mediated immune reactions in animal experiments. The treatment prolongs survival of allotransplants, while the effect on humoral immunity is less apparent.

There were great expectations for ALG as an agent to prevent transplant rejection in man. Unfortunately this has not come true. It has been assumed that treatment with ALG would decrease the risk of acute rejection of transplanted solid organs. ALG is therefore given together with other immunosuppressive treatment in connection with transplantation and threatening transplant rejection. These indications for ALG have not been generally accepted. ALG has been tried in GvH reactions following bone marrow transplantation and in various immunological diseases without any convincing effects. The usefulness is also limited by ALG being a heterologous protein which can give rise to antibodies in patients treated for more than two to three weeks.

**Pharmacological immunosuppression**

Most tumour inhibiting drugs with cytotoxic effects are immunosuppressive. Cytostatic drugs not only affect cells within the immune system but also other cells including those in the blood, since the metabolic processes inhibited by cytostatic drugs occur in many different types of cells (*Table 22.1*). Cytostatic drugs have a non-selective inhibiting effect on various immune functions. Therefore the use of cytostatics is an awkward and risky way of preventing undesired immunological reactions. These drugs should not be used more than absolutely necessary and mainly in life-threatening diseases and diseases which, without treatment, result in severe invalidism.

Cytostatics and other drugs used for immunosuppression are listed in *Table 22.2*. Only two cytotoxic drugs have been studied in detail as to their immunosuppressive activity, 6-mercaptopurine with its imidazole derivative azathioprine and cyclophosphamide (*Table 22.2*).

*Azathioprine and 6-mercaptopurine*

6-Mercaptopurine was one of the first immunosuppressive drugs to be used. Azathioprine was synthesized to prolong the effect of the rapidly inactivated 6-mercaptopurine and to decrease liver toxicity. These drugs are antimetabolites affecting DNA synthesis of cells (*Table 22.2*) and preventing the proliferative phase of an immune response. The antigen binding of the lymphocytes is possibly also blocked (*Table 22.1*).

In animal experiments the IgG antibody production is inhibited, while the IgM response is relatively unaffected. The drugs decrease delayed hypersensitivity reactions and prolong the survival of transplants, primarily depending on an anti-inflammatory effect. Azathioprine prevents proliferation and release of monocytes from bone marrow, resulting in decreased numbers in the blood and in inflammatory exudates.

Azathioprine has become the most widely used immunosuppressive cytotoxic agent in man, in spite of the fact that its immunosuppressive activity is weak. In the doses used, 1–3 mg/kg daily, the primary and secondary immune responses are not inhibited. The number of lymphocytes in the blood decrease after long-term treatment. Azathioprine has a strong anti-inflammatory effect which possibly can explain its capacity to suppress cell-mediated immunity. Azathioprine is usually used together

**TABLE 22.2. Immunosuppressive measures**

*I Non-specific immunosuppression*
A.    Chemical agents
    (1) Alkylating agents: cyclophosphamide, chlorambucil
    (2) Antimetabolites:
    (a) Folic acid antagonists: methotrexate
    (b) Purine analogues: 6-mecaptopurine, azathioprine, 6-thioguanine
    (c) Antipyrimidines: 5-fluorouracil
    (3) Metaphase inhibitors: vincristine, vinblastine, podophyllotoxin
    (4) Antibiotics: actinomycins, chloramphenicol, mitomycin, puromycin
    (5) Glucocorticosteroids
    (6) Others: procarbazine, penicillamine, niridazole
B.    Antilymphocyte globulin (ALG)
C.    Ionizing irradiation
D.    Surgical measures: thymectomy, thoracic duct drainage, splenectomy

*II Specific immunosuppression*
Immunosuppression with antibody or antigen

with glucocorticoids to prevent transplant rejection and in several immunological, as well as inflammatory diseases. Its toxicity is low.

*Cyclophosphamide*

Cyclophosphamide is the most widely used immunosuppressive agent in the group of alkylating substances (*Table 22.2*). The alkylating drugs bind to nucleic acids and proteins, inhibiting DNA synthesis. Cyclophosphamide also damages resting cells, including antigen reactive lymphocytes, which is important for its immunosuppressive effect (*Tables 22.1* and *22.2*). Cyclophosphamide given before the antigen, stimulates delayed-type hypersensitivity reactions in the skin. The reaction is inhibited if cyclophosphamide is given after the antigen. Similar effects have been described using azathioprine and other cytostatic drugs.

The treatment of patients with cyclophosphamide causes lymphocytopenia and inhibits the antibody response and cell-mediated immunity. Cyclophosphamide seems to influence B lymphocytes more than T lymphocytes. Since cyclophosphamide blocks secondary and established immune responses in man it is an effective immuno-suppressive agent useful in severe and acute immunological diseases.

*Methotrexate*

Methotrexate is an antimetabolite which has been used for many years against tumours (*Table 22.2*). The drug binds to dihydrofolate dehydrogenase inhibiting the conversion of folic acid to tetrahydrofolic acid. As a result DNA synthesis and cell proliferation is blocked. Methotrexate inhibits the proliferative phase of the immune response more efficiently if it is given just after the antigen. The drug also decreases the inflammatory response. The immunosuppressive effect of methotrexate in man has not been well studied but seems to be similar to that of azathioprine. The risk of liver damage limits its use in long-term treatment.

## Glucocorticoids

Glucocorticoids are the main drugs for symptomatic treatment of inflammatory diseases with or without known immunological background. There are large variations in the immunosuppressive effect of glucocorticoids in various species. Mice and rats belong to cortisone-sensitive species, whereas man and guinea pigs are cortisone-resistant.

A single moderate dose of glucocorticoids decreases the level of circulating lymphocytes and monocytes to approximately 20% of the original value within four hours. The level returns to normal after 24 hours. Both B and T lymphocytes decrease, probably due to a redistribution of the cells, many of which seem to move to the bone marrow (*Table 22.3*). During long-term treatment with low doses, there is no lymphocytopenia. The monocytopenia which occurs after a single dose is probably explained by a decreased release from the bone marrow.

Glucocorticoids act at several different levels in the immune response (*Table 22.3*). The redistribution of the macrophages and lymphocytes can decrease the possibility of the contact between the cells necessary for an optimal immune response. There is evidence that the degradation of antigen and its presentation to antigen reactive lymphocytes by macrophages is changed. Synthesis of macromolecules and activation of B and T lymphocytes is inhibited by high concentrations. The B lymphocytes are sensitive to glycocorticoids just after the exposure to antigen. Glucocorticoids decrease the primary immune response, but do not impair an already established antibody production. They diminish the capacity of suppressor T lymphocytes to block the differentiation of B lymphocytes to antibody producing plasma cells. Recent data indicate that activated lymphocytes may be lysed by glucocorticoids even in man.

Glucocorticoids are mainly used because of their anti-inflammatory effect (*Tables 22.2* and *22.3*). They counteract vasodilatation and decrease vascular permeability, diminishing the tendency for oedema and other results of inflammation. Glucocorticoids have a number of effects on the monocyte–macrophage system. Monocytes

**TABLE 22.3. The effect of glucocorticoids on immune response and inflammation in man**

*Effects on lymphocytes*
Cause lymphopenia (mainly T cells) depending on redistribution with increase of lymphocytes in the bone marrow.
Inhibit stimulation with concanavalin A and in allogenic and autologous MLR.
Lyse activated lymphocytes.
Inhibit production of interleukin-2 and other mediators.
Inhibit delayed hypersensitivity, mainly through its anti-inflammatory effects.
In moderate doses no effect on antibody production.
High dose over a long period inhibits antibody synthesis and increases catabolism of IgG.
Can increase Ig production by inhibition of suppressor cells.
No effect on antigen–antibody binding.

*Effects on monocytes and granulocytes*
Cause monocytopenia.
Inhibit phagocytosis and bactericidal effect (high dose).
Decrease chemotaxis.
Decrease aggregation in inflammatory exudates.
Inhibit release of lysosomal enzymes and interleukin-1.
Inhibit production of prostaglandins, thromboxanes and leukotrienes.

*Effects on complement*
Counteract vasodilatation and the increased vascular permeability caused by anaphylatoxins (C3a, C5a).
High doses increase complement activation.

in the blood decrease during treatment and the cells become less sensitive to MIF and other lymphokines. The response of the macrophages to chemotaxis decreases with less accumulation in inflammatory sites. Large doses decrease the phagocytic capacity of the macrophages, partly due to diminishing numbers of Fc receptors on the cell surface. The bactericidal and fungicidal activity also decreases.

Granulocytes are less affected than monocytes by glucocorticoids. Neutrophilic granulocytes in the circulation increase during treatment. Phagocytosis and bactericidal capacity is unchanged but chemotaxis and migration of granulocytes into inflammatory exudates decrease.

Glucocorticoids inhibit the production and liberation of inflammatory mediators. Thus the release of histamine from basophilic cells is prevented. Production of prostaglandins, thromboxanes and leukotrienes is inhibited by blocking the phospholipase which liberates arachidonic acid from phospholipids (*see* chapter 17).

Complement factors and their function is not influenced by glucocorticoids. In normal doses the drugs rather counteract the vasodilatation and vascular permeability increase induced by C3a and C5a (cf. chapter 20).

No difference has been established between various glucocorticoids as to their immunosuppressive or anti-inflammatory effects. Dexamethasone gives more pronounced lymphocytopenia than equivalent doses of other glucocorticoids, probably due to its longer half-life.

Only anti-inflammatory effects are utilized in regular maintenance therapy with glucocorticoids in doses around 7.5–15 mg prednisolone daily. If an efficient immuno-suppression and inhibition of inflammation and phagocytosis is required, it is important to give high doses. This can be motivated in life-threatening immunological diseases like immune haemolytic anaemia, immunological thrombocytopenia, acute SLE and transplant rejection.

### Cyclosporine A

Cyclosporine A is a new and potent immunosuppressive drug with little toxicity for blood-forming cells. The drug is purified from a fungus and is a cyclic endecapeptide with a molecular weight of approximately 1200. It inhibits primary and secondary antibody production as well as cell-mediated immune reactions in experimental animals. Its effect on the immune response is reversible and optimal if given about the same time as the antigen. Phagocytosis by granulocytes and macrophages, as well as their bactericidal function are not affected by cyclosporine A, which seems to be a selective inhibitor of lymphocyte functions.

The results in experimental allotransplantation are remarkably good. In man cyclosporine A seems to improve the organ survival after transplantation of kidney, liver and bone marrow. It reduces the need for treatment with cortisone. Cyclosporine therapy decreases the risk of GvH reactions after bone marrow transplantation.

The dose dependent side effects are dominated by liver and kidney damage. Monitoring of the serum concentration of the drug seems a promising measure to minimize the side effects. Cyclosporine A selectively inhibits T lymphocytes. Activation of T lymphocytes with antigen, mitogen and allogenic cells is prevented. The T cell-dependent antibody response and mitogen induced immunoglobulin synthesis is also sensitive to cyclosporine A. The effect on T cell-dependent B cell responsiveness is less evident. The mechanism for the inhibition of T cells by cyclosporine is not clear. A growing body of evidence suggests that cyclosporine A prevents the generation and/or release of interleukin-1 from antigen-presenting macrophages and interleukin-2 from activated T cells, resulting in inhibition of the cell proliferation.

*Aphaeresis*

Aphaeresis is a new therapeutic principle used for immunosuppression. Heparinized blood is led through a centrifuge which continuously separates plasma from blood cells. The plasma is taken away while the blood cells together with a plasma substitute is returned to the patient (plasmaphaeresis). With continuous centrifugation lymphocytes can also be selectively eliminated from the blood (lymphaphaeresis). Using a dialysis membrane letting through proteins with molecular weight up to $1 \times 10^6$, plasmaphaeresis can be made even more selective.

Plasmaphaeresis offers an efficient treatment for severe immunological diseases such as Goodpasture's syndrome, cryoglobulinaemia, acute attacks of SLE and myasthenia gravis. Each plasmaphaeresis eliminates about 4 litres. The immunoglobulins decrease by about 20%. Antibody titres are lowered, as well as complement factors and other mediators of inflammation. Combination with a cytostatic immunosuppressive agent like cyclophosphamide is usually required for efficient treatment. Lymphaphaeresis eliminates up to $10^{10}$ lymphocytes per treatment, inhibiting various T cell-mediated immune functions. Lymphaphaeresis has been tried for the treatment of rheumatoid arthritis in man.

## Side effects of treatment with immunosuppressive drugs

Cyclophosphamide, which is the most efficient immunosuppressive drug in man has more severe side effects than other cytostatics. Active metabolites excreted via the kidneys can induce haemorrhagic cystitis and urinary bladder fibrosis with a risk of development of bladder cancer. Hair loss is a common and psychologically disturbing side effect. The hair grows again when the treatment is discontinued. The risk of persistent sterility due to azoospermia or anovulation is high. Bone marrow depression can occur during treatment with cyclophosphamide or other cytostatic drugs and motivates repeated blood controls.

The side effects of azathioprine cause fewer problems than those of the alkylators. Allopurinol interferes with the excretion of azathioprine and 6-mercaptopurine in the kidneys requiring the doses of these cytostatic drugs to be reduced by one-third.

Methotrexate is strongly liver toxic. During long-term treatment the liver changes can turn into fibrosis and cirrhosis. The risk of liver damage decreases if the methotrexate is given once a week. Ulceration of mucosal membranes and hair loss are rather disturbing side effects.

Treatment with glucocorticoids or cytostatic drugs increases the risk of infection. An immunosuppressed patient is also sensitive to opportunistic infections, which can be difficult to diagnose and may cause life-threatening infections. One example is pneumonia due to *Pneumocystis carinii*, also seen in patients with certain T cell immunodeficiencies. Treatment every second day with glucocorticoids seems to decrease the risk of adverse effects, but also decreases the therapeutic efficiency in immunological diseases.

Treatment with immunosuppressive cytostatic drugs, especially alkylating agents increases the risk of malignant tumours. The incidence of tumours in patients with transplanted kidneys treated with azathioprine and prednisolone has been estimated at

5%, with a relative risk 80 times greater than a normal population. The increase is primarily due to B cell lymphoma of non-Hodgkin type with an incidence which is 350 times greater than expected. About half of the lymphomas start in the central nervous system. Recent findings demonstrate that the tumours are mostly due to polyclonally proliferating B cells stimulated by EB virus. Recently a number of cases of acute myeloblastic leukaemia have been noted in patients treated with cyclophosphamide or other alkylating agents for more than two years. Acute myeloblastic leukaemia is rare in kidney transplanted patients treated with azathioprine and corticosteroids. The risk of developing acute myeloblastic leukaemia in patients with Hodgkin's lymphoma is 5–10% after treatment with ionizing irradiation and cytostatic drugs. The tumour frequency increases with the time after treatment. It is still unknown how long after the treatment tumours can still occur. Against this background alkylating immuno-suppressive agents should be used with great caution for diseases with a good long-term prognosis.

Cytostatic treatment during pregnancy usually increases the risk of abortion and malformations. Normal pregnancies have been seen, however, in patients treated with azathioprine after renal transplantation.


## Bibliography

BACH, J. F. (1975). *The Mode of Action of Immunosuppressive Agents*. North Holland Publ. Co., Amsterdam.

GERBER, N. L. and STEINBERG, A. D. (1976). Clinical use of immunosuppressive drugs. *Drugs*, 11, 14 and 90.

MITCHELL, M. C. and FAHEY, J. L. (eds.) (1984). Immune suppression and modulation. *Clinics in Immunology and Allergy*, 4, 197.

MÖLLER, G. (ed.) (1982). Immunosuppressive agents. *Immunol. Rev.*, 65.

SALAMAN, J. R. (ed.) (1981). *Immunosuppressive Therapy*. MTP Press Limited, Lancaster, England.

SCHEIN, P. S. and WINOKUR, S. H. (1975). Immunosuppressive and cytotoxic chemotherapy: Long-term complications. *Ann. Int. Med.*, 82, 84.

# Blood group serology for clinical use

**Bengt Löw**

This brief review of practical blood group serology provides a basis for blood transfusions as performed in clinical practice.

## Sampling

Errors in connection with sampling, laboratory investigations and registration of names and results is a major risk factor in blood transfusion work. For this reason patient identity is important when taking blood for blood group serological analysis. Before taking the blood sample, test tubes and forms must be prepared. The patient's first and surname as well as birthdate must be noted on the labels. Just before the venepuncture the patient is asked to give his name and date of birth. If he is unable to do so (e.g. due to unconsciousness) it is necessary to secure his identity in some other way. When it has been secured the venepuncture is performed with 8–10 ml of blood without addition taken from adults and at least 5–6 drops of capillary blood in 2 ml sterile 3.8% sodium citrate solution from infants.

Since one of the objectives of the compatibility test is to reveal mistakes in sampling for blood grouping, it is unacceptable except in urgent situations to obtain the blood sample for cross-matching at the same time as the sample for blood grouping.

## Methodology for blood group serologic analyses

As mentioned in chapter 9, IgM antibodies, for instance those occurring naturally within the ABO system, agglutinate red cells in saline. In contrast IgG antibodies do not agglutinate cells in saline. To demonstrate agglutination with IgG antibodies the antiglobulin test (Coombs' test), tests with enzyme-treated red blood cells, or tests in high molecular media can be used.

### Antiglobulin test (Coombs' test)

To demonstrate IgG antibodies with this method, the antibodies first have to react with and attach to red blood cells. The erythrocytes are 'sensitized' with the antibodies. Unattached IgG antibodies are eliminated by washing the red cells in 0.9% saline three to four times before the addition of antihuman globulin serum. Antiglobulin serum added to the sensitized red blood cells causes agglutination. The incubation takes place at 37°C in 0.9% saline for one hour, or in sodium chloride solution of lower ionic strength (LISS*, low ionic salt solution) for 5–10 minutes. The antigen–antibody reactions are enhanced up to 1000 times in LISS.

This *indirect antiglobulin test (Coombs' indirect test)* is performed in the following steps and is used to demonstrate free antibodies in serum.

(1)    Sensitization of red blood cells with the IgG antibodies to be determined.
(2)    Washing of the sensitized red blood cells.
(3)    Addition of antihuman globulin serum, resulting in agglutination.

The antiglobulin serum can be directed against other immunoglobulin classes than IgG and/or against complement factors. Antiglobulin serum against C3 and C4 can be utilized to enhance antiglobulin reactions with complement-binding blood group antibodies.

In certain types of haemolytic anaemia, for instance acquired haemolytic anaemia in adults and haemolytic disease of the newborn where the mother is immunized, the sensitization takes place in the circulation. To demonstrate this sensitization, i.e. that the antibodies have already reacted with and attached to the erythrocytes, the patient's red blood cells are washed and the antiglobulin serum is added. This reaction occurs directly without previous incubation of the patient's antibodies and erythrocytes and is therefore called the *direct antiglobulin test (Coombs' direct test)*.

### Enzyme test

Certain proteolytic enzymes (trypsin, pepsin, bromelin, ficin, etc.) decrease the surface charge of the erythrocytes (chapter 9) so that they can be agglutinated by the IgG antibodies. The enzymes are first added to the red blood cells and incubated at 37 °C. After washing of the enzyme-treated red blood cells, the test serum is added and the antigen–antibody reaction takes place. This method is called a *two-step enzyme method* and is very sensitive. A *one-step enzyme method* is performed with simultaneous addition of erythrocytes, enzyme and test serum. This is much simpler, but less sensitive than the two-step method.

### Tests in high molecular weight medium

The required change in surface charge can also be induced by the suspension of the red blood cells in certain high molecular weight media such as albumin, gelatin, dextran, polyvinylpyrollidone (PVP), etc. The most commonly used is 20–30% bovine albumin solution.

The serological investigations performed before blood transfusion usually consist of the following:

(1)    blood grouping,
(2)    antibody determination,
(3)    compatibility testing.

Routine blood grouping includes antigen determination within the ABO and Rh systems.

---

* LISS: 180 ml *solution 1*, +20 ml *solution 2*, +800 ml *solution 3*, pH 6.7 μ 0.03. *Solution 1:* NaCl 0.17 M; *solution 2:* phosphate buffer 0.15 M, pH 6.7; *solution 3:* 0.3 M glycine to pH 6.7 with 0.1 M NaOH.

## ABO grouping

ABO grouping includes

(1)  analysis of the erythrocytes with anti-B and anti-A test sera, in certain cases with AB serum,
(2)  analysis of the serum with known red cells, usually $A_1$, $A_2$ and B.

The two analyses should always be performed when possible. If whole blood cannot be obtained two tests on the cell suspension should be made instead, using known test sera. The test sera should, if possible, be from different batches in these two tests. This latter technology must be used in blood grouping of newborn and young infants, since ABO antibodies are not present in sufficient titres until after the age of one.

Manufacturers of anti-B and anti-A test sera obtain these from individuals with high levels of the actual antibodies. Monoclonal antibodies from mice have shown a high quality and are increasingly being used as ABO test sera.

Test sera can be stained to avoid confusion: Anti-B yellow, anti-A blue or green and AB serum red. Test erythrocytes of $A_1$-, $A_2$- and B-type are obtained from individuals with these subtypes.

For blood grouping red cells and serum are separated and a red blood cell suspension is made. The red cells are washed by suspension in 0.9% saline, followed by centrifugation and preparation of a 3–5% suspension in saline. The red cell suspensions from the individual to be blood grouped and from test erythrocyte donors are prepared similarly. *Tables A1.1* and *A1.2* show the principle for ABO grouping and give the results of the examination of the four ABO groups with test sera and test cells. The investigation can, in practice, be performed so that equal parts (e.g. one drop) of serum and erythrocytes are mixed on a glass slide, on a special test plate, or in a test tube. The reaction takes longer if it is performed in a tube (60 minutes), than on a test plate (20 minutes), or on a glass slide (5 minutes). The reaction in the test tube can be enhanced by brief centrifugation at low speed. ABO grouping is performed at room temperature and reading is done macroscopically. Weak or doubtful reactions must be controlled in the microscope.

**TABLE A1.1. Investigation of erythrocytes**

| Sample no. | Anti-B | Anti-A | AB serum | Result |
|---|---|---|---|---|
| 1 | − | + |  | A |
| 2 | + | − |  | B |
| 3 | − | − |  | O |
| 4 | + | + | −[a] | AB |

[a] Motivated on p. 259

**TABLE A1.2. Investigation of sera**

| Sample no. | $A_1$-erythrocytes | $A_2$-erythrocytes | B-erythrocytes | Results |
|---|---|---|---|---|
| 1 | − | − | + | A |
| 2 | + | + | − | B |
| 3 | + | + | + | O |
| 4 | − | − | − | AB |

**Rh grouping**

Test sera for Rh grouping (D grouping) can be obtained from individuals immunized by transfusion or pregnancy. Most laboratories routinely use IgG antibodies and only in special circumstances are the rarely found IgM antibodies used as test serum.

The methods for Rh grouping commonly used are:

(1)  tube method with 3% erythrocyte suspension in physiological saline;
(2)  'rapid slide' method, using a heavy suspension on a glass slide with the addition of physiological saline.

The first method is better than the rapid slide technique for large numbers of samples, but cannot be read without centrifugation for at least $1\frac{1}{2}$–2 hours. For this reason the rapid slide method is mostly used for urgent tests since reading can be done after 2 minutes.

*Test-tube method*

Either IgM or IgG antibodies can be used for this method. The one-step enzyme method with papain is often applied. Immediately before use a 1% solution of papain* is mixed with IgG anti-D. The serum enzyme solution is then employed as test serum. The ready-made enzyme serum solution can be used during the day it is prepared, but has to be kept frozen. It is suitable always to include a known D-positive and a known D-negative blood sample as controls.

For the tube method small microtest-tubes of glass or plastic, about $0.6 \times 7$ cm are used with 0.01–0.02 ml test serum containing IgM or IgG antibodies together with papain as mentioned above, added with a special Pasteur pipette. The same amount of a 3% suspension in 0.9% saline of the erythrocytes to be investigated is also added and the content is mixed. The pipette is carefully washed between every sample. The tubes are incubated at 37°C for $1\frac{1}{2}$–2 hours.

Reading of the sediment can first be made macroscopically. A positive reaction gives a tough sediment, somewhat wrinkled with an irregular contour. A negative reaction gives a homogeneous sediment, sharply delineated and less spread, but easily floating out. The final reading should always be made microscopically by carefully sucking up the sediment in a Pasteur pipette, putting it on a microscope slide.

*'Rapid slide' method*

A large drop of carefully tested IgG anti-D serum is put on a labelled microscopic slide on a lightbox which keeps the glass at about 37 °C. At the other end of the same glass slide is put one drop of control serum, which is not the anti-D serum but only the special sera and substances used to dilute the serum for the rapid slide test (albumin, dextran, AB serum). The same volume of a 50% erythrocyte suspension is added. The red blood cells are suspended in their own serum or plasma, saline may not be used. The sample is mixed with a glass rod giving the fluid a diameter of about 2 cm. The sample is rocked a few times and this is repeated four to five times per minute. The final reading is made macroscopically after 2 minutes.

Rh-negative (D-negative) erythrocytes are not agglutinated but the suspension can have a fine granular appearance, especially if the investigated blood has a high sedimentation rate. The control serum must always give a negative reaction. If

* Papain: 1 g papain (papain soluble 1:350 Merck) + 0.485 g cysteine hydrochloride to 100 ml in 1/15 M phosphate buffer.

agglutination appears in the control serum, the sample must be further analysed.

Blood from certain individuals occasionally gives a very weak positive reaction with the saline/papain method. These individuals can be shown to belong to the Rh group $D^u$. $D^u$ designates a patient who has the D antigen in lower amounts than normal D-positive individuals. $D^u$ erythrocytes can therefore react positively with certain anti-D sera and negatively with others. For this reason persons belonging to the $D^u$ group can occasionally be reported as D-negative. To definitely secure the Rh-positivity an antiglobulin test is recommended.

Those individuals whose erythrocytes are not agglutinated by anti-D serum can as recipients of blood transfusions be regarded as Rh-negative. If the typing concerns a blood donor, the erythrocytes ought to be investigated with anti-C and anti-E according to the recommendations of the World Health Organization (WHO) for typing of blood donors. If a positive result is obtained on testing with anti-C and/or anti-E, but negative results on testing with anti-D, the donors are regarded as Rh-negatives when given blood transfusions or when pregnant, while they are seen as Rh-positive when being blood donors.

### Antibody investigation

Before a planned blood transfusion it is necessary to know well in advance if a patient has irregular antibodies which may limit the possibilities of obtaining sufficiently compatible blood. Therefore an antibody analysis is performed. The principle is to use test red cells with known antigens and to search for antibodies against them in the patient's serum. The test cells should be selected so that they contain as many different blood group antigens as possible. Depending on which antigens the test erythrocytes carry and which antibodies one needs to look for, the number of different test erythrocytes must be determined. For antibody investigation the previously mentioned methods (p. 253) are utilized to obtain agglutination with IgM and IgG antibodies.

### Compatibility testing (cross-matching)

Before each blood transfusion, compatibility testing should be performed in addition to blood typing and possibly antigen investigation. Compatibility tests in physiological saline were previously often the routine. They could prevent the severe transfusion reactions caused by ABO incompatibility, but antibodies within other blood group systems could not always be detected with these methods.

As a result a few cases of blood transfusion reactions of a haemolytic type could occur in spite of no incompatibility found by the test in saline. Therefore compatibility testing should be performed to discover incompatibility due to IgG antibodies, using for instance the indirect antiglobulin test. This is especially important if the recipient previously has been transfused, has had injections of blood, or has been pregnant. Patients with haemolytic anaemia belong to this risk group, as do patients from which no history of transfusion can be obtained, for example because of unconsciousness.

*Compatibility testing of red cells in saline at room temperature*

The patient's serum, undiluted or diluted 1/5, is mixed with equal parts of a 3% red cell suspension. The 1/5 dilution is used to avoid immune haemolysis being erroneously interpreted as a negative reaction. The patient's serum is used as a control, undiluted as well as diluted 1/5, against a suspension of the patient's own erythrocytes. The reading is always microscopical after 10 minutes on a glass slide, after 20 minutes on a plate, or one hour in a test-tube without centrifugation. In urgent cases the sample can be read almost directly after centrifugation. No agglutination whatsoever may appear in diluted or undiluted serum. Not even very strong aggregation due to rouleaux formation appears in the serum dilution 1/5. If the compatibility test shows agglutination the first measure is to repeat the ABO typing of the donor as well as the recipient.

*Compatibility testing with indirect antiglobulin test (Coombs' test)*

In the indirect antiglobulin test equal parts (at least 0.2 ml) of serum are incubated with a 5% erythrocyte suspension in physiological saline, or in a solution with lower ionic strength (LISS). After washing in saline three to four times, the antiglobulin serum is added to the test-tube and the sample is read after short centrifugation. The erythrocytes and reagents can also be mixed on a microscope slide. Reading is then done after 10 minutes at room temperature, usually microscopically. Positive sensitized and negative control erythrocytes should also be included in the antiglobulin test.

**Sources of error in blood group serological tests**

The most common errors in blood group tests are made on sampling and registration. The rules to follow to avoid such errors have been reviewed above.

In addition to these errors problems can appear due to technical or biological variations. The problem consists of either an unexpected negative or an unexpected positive reaction.

*Causes of unexpected negative reactions*

(1)  Test serum not added.
(2)  Weakened test serum.
(3)  Erroneous methodology, e.g. wrong reaction time, incorrect reaction milieu.
(4)  Surplus of antigen through the use of too strong a suspension of erythrocytes, which absorbs out the antibodies, but does not result in agglutination.
(5)  Using too old or improperly kept cells, the blood group antigens can be weakened or destroyed. An example of such a sensitive antigenic structure is the Kell antigen.
(6)  Haemolysis can occur if complement-binding antibodies are permitted to react with active complement. The lack of agglutination can be erroneously interpreted as a negative reaction. Anti-A, or anti-B, anti-Le$^a$ and anti-Jk$^a$ are examples of complement-binding antibodies. Agglutination is then obtained after heat activation of the serum complement.
(7)  Surplus of antibodies can bind most of the antigen determinants and a weakened agglutination, possibly total lack of agglutination, may result from the prozone phenomenon (cf. chapter 4). In this situation the antiglobulin test becomes positive.
(8)  ABO antibodies may be absent in the investigated sample. Neonates usually lack A and B agglutinins. In older individuals and in certain diseases, e.g. hypogamma-globulinaemia, they may have very low titres or be totally deficient. In such cases the ABO group is checked by repeated typing of the patient's erythrocytes with test serum.

*Causes of unexpected positive reactions*

(1)  Pseudo-agglutination due to rouleaux formation may occur in patients with high sedimentation rates, hypergammaglobulinaemia, or after infusions of dextran. The characteristic appearance of red cell rouleaux is easily recognized. If serum is diluted with physiological saline they vanish or are weakened, but real agglutinates persist.

(2)  Coagulated plasma containing red blood cells can appear in serum due to delayed coagulation. This can usually be differentiated from agglutination microscopically. The addition of thrombin to such a sample can enhance the coagulation.

(3)  Panagglutinable red blood cells due to an infected blood sample (Tomsen phenomenon). Such red cells are agglutinated by old sera. Serum from an AB individual can be used as a control serum (*Table A1.1*) in ABO typing and can differentiate blood group AB cells giving a negative reaction from panagglutinable cells which give a positive reaction.

(4)  Irregular specific antibodies, such as anti-$P_1$, anti-M, anti-N, anti-Le$^a$, etc., as well as non-specific cold-agglutinins (anti-I) of IgM-type. They have a temperature optimum at $4\,°C$ but also often react at room temperature. If the agglutination is totally absent at $37\,°C$ the antibodies are probably without clinical significance.

(5)  In an individual who is A or AB, the serum can react with A blood cells. This may be due to the fact that an $A_2$ or $A_2B$ individual has an anti-$A_1$ in the serum, or an $A_1B$ individual has an anti-H. The cells of such individuals should be subtyped for $A_1$ and $A_2$ and their sera should be tested against $A_1$-, $A_2$- and O-cells, preferably at the temperature optimum of $4\,°C$.

The unexpected negative and positive results described above can often be directly explained if adequate controls have been included in the testing. Positive as well as negative control serum and control red cells are essential and should not be omitted. Each case of significant transfusion reaction should be clarified. Blood samples from the donor as well as the recipient should be taken before each blood transfusion and kept in the refrigerator to be available for investigation after a reaction. A sample taken after transfusion can be difficult to evaluate serologically due to the added donor blood.

## Bibliography


DUNSFORD, J. and BOWLY, C. C. (1967). *Techniques in Blood Grouping*. Oliver & Boyd, Edinburgh.

MOLLISON, P. L. (1979). *Blood Transfusion in Clinical Medicine*, Blackwell, Oxford.

MOORE, H. C. and SIPES, B. R. (1977). The effects of ionic strength on antibody uptake with special reference to the antiglobulin test. In Pollack, W., Mollison, P. L. and Reiss, A. M. (eds): *The Nature and Significance of Complement Activation*. The second international Symposium sponsored by the Ortho Research Institute of Medical Sciences, Raritan, New Jersey, USA.

# Immunological diagnosis of immunodeficiencies and immunological diseases

**Lars Å. Hanson and Renée Norberg**

This is a brief review of some diagnostic possibilities in the work up of patients with suspected immunodeficiencies, or immunological diseases. Explanations of abbreviations used and a bibliography can be found at the end of the appendix.

## Immunological investigations in cases of increased sensitivity to infections

First it is useful to decide whether or not the patient really has an increased frequency of infections. In an adult it is acceptable to have two to three upper respiratory tract infections per year and in children as many as six to seven. If the patient has more infections than seems normal his profession and living conditions should be analysed. Heavy smoking, or an unusual exposure to infectious agents may explain at least part of the problem.

The nature of the infections also gives useful information. An increased frequency of bacterial infections is primarily seen in patients with antibody and complement deficiency syndromes, as well as phagocyte deficiencies. Recurrent sinusitis and/or otitis media as complications to upper respiratory infections and the occurrence of repeated severe bacterial infections like sepsis, or meningitis makes it mandatory to search for deficiencies in host defence.

Deficiencies in cell-mediated immunity are often seen early on as severe candida infections and also as infections with other commensals like *Pneumocystis carinii*. In AIDS it is very obvious that the impaired host defence is followed by the appearance of infections with various commensals as in a compromised host.

### I Deficiencies in antibody-mediated immunity

*1. Quantitative: (A) Immunoglobulin determination*

*Method:* For IgG, IgA, IgM and IgD usually simple radial immunodiffusion (Mancini) or electroimmunoassay techniques are used (the 'rocket method' by Laurell), but automated densitometry is also employed. For IgE the radioimmunosorbent test (RIST, *Figure A2.1A*). As a solid phase paper with attached anti-IgE antibodies is now usually used. These bind IgE in the serum to be tested. This IgE is measured with radioactively labelled anti-IgE. The paper-RIST is called PRIST.

Immunosorbent  Serum sample  IgE labelled
particle with  with IgE  with $^{125}$I
attached IgE

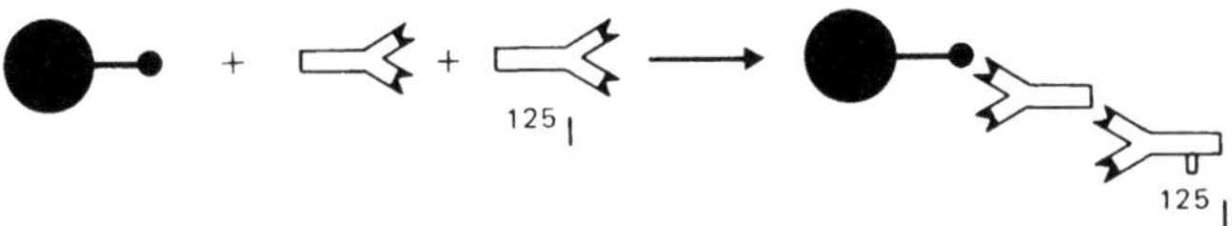

Immunosorbent  Serum sample  Anti-IgE
particle with  with reagins  labelled
attached allergen (IgE)  with $^{125}$I

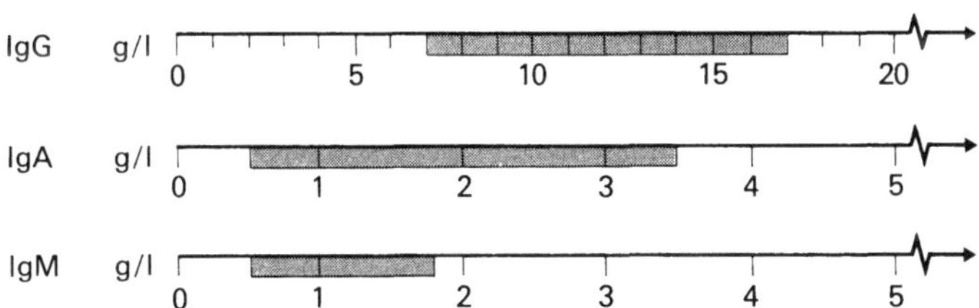

*Figure A2.1*  A. Radioimmunosorbent test (RIST) for quantitative determination of IgE. Anti-IgE attached to a solid phase reacts with IgE in a serum sample in competition with IgE labelled with $^{125}$I. The more IgE there is in the investigated serum sample, the more iodine labelled IgE can attach to the solid phase. B. Radioallergosorbent (RAST) for quantitative determination of reaginic IgE antibodies. The allergen is attached to a solid phase and reacts with the serum sample, binding the allergen specific reaginic antibodies in this serum. Since the reaginic antibodies are of the IgE class, they can be measured by addition of an iodine labelled anti-IgE. The more reaginic antibodies there are in the serum sample, the more radioactive anti-IgE will attach to the solid phase

*Figure A2.2* Normal levels for IgG, IgA and IgM in adults

*Evaluation:* Normal values vary with age: for IgG, IgA, IgM and IgD (*see Figure 2.7*, p. 29) WHO provides standards. Normal levels for adults are shown in *Figure A2.2*.

Normal levels of IgE in adults 13.2 kU/l ($\pm$ 2 s.d.: 1.53–114 kU/l) as related to a WHO standard. One international unit corresponds to about 2.5 ng.

An international standard for quantification of secretory IgA (11S) is still lacking. The use of serum IgA as standard (mainly 7S) gives much too low values for secretory IgA, especially with the Mancini technique. The presence of aggregates in the standard for serum IgG may also be a cause of error. An abnormal distribution of immunoglobulins within one immunoglobulin class, for instance redistribution between IgG subclasses or the appearance of a monoclonal component can give incorrect values. The standard is then no longer representative.

Selective deficiencies in single subclasses of IgG, e.g. IgG2, can easily be overlooked since serum IgG may be normal. Mean $\pm$ 2 s.d. for IgG1: $1.55 \pm 4.90$, IgG2: $3.80 \pm 3.00$, IgG3: $0.73 \pm 0.52$, IgG4: $0.55 \pm 1.26$, determined with Mancini or Laurell technique.

The method error for simple radial immunodiffusion is about 10%, for electro-immunoassay somewhat less.

### (B) Determination of B lymphocytes in blood

*Method:* Identification of the immunoglobulin receptors on B lymphocytes by means of immunofluorescence. Normal frequency is about 5% (1–9%) according to one study and $7 \pm 4$% according to another. Other surface structures such as Fc receptors, C3 receptors and DR antigens can also be used. The latter two can in addition be employed as maturation markers for B lymphocytes. Fc and C3 receptors are present on monocytes and certain T lymphocytes as well. The receptors for Epstein–Barr virus are only present on B lymphocytes.

*Evaluation:* Low frequency of B lymphocytes suggests antibody deficiency syndrome, but in some cases of common variable immunodeficiency there are increased numbers of immunoglobulin positive cells. In selective IgA deficiency there are IgA-containing B lymphocytes, apparently with a maturation inhibition. In certain forms of immunodeficiency maturation defects of B lymphocytes can be detected by the absence or presence of surface structures such as C3 receptors and DR antigens. Surface markers, as well as the presence of Ig in the lymphocyte cytoplasm can be used for classification of the immunodeficiency.

*2. Qualitative:* (*A*) *Demonstration of alloagglutinins* (anti-A and anti-B) *and antibodies* against various micro-organisms

(*B*) *Demonstration of antibody response* against various vaccines.

All live vaccines (BCG, live mumps and polio vaccines, as well as measles, rubella and yellow fever vaccines) should be avoided in patients with a possible immunodeficiency. Antibody determination before and after one to two weeks of one to two doses of inactivated polio vaccine, pneumococcus, typhoid vaccines, diphtheria or tetanus toxoid, etc. permits evaluation of the patient's capacity to produce antibodies.

(*C*) *Biopsy of lymph glands, intestine or bone marrow* can contribute to the diagnostic work up by demonstration of antibody-producing cells. A regional lymph gland should preferably be obtained a few days after the antigen stimulation. Bone marrow should normally contain 1–2% plasma cells, less before the age of three years. Intestinal biopsy can be easier to evaluate from this point of view.

## II   Deficiencies in cell-mediated immunity

*1. Quantitative:* (*A*) *Demonstration of lymphopenia* in peripheral blood, usually under $1$–$1.5 \times 10^9$ cells/l (1000–1500 cells/mm$^3$).

(*B*) *Determination of T lymphocytes* in the blood.

*Method:* T lymphocytes bind sheep red blood cells, forming rosettes of erythrocytes around the T lymphocytes. The normal value is about 50–85% of the lymphocytes in the blood according to one study, $66 \pm 11$% according to another.

T lymphocyte populations can now be characterized by means of monoclonal antisera. Pan T reagents show with blood lymphocytes normally $72 \pm 9$% with OKT3 and $72 \pm 7\%$ with Leu 1. T helper/T inducer cells show with OKT4 $43 \pm 10\%$ and with Leu 3 $45 \pm 10\%$. T suppressor/T cytotoxic cells show with OKT8 $21 \pm 7\%$ and with Leu 2 $28 \pm 8\%$. The ratio T helper/T suppressor cells is around 2 with a range of 1.2–2.2.

*2. Qualitative: (A) In vitro testing of T lymphocyte function*

*Method:* (a) *Lymphocyte stimulation* non-specifically with phytohaemagglutinin and other mitogens, or specifically with antigens (e.g. tuberculin or candida antigen). This mainly reflects T lymphocyte functions. Lymphocyte stimulation can either be demonstrated morphologically by blast cell transformation, or by measurement of $^3$H-thymidine incorporation in the cells (chapter 7).

*(b) Demonstration of responsiveness of T lymphocytes to allogeneic cells*

*Method:* MLC, mixed lymphocyte culture. The patient's lymphocytes are exposed to lymphocytes from a normal individual. The normal cells have been exposed to mitomycin to stop their capacity to react. If the patient's lymphocytes are stimulated by the antigens on the foreign cells, increased $^3$H-thymidine uptake can be measured.

*Evaluation:* Standardization of these methods is not yet uniform for various laboratories.

*(B)* In vivo *testing of T lymphocyte functions*

*Method:* Skin testing with certain recall antigens normally releases delayed-type hypersensitivity reactions. Suitable antigens for intradermal injections are tuberculin, candida, tetanus, diphtheria, proteus, streptococcus, trichophyton and mumps antigens. In special cases the skin can also be sensitized with dinitrochlorobenzene (DNCB). On renewed exposure a delayed-type hypersensitivity reaction is normally produced in the form of contact eczema.

*Evaluation:* Positive reactions with erythema and induration are easy to read. The eczema induced by DNCB can be more difficult to evaluate. While positive reactions indicate the presence of functioning T lymphocytes, their failure to occur does not necessarily show that there is a T cell deficiency. About 80% of Swedish adults react to tuberculin, *Candida*, *Streptococcus* and mumps antigens, but only about 20% to trichophyton. About 95% can normally be sensitized with DNCB, but the frequency of positive reactions decreases with increasing age, which is also true for the other antigens.

*(C) Analysis of lymphocytes in biopsies* of lymph glands, intestine, bone marrow, blood and thymus.

## III  Deficiencies in non-specific host defence

*1. Complement*
*Method:* Determination of total complement by induction of haemolysis with fresh serum. Determination of C1q, C3, C4 and possibly C5 with radioimmunodiffusion, or electroimmunoassay. C1 esterase inhibitor which is deficient in hereditary angio-oedema, can also be determined. There are simple screening tests to detect deficiencies in the classical and alternative pathway for complement activation. If abnormalities are found in these, extended analyses should be performed by special laboratories for the various single components of the complement system (cf. chapters 5 and 20).

*Evaluation:* Normal value for total complement depends on the method used. Normal values for Clq: 76–136%, C4; 72–171%.

*2. Phagocytosis:*

(A) *Quantitative: Demonstration of granulocytopenia, agranulocytosis.*
(B) *Qualitative: Demonstration of phagocyte dysfunction.*

*Method:* Nitroblue–tetrazolium (NBT) test reveals a phagocytosis defect in patients with chronic granulomatous disease. The phagocytes of such patients lack the capacity to reduce NBT to insoluble dark blue formazan.

Special laboratories can also test for other phagocytosis functions: chemotaxis, bacterial engulfment, bactericidal activity and various enzyme functions in granulocytes such as NADH oxidase, glucose-6-phosphate dehydrogenase, glutathione peroxidase and leucocyte myeloperoxidase. The presence of lactoferrin can also be determined.

*Evaluation:* There are quantitative NBT but they are laborious and for clinical use it is sufficient to have a simplified, rapid semiquantitative modification. Absent reduction of NBT is characteristic for chronic granulomatosis, but can also be caused by neutropenia or an outdated blood sample. By stimulation of the phagocytes in the sample with endotoxin or by uptake of bacteria or latex particles, an enhancement of the reaction in normal individuals is achieved. In patients with an ongoing bacterial infection, there is spontaneously a large number of reducing granulocytes, which give an increased precipitation of formazan in a non-stimulated sample.

The clinical value of the determination of other granulocyte functions seems to be relatively limited at the present time.

(C) *C-reactive protein* (CRP) can easily be determined and is a useful indicator of infections and inflammatory conditions, especially neonatally, where it can be used for quick detection of the presence of life-threatening bacterial infections such as sepsis and/or meningitis. Its probable role as a phagocytosis-stimulator makes it of special interest in individuals with an increased frequency of infections.

*Method:* Quantification of CRP is performed with single radial-immunodiffusion or electroimmunoassay.

Demonstration of CRP by commercial slide agglutination tests is crude and easy to misinterpret, but it is also fast. It is useful to verify the result with a quantitative method. The agglutination test can, by employing three dilutions of the serum, be made semiquantitative. If properly adjusted it can indicate whether the sample is most probably negative, being less than 10–20 mg/l, doubtfully positive being 20–40 mg/l, or definitely positive being more than 40 mg/l.

*Evaluation:* With sensitive techniques CRP can be demonstrated in low concentrations in blood of normal individuals (< 10 mg/l). There is a very rapid increase within hours often to high levels (50–200 mg/l) in the presence of bacterial infection. When the infection is eliminated CRP returns much faster to normal levels than several of the other acute phase parameters, especially the sedimentation rate. CRP is therefore a very practical diagnostic test for ascertaining the presence of acute bacterial infections and can be used to monitor antibiotic treatment. CRP also gives a better evaluation of the disease activity in rheumatoid arthritis than the sedimentation rate.

A number of other parameters of definite or probable significance for the host defence against infections are usually not tested routinely in most laboratories— interferon, lysozyme and lactoferrin—although methods are available. The capacity to develop various forms of inflammation and the functional capacity of macrophages is not easily investigated.

*Summary of work-up of patients with increased frequency of infections*

When history and clinical findings give reasons to suspect a deficiency in host defence, the work-up may be planned with a clinical immunologist. Several of the suggested procedures are laborious and expensive and should only be used restrictedly.

The following primary tests could be carried our:

(1) Determination of IgA, IgG and IgM in serum.
(2) Differential counts of leucocytes in peripheral blood with determination of total numbers of granulocytes and lymphocytes per volume.
(3) Skin testing with tuberculin.
(4) Determination of antibody titres (anti-A, anti-B antibodies against streptolysin, staphylolysin, antibodies against *E. coli*, *Haemophilus influenzae*, pneumococci, etc.)

If required the further work-up can include:

(1) Lymphocyte stimulation with mitogens and antigens, possibly MLC.
(2) Skin test with further antigens, e.g. candida, streptococcus, mumps and trichophyton antigens; DNCB in special cases.
(3) Quantification of T and B lymphocytes in peripheral blood. Characterization of lymphocytes with monoclonal antisera.
(4) Determination of the antibody response after vaccination.
(5) Determination of IgE in serum, and secretory IgA in saliva.
(6) Lymph gland biopsy, possibly thymus and gut biopsy.
(7) Screening for deficiencies in the classic or alternative pathway of the complement system.
(8) Bone marrow investigation.
(9) NBT test and other phagocyte function tests.
(10) Possibly determination of lactoferrin and myeloperoxidase in granulocytes and capacity to produce interferon.
(11) CRP determination.


## Immunological investigation of allergic diseases and immune complex diseases

### I  Type 1—immediate type hypersensitivity reactions, atopic allergies

A careful history should always be the basis of the diagnosis. If the history is insufficient, the allergens suspected on the basis of the history are verified by

(1) In vitro *methods:* skins tests (possibly followed by provocation test).
(2) In vitro *methods:* Determination of IgE antibodies against the suspected allergens.

The diagnostic methods are based on the components that participate in the immediate type hypersensitivity reaction, allergen; IgE antibodies and the biologically active mediators.

*1. In vivo methods*

(*A*) *Skin testing.* The patient is exposed to the allergens that are believed to be the cause of his symptoms. This is usually performed as a prick test. A thin needle penetrates the epidermis through a drop of the allergen solution applied on the skin. If the patient is hypersensitive to this allergen, there is a weal and flare reaction within about 15 minutes.

(*B*) *Provocation* of the patient using the suspected allergen is made either by dropping the diluted allergen onto the mucous membranes of the eyes or nose, or by letting the patient inhale the allergen as an aerosol. Characteristic atopic symptoms appear in the hypersensitive patient within some 15 minutes. Symptoms appear in the form of conjunctivitis, obstruction of the nose and dyspnoea. Objective registration after bronchial provocation can be made by auscultation and determination of PEF (peak expiratory flow) or $FEV_1$ (forced expiratory volume in one second).

*Evaluation:* A positive skin test is not definite proof that the individual is allergic to the antigen used, although strong positive skin reactions primarily occur in those who have atopic symptoms from exposure to that allergen. If the skin testing and the typical history cannot define the role of an allergen, a provocation test can be used to verify the patient's problem. It should be observed that skin testing as well as provocation can cause transient allergic symptoms and even anaphylactic shock if one is not careful in using a sufficiently high dilution of the allergen in patients who may be very sensitive to that allergen. The risk with prick testing is much less than with intracutaneous testing. A negative test does not exclude an atopic allergy, especially not allergy to food.


*2. In vitro methods*

(*A*) *Quantification of IgE* with the radioimmunosorbent test (RIST or PRIST, *Figure A2.1A*).

(*B*) *Demonstration of specific reagins with the radioallergosorbent test* (*RAST*). With this method it is possible to quantify reaginic antibodies in a patient's serum which has been added to an allergen attached to a solid phase. The patient's IgE antibodies binding to the allergen are measured with a radioactively labelled anti-IgE (*Figure A2.1B*).

(*C*) *Demonstration of eosinophilia* in serum and secretion.

*Evaluation:* Quantification of IgE can be of use in cases of suspected atopic reactivity, where history and normal diagnostic work-up do not result in a clear diagnosis. However, it should be mentioned that IgE is clearly increased in about 60–70% of patients with allergic asthma, hay fever and atopic eczema. In patients with single attacks of urticaria there are often increased levels of IgE. Increased serum IgE is also seen in patients with helminthic infections and certain rare forms of immuno-deficiencies (Wiskott–Aldrich's syndrome and the hyper-IgE syndrome with eczema and recurrent infections).

Demonstrations of specific reagins *in vitro* with RAST has the same diagnostic value as the skin test, but can be more convenient—and more expensive. A typical history may be sufficient for diagnosis, although skin testing may be required as well. RAST can be used for verification.

It is true for specific *in vivo* and *in vitro* diagnosis of atopic allergies that it is no better than the quality of the allergen preparations used. It is important to use well characterized and standardized allergens, such preparations are now becoming available.

## II  Type 2—cytolytic or cytotoxic reactions

*Method:* In haemolytic anaemia caused, for instance by penicillin allergy antibodies mainly reacting with the penicilloyl group, can be demonstrated with an indirect haemagglutination technique. The Coomb's direct reaction can also be utilized.

*Evaluation:* Increased titres together with a typical history give a good basis for the diagnosis.

## III  Type 3—immune complex induced reactions

The aim is to demonstrate the antibodies, mainly IgG, which release these reactions, or to demonstrate deposits in tissues of the complexes in the form of antigen, antibody and/or complement factors, alternatively demonstration of circulating immune complexes.

*Method:*
(1) *In vivo:* Injection in the skin of the antigen may induce an Arthus' reaction (chapter 19).
(2) *In vitro:* Demonstration of IgG antibodies participating in immune complex reactions is often made with double immunodiffusion technique. Examples of precipitating antibodies which can be demonstrated and the antigens used, are given in chapter 19. More sensitive techniques, including radioimmunoassays, are being applied.
With immunofluorescence technique antigen and antibody, as well as complement factors may be demonstrated in tissues where immune complexes are deposited.

*Evaluation:* The Arthus' reaction occurs but cannot on its own be used as evidence of the presence of an immune complex induced disease. Precipitins in serum against for instance serum proteins from pigeons, or budgerigars in patients with a characteristic history of lung symptoms after exposure to these animals is diagnostically very helpful. On suspicion of allergic alveolitis one can look for precipitins against, e.g. *Cladosporium, Alternaria, Penicillium, Botrytis* and *Micropolyspora faeni.* Precipitating antibodies are seen in more than 90–95% of the cases, but are also seen in about 30% of healthy individuals. Higher titres of antibodies usually relate to the presence of symptoms. There are no quantitiative antibody determinations available of proven diagnostic value.

Particularly in patients with nephritis immunofluorescence studies of biopsies can be of great use.

*Demonstration of circulating antigen–antibody complexes*

*Method:* The most commonly used methods utilize the biological activity of the immune complexes to activate complement, to bind IgM rheumatoid factor (RF) and to react with receptors on cells.

*Anti-complement reactivity,* i.e. the spontaneous reaction of serum with the haemolytic system in a classic complement binding reaction can indicate the presence of soluble immune complexes. The reaction is quite non-specific, since a number of other substances can interfere with the complement reaction and give false positive results.

Several methods utilize the *reaction between immune complexes and C1q.* The usefulness of the methods is limited to those complexes which can bind complement *in vitro.*

Antigen–antibody complexes which already have bound C1q *in vivo* often give negative reactions, even if the binding of C1q seems to be reversible so that endogenously bound C1q can be exchanged for the C1q used in the test. With the C1q methods immune complexes of smaller sizes are not found, since C1q primarily reacts with immune complexes with a sedimentation coefficient of $\geqslant 19S$. The patient's serum may also contain substances, such as DNA and bacterial products which react with C1q causing erroneous positive results with the C1q techniques.

A number of different C1q methods have been developed. Most suitable from a diagnostic point of view are the methods in which the amount of immunoglobulin bound to C1q can be determined in RIA or ELISA. The C1q should be very pure, isolated from human serum and adsorbed to a solid phase. The C1q methods are usually sensitive and permit simultaneous analysis of large numbers of sera.

The reaction of *monoclonal IgM RF* with immune complexes containing IgG is a technique which so far has had little application. This is especially due to the fact that it is difficult to find suitable IgM RF. The method has shown great sensitivity, good reproducibility and relatively few false positive reactions.

In *conglutinin tests* the affinity of conglutinins (a bovine serum protein reacting with complement) to immune complexes that contain inactivated C3 fragment are exploited. The tests only reveal C3 binding complexes. The conglutinin, adsorbed to a solid phase, binds the complexes and the amount of immunoglobulin in the complexes is measured in RIA or ELISA.

*Reaction between receptors on cells and immune complexes*

Lymphoid cells from a cell line called 'Raji' with receptors for Fc, as well as C3b and C1q have been utilized. The Raji cell test is technically more complicated than other immune complex tests. The results agree well with those obtained in C1q tests.

In *thrombocyte aggregation tests*, thrombocytes from normal blood donors are used. The method only detects IgG complexes with a molecular weight above one million. The reaction is inhibited by IgM RF, but not by C1q. The test is sensitive but technically difficult. It is also quite expensive since large volumes of fresh blood are required for the preparation of thrombocytes. False positive reactions, due to the presence in the patient's serum of thrombocyte antibodies and other thrombocyte aggregating factors are common.

*Evaluation:* There is no method available for the determination of all kinds of circulating immune complexes. It is usually necessary to analyse serum from a patient by several different methods. For all methods in practical use it is correct to say that positive results give only indirect evidence for the presence of antigen–antibody complexes and immune complex diseases.

IgG aggregates appearing after improper treatment of serum, for instance heating to 56 °C for inactivation of the complement, or repeated freezing and thawing give positive results in all tests. There can also be other components in the serum which may induce false positive results.

## IV  Type 4—delayed type hypersensitivity reactions

*Method:*

(1)  *In vivo:* Contact test (epicutaneous test) on the skin can be used for a number of substances.

(2)  *In vitro:* Demonstration of T lymphocyte reactivity *in vitro* against the antigens nickel, cobalt and chromium holds promise for clinical use.

*Evaluation:* The characteristic delayed-type hypersensitivity reaction resulting from a contact test is usually easy to read and together with a careful history is a useful but not decisive diagnostic aid in cases of contact dermatitis. The experience with *in vitro* tests in this connection is limited.

## Immunological investigation of autoimmune diseases

### Connective tissue disease

*Antinuclear antibodies (ANA)*

*Method:* Determination of *antibodies against cell nuclei*—often incorrectly called antinuclear factors (ANF)—is the most commonly used immunological test. Screen for ANA by immunofluorescence (IF) techniques is usually performed with tissue from suitable animals such as rats or guinea pigs as the antigen.

In principle any tissue can be used, but usually parenchymatous organs such as liver or kidneys are employed. Various nuclear antibodies give different fluorescence patterns, mainly of three types: homogeneous, granular or nucleolar. To further investigate the specificity of the antibodies, various purified antigens must be employed (*Table A2.1*). In the LE cell test only antibodies against DNA histone are detected. This investigation does not give any information beyond that of the IF method.

*Evaluation:* Nuclear antibodies can be demonstrated in almost all patients with SLE. They also occur in many other conditions, especially other connective tissue diseases such as Sjögren's syndrome, systemic sclerosis, RA, juvenile RA (where the frequency is approximately 40%), chronic active hepatitis, etc., but also in many acute infectious diseases and in connection with some drugs. The frequency of nuclear antibodies in healthy controls increases with advancing age, especially in women.

Antibodies against *native, double stranded (ds) DNA* can be demonstrated almost exclusively in cases of SLE. Several different methods can be used, including immunofluorescence with the trypanosoma *Crithidia luciliae* as the source of DNA. Radioimmunological techniques, for instance the Farr test, can also be employed (*Table A2.1*).

Antibodies against *single stranded (ss) DNA* cannot be demonstrated in tissue sections. The determination must be performed after denaturation of DNA. The presence of antibodies against ssDNA is considered to be of no diagnostic use. A few cases of SLE have been described, however, where these were the only detectable autoantibodies.

Antibodies against *DNA protein* (DNA histone) are the most commonly found nuclear antibodies and are seen alone or together with other nuclear antibodies in a number of conditions. DNA histone is also usually the antigen, which coupled to latex particles is employed in commercial screening tests.

Antibodies against *histone* can be found in RA as well as in SLE and especially in drug-induced SLE where histone antibodies can be the only demonstrable antinuclear antibodies. Nuclear antibodies appear in 80–90% of all cases treated with procainamide or hydralazine during a long period of time (>three months). The frequency of SLE symptoms is considerably lower.

Antibodies against *RNAase sensitive extractable nuclear antigen* (nRNP) are found in SLE and systemic sclerosis, but are considered to be of diagnostic importance

**Table A2.1. Nuclear antibodies in connective tissue disease**

| Antigen | Type of nuclear fluorescence in tissue sections | Method of determination | Are found in | | | | | |
| --- | --- | --- | --- | --- | --- | --- | --- | --- |
| | | | SLE | MCTD | SC | SS | RA | CAH |
| Double-stranded DNA | Homogeneous | IF-*Chrithidia luciliae*; RIA | + | | | | | (+) |
| Single-stranded DNA | Negative | RIA | + | | + | + | + | + |
| Nucleoprotein (DNA histone) | Homogeneous | IF; LE-cells | + | | + | + | + | + |
| Histone | Homogeneous | IF; ID | +(drug induced) | | | + | + | |
| RNA protein, nRNP | Granular | IF; HA; ID | + | +++ | + | + | (+) | |
| RNA protein, Sm | Granular | IF; HA; ID | +(in 20–40%) | | | | | |
| Nucleolus | Nucleolar | IF | + | | + | + | | + |
| SS-A, Ro | Mostly negative | ID | + | | | + | | |
| SS-B, La | Granular | ID | + | | | | + | |
| Scl-70 | Granular | ID | | | +(only in approx 20%) | | | |
| Centromere | Negative | IF, cell in tissue culture | | | +(in so-called CREST-syndrome) | | | |
| Rheumatoid arthritis protein=RAP=RANA | Negative | IF, EBV infected lymphocytes; ID | | | | | +(also in other diseases and in healthy individuals) | |

IF = immunofluorescence technique, RIA = radioimmunological technique, ID = immunodiffusion, HA = haemagglutination, EBV = Epstein–Barr virus, SLE = systemic lupus erythematosus, MCTD = mixed connective tissue disease, SC = systemic sclerosis, SS = Sjögren's syndrome, RA = rheumatoid arthritis, CAH = chronic active hepatitis, CREST = Calcinosis–Raynaud phenomenon–oesophagus dysmotility–sclerodactylia–telangiectasia.

primarily in socalled mixed connective tissue disease (MCTD). This is a clinical syndrome characterized primarily by a very mixed flora of symptoms and the diagnosis must not only be based on the finding of antibodies.

Antibodies against the *Sm antigen* (the antigen is named after the patient in which the antibodies were first demonstrated) are believed to appear only in SLE. The frequency of positive cases is relatively low (20–30%). In serum from patients with Sjögren's syndrome (SS) there are often specific nuclear antibodies, *SS-A* and *SS-B*, which react with incompletely characterized RNA proteins. SS-A and/or SS-B antibodies are considered to appear in 60–70% of all patients with Sjögren's syndrome. The frequency is lower in other rheumatic diseases. Determination of SS-A and SS-B antibodies seems to be of diagnostic value mainly in the cases where the symptoms of Sjögren's syndrome are less obvious.

In RF-positive as well as RF-negative rheumatoid arthritis more than 90% of the patients have antibodies reacting with nuclear antigen from Epstein–Barr virus (EBV)-infected lymphoid cells. These antibodies *RAP* (rheumatoid arthritis precipitins) or *RANA* (rheumatoid arthritis nuclear antibodies) are also seen in normal individuals, but in lower titres. The determination of RAP is of no diagnostic use.

In systemic sclerosis there are antibodies giving granular nuclear fluorescence which react with an unknown antigen, called *Scl-1* or *Scl-70*. The antibodies are rare—the frequency is approximately 15%—but their presence is a strong support for a diagnosis of systemic sclerosis. In the socalled CREST syndrome, which is a more slowly progressing and less generalized variant of systemic sclerosis, there is an antibody reacting with *centromers* in chromosomes of cultured cells (Hep-2). The centromere antibodies are reported to appear in at least half of all CREST patients and in single cases of systemic sclerosis.

In polymyositis antibodies directed against soluble cellular constituents are detected by immunodiffusion in about 60% of the cases; the commonest of these, found in 25% of the patients, are antibodies to the socalled *Jo-1 antigen*.

Antibodies against *nucleoli* can be seen in all connective tissue diseases, especially in Sjögren's syndrome and systemic sclerosis, as well as in active hepatitis. It is of the same diagnostic use as nuclear antibodies in general.

*Determination of antibodies against cardiolipin*

*Method:* RIA or ELISA (Enzyme Linked Immunosorbent Assay) techniques.

*Evaluation:* Positive outcome in a substantial number of SLE patients, especially in those with thromboembolic manifestations.

*Determination of the 'lupus anticoagulant'*

*Method:* The capacity of test immunoglobulin to inhibit *in vitro* the kaolin clotting time of normal plasma. The antibodies react with negatively charged phospholipids.

*Evaluation:* The proportion of SLE patients with circulating lupus anticoagulant is unknown. The presence of lupus anticoagulant is correlated with increased frequency of thrombotic episodes and with repeated abortions.

*Determination of rheumatoid factor (RF)*

*Method:* Screening to detect RF can be made with one of the commercial RF tests based on the reaction between RF and aggregated IgG on a carrier such as latex particles. Positive reactions should be controlled with indirect haemagglutination techniques or in an ELISA or DIG ELISA modification. With the latter methods it is also possible to distinguish between RF of the IgM-, IgA- and IgG-classes if false positive reactions due to RF binding to the Fc part of the enzyme-conjugated anti-Ig antibodies are avoided. This can be done using the F(ab)2 of the defective antibodies.

*Evaluation:* Positive outcome in 85% of RA. There are often positive findings in other diseases of immunological origin. The determination of immunoglobulin class-specific rheumatoid factor agrees well with the test which are non-immunoglobulin class-specific and in addition it gives information about generalized symptoms, including vasculitis.

## Blood diseases

### Haemolytic anaemia

*Method:* Demonstration of *erythrocyte* antibodies with Coombs' direct and/or indirect test (*see* Appendix 1).
   *Comment:* Coomb's test can be positive even in cases without any sign of haemolysis.

### Pernicious anaemia

*Method:* Antibodies against *intrinsic factor* (*IF*) are demonstrated in RIA.
   *Evaluation:* IF antibodies can be demonstrated in almost all patients with pernicious anaemia. Determinations are technically difficult and do not add any further information for the diagnosis.

### Leucopenia and thrombocytopenia

*Method:* Antibodies reacting with *leucocytes*, or *thrombocytes* are demonstrable in IF or in agglutination tests.
   After isolation and homogenization of the patient's thrombocytes it has been possible to show immunoglobulin bound to the cells with an ELISA technique.
   For determination of cytotoxic antibodies against *lymphocytes* the serum is tested against a panel of B and T lymphocytes from different donors.

   *Evaluation:* The methods are still being evaluated and the results are not always of clinical relevance. Granulocytes, as well as thrombocytes have receptors for IgG Fc, which may result in positive agglutination reactions with sera containing IgG complexes of various kinds.

## Endocrine diseases

### Thyroid diseases

*Method:* Antibodies against *microsomal antigens* of thyroid cells can be demonstrated by IF with human thyrotoxic thyroid as antigen or by HA and complement binding reactions using thyroid microsomal antigens. *Thyroglobulin antibodies* are demonstrated in indirect haemagglutination (IHA), or ELISA against human thyroglobulin. *Thyroid-stimulating* antibodies (TSab) are demonstrated by measurement of the production of cyclic AMP from isolated human thyroid cell membranes in the presence of test antibodies or by showing the inhibition of test antibodies in the binding of $^{125}$I labelled thyroid stimulating hormone (TSH) to isolated membranes of thyroid cells.

*Evaluation:* Antibodies against cytoplasmic thyroid antigen are found in increasing frequency with age, especially in women. After 50 years of age thyroid antibodies in titres above 25 are not definitely pathological. Pathological titres are often seen in thyrotoxicosis, especially after treatment with $^{125}$I. In chronic thyroiditis there are often high titres against cytoplasmic thyroid antigens as well as thyroglobulin. The titres usually persist for over a year and then decrease. TSab can be demonstrated in almost all cases of thyrotoxicosis and indicates active disease.

### Addison's disease

*Method:* Antibodies against cells from the *adrenal cortex* can be demonstrated with IF with human adrenal tissue as the antigen.
*Evaluation:* 40–60% of patients with idiopathic disease have such antibodies. The frequency is highest in the early stages of the disease.

### Hypoparathyroidism–hypogonadism

*Method:* Antibodies can be demonstrated against the two organs using IF.
*Evaluation:* Antibodies are often found in early cases. The investigations are difficult to perform routinely due to the lack of human antigen.

### Diabetes mellitus

*Method:* Antibodies against the *islets of Langerhans* can be demonstrated with IF using human pancreas as the source of antigen.
*Evaluation:* Antibodies in low titres are found in high frequency at the onset of insulin-dependent diabetes. The findings are scientifically very interesting, but still lack clinical usefulness.

## Skin diseases

### Pemphigus vulgaris and pemphigoid

*Method:* Circulating antibodies are demonstrated by IF against *epithelium* from man or monkey. Direct IF is used on skin biopsies from patients with suspected disease.
*Evaluation:* Antibodies against the intracellular substance of the skin are demonstrable in all patients with pemphigus vulgaris, and against the basement membrane of the skin in all cases of pemphigoid.

### Dermatitis herpetiformis

*Method:* Direct IF on biopsies from affected skin.
*Evaluation:* The finding of IgA in the subepidermis supports the clinical diagnosis.

### Systemic lupus erythematosus (SLE) and discoid lupus erythematosus (DLE)

*Method:* Direct IF on biopsy from diseased and healthy skin.
*Evaluation:* In SLE there are often deposits of immunoglobulin and complement in healthy, as well as diseased skin, while in DLE there are changes only in diseased skin. Further diagnostic possibilities in SLE are listed under connective tissue diseases.

## Liver diseases

### Active chronic hepatitis

*Method:* Circulating antibodies against *smooth muscle* are routinely demonstrated by IF on rat tissue. Absorption with *actin* (purified from skeletal muscle) confirms the specificity.

*Evaluation:* Antibodies against actin are found in high titres ( > 100) in most cases of active chronic hepatitis (CAH). The titres show a certain relation to the course of the disease. Antibodies against smooth muscle, mostly of the IgM class, appear in low titres ( < 25) in about 5% of healthy controls and in a number of various conditions with or without clinically demonstrable liver engagement. Nuclear antibodies, usually in lower titres, are found in around half of the cases with active chronic hepatitis.

### Primary biliary cirrhosis

*Method:* Antibodies reacting with *mitochondria* are demonstrated by indirect IF.

*Evaluation:* Antibodies against mitochondria (AMA), type M2, are shown in almost all cases of primary biliary cirrhosis. The titres are usually high ( $^2$100). Lower titres of AMA evidently occur in single cases of other liver diseases (type M4) and in SLE, Sjögren's syndrome and systemic sclerosis (type M5). AMA type M5 can be differentiated from M2–M4 antibodies by their lack of reactivity with human gastric mucosa. Their presence is not related to any liver disease. M1 are rarely found, but occur in syphilis.

## Gastrointestinal diseases

### Atrophic gastritis

*Method:* Antibodies against *parietal cells* can be demonstrated by IF or by complement binding using mucosa from man, or mice as the antigen.

*Evaluation:* The investigation is of doubtful diagnostic value. Antibodies are often found without any clinically relevant symptoms and a negative finding can even be seen in patients with a definite diagnosis.

## Myasthenia gravis

*Method:* Antibodies against *acetylcholine receptors* are determined with RIA by measurement of the inhibition of the patient's antibodies on the binding of radio-actively labelled α-bungarotoxin to acetylcholine receptors prepared from human muscle.

*Evaluation:* The receptor antibodies are demonstrated in more than 90% of the patients. The specificity is high, but the titres show little relation to the clinical activity of the disease. These antibody determinations can only be performed in special laboratories.

## Bibliography

### Methods

*Single radial immunodiffusion*
MANCINI, G. *et al.* (1965). Immunochemical quantitation of antigens by single radial immunodiffusion. *Immunochemistry,* **2,** 235.

*Quantitative immunoelectrophoresis*
AXELSEN, N. H. (ed.)(1983). Handbook of immunoprecipitation in gel technique. *Scand. J. Immunology*, **17**, Suppl. 10.
*RIST*
WIDE, L. and PORATH, J. (1966). Radioimmunoassay of proteins with the use of Sephadex-coupled antibodies. *Biochim. Biophys. Acta*, **130**, 257.
*RAST*
WIDE, L. *et al.* (1967). Diagnosis of allergy with an *in vitro* test for allergen antibodies. *Lancet*, **II**, 1105.
*Skin testing of atopic allergies and standardization of allergens*
AAS, K., BACKMAN, A., BELIN, L. and WEEKE, B. (1978). Standardization of allergen extract with appropriate methods. The combined use of skin prick testing and radioallergosorbent test. *Allergy*, **33**, 130.
*Testing of contact dermatitis*
FISHER, A. A. (1967). *Contact Dermatitis*. Lea & Febiger, Philadelphia.
*Investigation of immunodeficiencies*
WHO Committee (1983). Primary immunodeficiency diseases. *Clin. Immunol. Immunopath.*, **28**, 450.
STIEHM, E. R. and FULGINITI, V. A. (eds) (1980). *Immunologic Disorders in Infants and Children* (2nd edn). Saunders, Philadelphia.
*General*
WEIR, D. M. (ed.) (1978). *Handbook of Experimental Immunology*. Blackwell, Oxford.
LACHMANN, P. J. and PETERS, D. K. (eds) (1982). *Clinical Aspects of Immunology*, vol. I–II, 4th edn, Blackwell Scientific Publications, Oxford.
TAN, ENG (1982). Autoantibodies to nuclear antigens. *Advances in Immunology*. Vol. 33, Ed. by Henry, G. Kunkel and Dixon, F. J. Academic Press, New York.
WILLIAMS, R. C. Jr. (1980). *Immune Complexes in Clinical Experimental Medicine*. Harvard University Press, Cambridge, USA and London, UK.
ZUBLER, R. H. and LAMBERT, P. H. (1977). In *Recent Advances in Clinical Immunology*. R. A. Thompson, (ed.). Churchill Livingstone, Edinburgh, London and New York.
*Normal levels and standardization*
BAZAREL, M. and HAMBURGER, R. N. (1972). Standardization and stability of immunoglobulin E (IgE). *J. Allergy Clin. Immunol.*, **49**, 189.
ROWE, D. S. *et al.* (1970). A research standard for human serum immunoglobulins IgG, IgA and IgM. *Bull. WHO*, **42**, 535.
ROSE, D. S. *et al.* (1970). A research standard for human serum immunoglobulin D. *Bull. WHO*, **43**, 607.
ROWE, D. S. *et al.* (1970). A research standard for human serum immunoglobulin E. *Bull. WHO*, **43**, 609.
ROWE, D. S. (1973). Concentration of serum immunoglobulins in healthy young adult males estimated by assay against the international reference preparation. *Lancet*, **II**, 1232.

# Glossary

**Lars Å. Hanson and Hans Wigzell**

**ADCC (antibody dependent cellular cytotoxicity)**   Antibodies against the target cells will be linked via Fc receptors to cytotoxic cells which destroy the target cells. *See also* K cells.

**Acquired immunity**   Immunity appearing in an individual who has developed an immune response after an infection or vaccination.

**Active immunization**   Giving antigen to an individual in such a way that he will develop an immune response against that immunogen (*see also* Vaccination).

**Adjuvant**   Substance which together with an antigen will increase the immune response against that antigen.

**Adoptive immunity**   Transfer of immunity from one individual to another using immunocompetent cells from the immunized donor. *See also* Passive immunity.

**Affinity**   The binding constant between the antigen binding site of an antibody and an isolated hapten or determinant present on an antigen.

**Agglutination**   A clumping of cells or particles upon reaction between antigens present on the cells or the particle (agglutinogens) and antibodies (agglutinins) directed against the former. Agglutination of red blood cells is called haemagglutination.

**Allergen**   An antigen which will give rise to the production of the special types of antibodies, reagins or IgE, which will fix to mast cells and basophil granulocytes, and which upon contact with the allergen will then give rise to a rapid hypersensitivity reaction.

**Allergy**   According to von Pirquet's original definition (1906) this means the changed capacity of the body to react against a renewed contact with the same antigen. It is still used by many in this original connotation and would then comprise all specific immune reactions. The most frequent use of the term nowadays, like in this book, is however to mean only certain hypersensitivity reactions provoked by immunological mechanisms such as atopic diseases, anaphylactic chock, drug allergies and contact allergies.

**Alloantigen**   An antigen the structure of which is determined by a gene locus which within the same species may exist in two or more allelic forms. When the substance is transferred from one individual to another lacking the same allele, this will give rise to an immune response. The term is derived from the Greek 'allos' = someone else. Previously used synonym for allogen is isoantigen. Serum proteins that exist in different forms are called allotypes. Such allotypes exist for instance among the immunoglobulins.

**Alloantibody**    Meaning antibody directed against alloantigen. Previously used synonym—isoantibody. Examples of alloantibodies are the alloglutinins, such as anti-A and anti-B directed against the blood group antigens A and B. Previously used synonym, isoagglutinin. *Allogen* means of foreign origin. Is used in transplantation immunology to denote material from genetically different individuals belonging to the same species. *Allograft* means transplant from genetically different individuals of the same species.

**Allograft rejection**    Rejection reaction against a transplant from genetically different individuals of the same species. The immune response of the recipient against histocompatibility antigens of the donor which are lacking in the recipient will cause this reaction.

**Alloimmunization**    Immunization of one individual with an alloantigen, i.e. an antigen of the same species but being a genetic variant which is lacking in the individual. Previously used synonym, isoimmunization. Examples: Rh immunization, ABO immunization.

**Allotype**    *See* Alloantigen.

**Anaphylatoxin**    Activation of complement will result in the creation of the fragments C3a and C5a which function as anaphylatoxins, i.e. they will induce anaphylaxis, a generalized hypersensitivity reaction of the rapid type. The symptom picture is called anaphylactic shock. Anaphylaxis was used already in 1902 by Richet to mean a generalized hypersensitivity reaction in dogs.

**Anamnestic immune response**    *See* Secondary immune response.

**Antigen**    Substance which is recognized by the organism by specific receptors on the surface of immunocompetent T and B lymphocytes and their soluble products. Upon reaction between antigen and receptors there will be either induction of immune response or of tolerance. The antigens have a stable conformation and are normally macromolecules. Antigenic features are called antigenicity and are frequently used to define the capacity to react with the effector mechanisms of the immune response. The ability to induce an immune response is called immunogenicity and that to induce tolerance tolerogenicity.

**Antigenic determinant**    The specific part of a structure of an antigen which will induce an immune response, i.e. will fit to the receptors on T and B lymphocytes and will also be able to react with the antibodies produced.

**Antibody**    After exposure to antigen specific cells (B lymphoblasts and plasma cells) will start to produce proteins at high rate, being of a characteristic structure, i.e. consist of peptide chains of two types, H and L chains. These proteins, antibodies, have areas (binding sites) which specifically fit to and can bind the antigen which has induced the production of that antibody. The circulating humoral antibodies constitute one of the two effector mechanisms of the immune response. Antibody active proteins are frequently called immunoglobulins (q.v.).

**Antiserum**    Serum which contains antibodies against a particular antigen. This frequently means serum from an immunized animal.

**Antitoxin**    Antibody against a toxin. This can be neutralized and detoxified by this antibody.

**Arthus' reaction**    A local inflammatory vasculitis induced by complement which has been activated by antigen–antibody complexes created by locally inoculated antigens reacting with precipitating antibodies. Chemotactic factors will then be generated and they will attract granulocytes which will contribute to the tissue damage.

**Association constant**    A reaction between antibody and hapten which comprises a measure of affinity.

**Atopy**   Allergic diseases caused by the immediate type of hypersensitivity reaction which will appear in individuals carrying a hereditary disposition. Examples: hay fever, urticaria, asthma.

**Autoantibody**   Antibodies directed against cell components (autoantigens).

**Autoantigen**   Substance made by the cells of the body against which the same body has started to react against in an immunological manner.

**Autoimmunity**   Condition in which the immune response will exist against antigens in the body's own tissues.

**Autologous**   Derived from the same individual.

**Avidity**   The total binding strength between all available binding sites of an antibody molecule and the corresponding determinants present on an antigen. Avidity and affinity have sometimes been used in a synonymous manner which is truly erroneous.

**B lymphocyte**   Lymphocytes using immunoglobulins as receptors for antigen in the cell surface. These cells can upon adequate stimulation produce and release antibodies with the same specificity as the receptor molecules. The cells may undergo differentiation to plasma cells.

**Bence-Jones' protein**   Free monoclonal light chains of immunoglobulin molecules.

**Binding site**   The part of the antibody molecule which will specifically bind antigen.

**Booster dose**   A repeated dose of antigen, e.g. a vaccine, which will induce a secondary immune response (q.v.).

**Cell-mediated immunity**   Immunity mediated by antigen-stimulated T lymphocytes which consist of one part of the two specific effector mechanisms of the immune response. An antigen non-specific cell-mediated immunity can also be mediated by, for instance, macrophages but is then frequently recruited by specific components from B cells or T cells.

**Clone**   Progenitor cells and their daughter cells express all the same genes normally and are thus identical. They belong to the same clone. If this is a B lymphocyte clone, they will normally produce identical antibodies, i.e. monoclonal antibodies.

**Complement**   A system of at least 11 serum components which can be activated upon the reaction between antigen and antibody. Upon activation complement can mediate a series of important biological functions such as lysis of bacteria and other cells, histamine release, chemotaxis and increase of phagocytosis which all will lead to inflammation. Complement can also be activated by an alternative pathway which does not require an antigen–antibody reaction.

**Cross-reaction**   Antibodies against an antigen A can react with other antigens if the latter has one or more determinants identical with the determinants present on the antigen A or carry one or more determinants which are structurally very similar to the determinants present on antigen A.

**Cytotoxic T lymphocytes**   A subpopulation of activated T lymphocytes which will kill target cells carrying surface antigens which fit antigen-specific receptors present on such T cells. This reaction does not require antibody molecules.

**Delayed type hypersensitivity reaction**   A hypersensitivity reaction which is caused by a reaction between the stimulated T cells and corresponding antigens. Upon injection of antigen in the skin there will appear after 12–48 hours a characteristic redness and induration. A typical example of this is the tuberculin reaction. This kind of reaction is also involved in the creation of allergic contact eczema.

**Epitope**   Has the same meaning as antigenic determinant.

**Fc receptor**   Immunoglobulin class specific receptor for the Fc-part of different immunoglobulin molecules. Will exist on the surface of cells of various types.

**Graft-versus-host reaction**   An immune response directed against the histocompatibility antigens of a host by inoculated immunocomponent cells which have been transferred into the individual from a foreign donor. The graft-versus-host reaction will frequently give rise to disease in the individual in whom it does occur. A shorter term is GVH.

**Haemagglutination**   *See* Agglutination.
**Hapten**   A low molecular weight substance which alone can react with the effector systems of the immune response (humoral antibodies). In order to be immunogenic, haptens need to be aggregated or to react with larger molecules.
**Heteroantigen**   Antigen from one species which upon transfer to an individual of another species, will give rise to an immune response. Synonymous with xenoantigen.
**Heterologous**   Derived from another species.
**Histocompatibility antigens**   Genetically determined cellular antigens which upon transplantation between genetically different individuals will cause an immune response. Such an immune response can cause a rejection and destruction of the transplant. These antigens are therefore also called transplantation antigens, e.g. the HLA system in man.
**Humoral immunity**   Immunity immediated by circulating humoral antibodies.
**Hybridoma technology**   Fusion between an antibody forming cell and a malignant myeloma cell will result in a continuously growing cell clone which can produce antibodies of a single specificity, i.e. monoclonal antibodies.
**Hypersensitivity reaction**   *See* Allergy as well as immediate and delayed-type hypersensitivity.

**Ia antigens**   Gene products in the mouse which are detectable by immunological reactions, for instance serology or MLC. Ia antigens belong to the socalled class II MHC antigens and are identical to the MHC linked IR gene products. Corresponding gene loci in man are HLA-D/DR, DC and SB.
**Idiotope**   An antigenic determinant of the variable part of an antibody which will separate this antibody from other antibodies.
**Idiotype**   The collective name for all idiotopes on one antibody molecule.
**Immediate-type hypersensitivity**   A reaction which is caused by the release of biologically active substances (leukotrienes, histamines, etc.) from mast cells or basophil granulocytes where IgE antibodies fixed to the surfaces of these cells have reacted with their specific antigen (allergen). Immediate type hypersensitivity reactions can be transferred from one individual to another with IgE antibody containing serum. Upon injection of allergen into the skin, the presence of IgE antibodies will result in a characteristic blister and redness at the site of inoculation within minutes. Immediate type hypersensitivity reactions are responsible for the symptoms of atopic diseases such as asthma, hay fever, etc.
**Immune antibodies**   Antibodies produced after antigen stimulation.
**Immune complex**   Complexes created by antigen–antibodies which, by complement activation in certain situations, can produce tissue damage (glomerulonephritis, vasculitis, etc. *See also* Arthus' reaction and serum sickness).

**Immune cytolysis**  Reaction caused by complement activated by antibodies which have reacted with antigens present on the surface of the cell. The cell will then rupture, i.e. become lysed. If the target is an erythrocyte, this is called haemolysis, and in the case of a bacteria; bacteriolysis. When the reaction is used to prove the presence of antibodies against nucleated cells it is called a cytotoxicity test.

**Immune defect**  Primary or secondary defect in one or both of the effector mechanisms of the immune response, i.e. in the antibody-mediated or cell-mediated immune reaction.

**Immune prophylaxis**  Prophylaxis of disease via active immunization (vaccination) or passive immunization (addition of immune serum and immunoglobulin).

**Immune reaction**  Specific reaction between antigen and antibody or antigen and T lymphocyte.

**Immune response**  The result of contact between antigen and immunocompetent cells. This contact will cause cell proliferation and differentiation among the immuno-competent cells. B cells will differentiate into plasma cells and produce humoral antibodies directed against antigen. T lymphocytes will become cytotoxic or in other ways aggressive towards the antigen and may, in addition, produce lymphokines which will non-specifically activate macrophages.

**Immunity**  Used to define the protection against infection which will appear after a previous infection caused by the same microbial organism or after vaccination. The term originally comes from the Latin, *muni*, which means exempt from common service.

**Immunocompetent cells**  Lymphoid cells which via specific receptors for antigen have the capacity to react against immunogens and then develop tolerance or immune response patterns.

**Immunogenicity**  The capacity of an antigen to induce immune response. The antigen will then function as an immunogen.

**Immunoglobulins**  Antibody-active proteins. The original definition gammaglobulin is still used in some clinical situations. Strictly speaking, gammaglobulin however only comprises molecules which have that electrophoretic mobility.

**Immunological diseases**  Collective term for diseases completely or partly caused by immunological reactions. Examples are allergic diseases, transfusion complications, alloimmunization, immune complex and autoimmune diseases.

**Immunological enhancement**  Specific prolongation of transplanted tissue in a foreign individual who has been immunized against tissue before or alternatively been treated with antiserum directed against the transplant. The phenomenon was originally observed in experiments with certain tumours in mice which could normally not grow in foreign mice strain but were able to do so if the recipient individual was preimmunized against the tumour tissue. Enhancement exists predominantly because of the existence of humoral antibodies directed against the transplant in the recipient individual.

**Immunological specificity**  Effector mechanisms in an immune response, that is humoral antibodies and antigen-specific T lymphocytes will normally only react with the antigen which has been used in its induction.

**Immunological tolerance**  Specific loss or capacity to react immunologically against a defined antigen. Tolerance can occur in a natural form or be acquired. Synonym: immune paralysis.

**Immunosuppression**  The term is normally used for non-specific suppression of the capacity of an individual to develop an immune response. This is normally achieved in the clinic via treatment with cytostatic drugs, corticosteroids, radiation, anti-lymphocyte serum or via the drainage of lymphocytes from ductus thoracicus.

Treatment of an individual with such agents to suppress the capacity to respond immunologically is called immunosuppressive therapy. Specific immunosuppression will also include immunological tolerance and immunological enhancement.

**Incomplete antibody**  Situations where antibodies react with for instance erythrocytes without causing any secondary manifestation of the antigen–antibody reaction such as agglutination or haemolysis. The term is not a suitable one as the antibodies are structurally and functionally complete but are unable to produce the ordinary secondary manifestations of the antigen–antibody reaction due to the localization and concentration of the surface antigens.

**Indirect agglutination**  Agglutination of particles with antibodies directed against antigens which have been brought to the surface of such particles. The term is synonymous with passive agglutination.

**IR genes**  Immune response genes. Defining genes the products of which will selectively influence the capacity of an individual to respond against a defined antigen. Many different IR genes exist with the most important being linked to either the MHC or Ig loci.

**Isoantibody**  *See* Alloantibody.

**Isoantigen**  *See* Alloantigen.

**Isoimmunization**  *See* Alloimmunization.

**Isotype**  An antigenic variant which exists in all individuals of the same species.

**K cells**  The term is used to define cells with the capacity to mediate antibody-dependent cell-mediated cytotoxicity. The cells carry in the cell membrane Fc-receptors for IgG in particular. Among cells with the K cell capacity are T lymphocytes, NK cells, monocytes and granulocytes. *See also* ADCC.

**Killer T cells**  T lymphocytes which, after a specific antigen stimulation, have developed cytotoxic capacity for target cells carrying the antigen on the surface.

**Langerhans cells**  Macrophage-like cells which create a network particularly in the skin. The human Langerhans cells carry HLA-D/DR antigens on the outer membrane and are able to bind antigen and present it to T lymphocytes in the skin.

**Lymphokines**  Substances released predominantly from T lymphocytes after reaction with the specific antigen. Lymphokines are biologically highly active and will cause chemotaxis and activation of macrophages and other cell-mediated immune reactions. Gamma-interferon is a lymphokine.

**M components**  Immunoglobulins which appear in an increased concentration in the serum or the urine, for instance in the disease macroglobulinaemia (Waldenström's disease) and multiple myeloma. M components can also exist in completely healthy individuals. M components are monoclonal and may consist of IgG, IgA, IgM, IgE heavy chain-like proteins or light chains (Bence-Jones' proteins). A synonym for M component is paraprotein.

**Monoclonal antibodies**  Antibodies produced by a cellular clone are all identical, i.e. monoclonal.

**Natural antibodies**  Antibodies which appear without known cause. In most cases they probably reflect the response to antigenic stimulation, for instance from food or intestinal bacteria.

**Natural immunity**  Non-specific resistance against infection which is not dependent upon immunization by infection or vaccination.

**Natural killer cells**   NK cells are spontaneously occurring lymphocyte-like cells of non-conventional non-T/non-B type with cytolytic capacity against certain tumour cell types and immature, normal cells.

**Opsonin**   Antibody which will add to the phagocytosis of bacteria by reaction with the surface of the bacteria causing complement activation. Even other substances such as, for instance C reactive protein, can have a phagocytosis-stimulating impact.

**Passive immunity**   Immunity in one individual by the administration of antibodies created in another individual. The term also covers the administration of immuno-competent cells from one individual, but here normally the term adoptive immunity (q.v.) is used.
**Plasma cell tumour**   Normally produces monoclonal immunoglobulin which can be seen as an M component in the blood.
**Polyclonal immunoglobulins**   Antibodies against the same antigen produced by different cell clones are thus heterogeneous and are called polyclonal. Certain antigens which stimulate many B lymphocytes (polyclonal stimulation) will cause the production of polyclonal immunoglobulin.
**Precipitation**   The reaction of insoluble complexes via the reaction between antigen and antibody.

**Reagin**   Antibody with a special tendency to be bound to mast cells in the skin or the mucosa and to basophil granulocytes. Upon reaction between reagin and the corresponding antigen (here called allergen) a rapid hypersensitivity reaction is induced via release from the cells of histamine, leukotrienes and other biologically active substances. Reagins belong to immunoglobulin class E. Reagins are also called skin sensitizing or homocytotrophic antibodies.

**Secondary immune response**   Defines the more rapidly appearing and strong immune response that is seen in an individual which has previously been in contact or immunized with the same antigen.
**Serum sickness**   Disease caused by circulating immune complexes created by inoculated antigen (often serum from another species) and antibodies created in the organism against this foreign protein. Tissue damages may be caused by the activated complement system creating inflammatory reactions in the tissues where the immune complexes have been exposed.
**Syngeneic**   The word means of identical genetic constitution. Synonym is isogeneic.

**T helper cells**   T lymphocytes with specific capacity to help other cells such as B lymphocytes to make antibodies against thymus-dependent antigens. T helper cells are also required for the induction of other T lymphocyte activities. Synonym is T inducer cell.
**T suppressor cells**   T lymphocytes with specific capacity to inhibit T helper cell function in particular.
**Thymus-dependent antigens**   Antigens that require T helper cells to be present in order to provoke significant antibody production. Protein antigens are normally thymus-dependent antigens.
**Thymus-independent antigens**   Antigens that do not require the participation of T helper cells in order to induce significant antibody production. Polysaccharide antigens are frequently thymus-independent.

**Tolerance**   *See* Immunological tolerance.

**Tolerogen**   Substance which will provoke a specific non-reactivity in immuno-competent cells.

**Transfer factor**   Cellular fraction from lymphocytes which has been claimed to be able to transfer delayed-type hypersensitivity reactions and possibly other cell-mediated reactivity from immune to non-immune individuals.

**Transplantation antigen**   *See* Histocompatibility antigen.

**Vaccine**   Antigen preparation of a microbial organism which upon transfer to an individual will produce an immune response leading to immunity. Active immunization of an individual with such an antigen is called vaccination. The original meaning of the word comes from the Latin 'vacca' meaning cow due to the use of cowpox viruses in the initial vaccine against smallpox. For historical reasons the word vaccine is now used despite the fact that it has no direct link with cows in most circumstances.

**Valency**   The number of binding sites for antigen determinants on an antibody or the number of determinants present on an antigenic molecule.

# Index

Printed in France by Amazon
Brétigny-sur-Orge, FR

48269741R00172